6.5.00

Rehabilitation
SOURCEBOOK

Health Reference Series

First Edition

Rehabilitation
SOURCEBOOK

*Basic Consumer Health Information about
Rehabilitation for People Recovering from
Heart Surgery, Spinal Cord Injury, Stroke,
Orthopedic Impairments, Amputation,
Pulmonary Impairments, Traumatic Injury,
and More, Including Physical Therapy,
Occupational Therapy, Speech/Language
Therapy, Massage Therapy, Dance Therapy,
Art Therapy, and Recreational Therapy;
Along with Information on Assistive and
Adaptive Devices, a Glossary, and Resources
for Additional Help and Information*

Edited by
Dawn D. Matthews

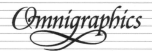

615 Griswold • Detroit, MI 48226

Bibliographic Note

Because this page cannot legibly accommodate all the copyright notices, the Bibliographic Note portion of the Preface constitutes an extension of the copyright notice.

Beginning with books published in 1999, each new volume of the *Health Reference Series* will be individually titled and called a "First Edition." Subsequent updates will carry sequential edition numbers. To help avoid confusion and to provide maximum flexibility in our ability to respond to informational needs, the practice of consecutively numbering each volume will be discontinued.

Edited by Dawn D. Matthews

Health Reference Series

Karen Bellenir, *Series Editor*
Peter D. Dresser, *Managing Editor*
Joan Margeson, *Research Associate*
Dawn Matthews, *Verification Assistant*
Margaret Mary Missar, *Research Coordinator*
Jenifer Swanson, *Research Associate*

Omnigraphics, Inc.

Matthew P. Barbour, *Vice President, Operations*
Laurie Lanzen Harris, *Vice President, Editorial Director*
Kevin Hayes, *Production Coordinator*
Thomas J. Murphy, *Vice President, Finance and Comptroller*
Peter E. Ruffner, *Senior Vice President*
Jane J. Steele, *Marketing Consultant*

Frederick G. Ruffner, Jr., Publisher

© 2000, Omnigraphics, Inc.

Library of Congress Cataloging-in-Publication Data

Rehabilitation sourcebook : Basic consumer health information about rehabilitation for people recovering from heart surgery . . . / edited by Dawn D. Matthews. — 1st ed.
   p.cm. — (Health reference series)
  Includes bibliographical references and index.
  ISBN 07808-0236-5 (lib. bdg. : acid-free paper)
  1. Medical rehabilitation—Popular works. I. Matthews, Dawn D.
  II. Health reference series (Unnumbered)
RM930 .R3665 1999
362.1'786'0973—dc21   99-045827

∞

This book is printed on acid-free paper meeting the ANSI Z39.48 Standard. The infinity symbol that appears above indicates that the paper in this book meets that standard.

Printed in the United States

Table of Contents

Part III: Assistive and Adaptive Devices Used during Rehabilitation

Part IV: The Role of Family in the Rehabilitation Process

Part V: Financial Considerations

Part VI: Common Disorders and Specific Issues in Rehabilitation

Part VII: Additional Help and Information

Preface

About This Book

People do not typically anticipate the need for physical rehabilitation services. As a result, it is an area with which most are unfamiliar, filled with new terminology, anxiety, and uncertainty about the future. Yet, every year an estimated 38 million Americans experience conditions that limit their daily activities, including chronic physical health disorders, injuries, and impairments.

This *Sourcebook* contains information about the most common conditions causing the need for rehabilitation and the different types of rehabilitation services available to treat these conditions. It provides helpful information about choosing the right rehabilitation program, offers tips on choosing assistive equipment to help in recovery and adaptation to daily living, and includes a glossary of related terms and a list of resources for further help and information.

How to Use This Book

This book is divided into parts and chapters. Parts focus on broad areas of interest. Chapters are devoted to single topics within a part.

Part I: Rehabilitation Basics offers information about the rehabilitation process and the professionals who work in the rehabilitation field, as well as helpful information on selecting a rehabilitation program.

Part II: Types of Rehabilitation Therapy explains the different types of available rehabilitation programs, including physical, occupational, massage, movement, art, and recreation therapies.

Part III: Assistive and Adaptive Devices Used during Rehabilitation gives informative advice on the selection and performance of wheelchairs, walkers, and other assistive and adaptive equipment, as well as information on adapting homes and workplaces for daily living.

Part IV: The Role of Family in the Rehabilitation Process discusses the problems encountered by the family and friends of an individual receiving rehabilitation services.

Part V: Financial Considerations contains information about managed care, social security, and Medicaid as they relate to rehabilitation.

Part VI: Common Disorders and Specific Issues in Rehabilitation discusses the common disorders causing the need for rehabilitation, including traumatic injuries, spinal cord injuries, hip and knee replacement, broken bones, communication disorders, respiratory disorders, burns, stroke, and heart disease.

Part VII: Additional Help and Resources includes glossaries of important terms, and resources for further help and information.

Bibliographic Note

This volume contains documents and excerpts from publications issued by the following government agencies: Agency for Health Care Policy and Research (AHCPR), Department of Health and Human Services (DHHS), Health Care Financing Administration (HCFA), National Institute of Handicapped Research (NIHR), National Institute on Deafness and Other Communication Disorders (NIDCD), National Institute on Disability and Rehabilitation Research (NIDRR), National Rehabilitation Information Center (NARIC), Rehabilitation Services Administration (RSA), Social Security Administration (SSA), and the U.S. Administration on Aging (AoA).

In addition, this volume contains copyrighted articles from The American Hospital Association, Brain Injury Association of Kansas and Greater Kansas City, Lippincott - Raven Publishers, *AbleData*, American Academy of Physical Medicine and Rehabilitation, American Art Therapy Association, American Occupational Therapy Association,

American Physical Therapy Association, American Speech-Language-Hearing Association, Assistive On-Line Web Group, Assistive Technology On-Line, Gerald M. Carter, Clinical Reference Systems, American Dance Therapy Association, Disability Statistics Centers, *Johns Hopkins Health After 50*, *Journal of Burn Care & Rehabilitation*, *Journal of Prosthetics and Orthotics*, Manisses Communications Group, Inc., Medical Economics, Medscape Respiratory Care, *Male Health Weekly Plus*, National Easter Seal Society, National Rehabilitation Hospital Research Center, Siskin Hospital for Physical Rehabilitation, and *Work: A Journal of Prevention, Assessment, & Rehabilitation*,

Full citation information is provided on the first page of each chapter. Every effort has been made to secure all necessary rights to reprint the copyrighted material. If any omissions have been made, please contact Omnigraphics to make corrections for future editions.

Acknowledgements

Thanks to Terry Murray for giving me a great head start on this Sourcebook, to Maria Franklin, Joan Margeson, and Jenifer Swanson for their patience as I "learn the ropes," and to Karen Bellenir for her endless supply of encouragement.

Note from the Editor

This book is part of Omnigraphics' *Health Reference Series*. The series provides basic information about a broad range of medical concerns. It is not intended to serve as a tool for diagnosing illness, in prescribing treatments, or as a substitute for the physician/patient relationship. All persons concerned about medical symptoms or the possibility of disease are encouraged to seek professional care from an appropriate health care provider.

Our Advisory Board

The *Health Reference Series* is reviewed by an Advisory Board comprised of librarians from public, academic, and medical libraries. We would like to thank the following board members for providing guidance to the development of this series:

Nancy Bulgarelli, William Beaumont Hospital Library, Royal Oak, MI

Karen Imarasio, Bloomfield Township Public Library, Bloomfield Township, MI

Karen Morgan, Mardigian Library, University of Michigan-Dearborn, Dearborn, MI

Rosemary Orlando, St. Clair Shores Public Library, St. Clair Shores, MI

Health Reference Series *Update Policy*

The inaugural book in the *Health Reference Series* was the first edition of *Cancer Sourcebook* published in 1992. Since then, the *Series* has been enthusiastically received by librarians and in the medical community. In order to maintain the standard of providing high-quality health information for the lay person, the editorial staff at Omnigraphics felt it was necessary to implement a policy of updating volumes when warranted.

Medical researchers have been making tremendous strides, and the challenge to stay current with the most recent advances is one our editors take seriously. Each decision to update a volume will be made on an individual basis. Some of the considerations will include how much new information is available and the feedback we receive from people who use the books. If there's a topic you would like to see added to the update list, or an area of medical concern you feel has not been adequately addressed, please write to:

Editor
Health Reference Series
Omnigraphics, Inc.
615 Griswold
Detroit, MI 48226

The commitment to providing on-going coverage of important medical developments has also led to some technical changes in the *Health Reference Series*. Beginning with books published in 1999, each new volume will be individually titled and called a "First Edition." Subsequent updates will carry sequential edition numbers. To help avoid confusion and to provide maximum flexibility in our ability to respond to informational needs, the practice of consecutively numbering each volume will be discontinued.

Part One

Rehabilitation Basics

Chapter 1

Health Conditions and Impairments—A Statistical Overview

Approximately 38 million Americans with disabilities report a total of 61 million disabling conditions—any chronic health disorder, injury, or impairment that contributes to a person's being limited in social or other activities. This figure comprises 42 million chronic conditions classified as physical health disorders, 16 million as impairments (such as orthopedic and sensory impairments, paralysis, learning disabilities, and mental retardation), 2 million as mental health disorders, and about 1 million injuries that are not classified as impairments.

This abstract presents data on the prevalence of disabling conditions among the civilian non-institutionalized population of the United States. The data are obtained from the National Health Interview Survey (NHIS), a continuing national household survey consisting of 49,401 household interviews with 128,412 people in 1992. In the NHIS, disability is defined as a limitation in social or other activity that is caused by a chronic mental or physical disorder, injury, or impairment.

Impairments are deficits of bodily structure or function, either congenital in origin or acquired from a past or ongoing disorder or injury. Impairments include deficits of senses (vision, hearing, and sensation) or speech, absence of limbs or other anatomy, learning disabilities, deformities, paralysis, and other orthopedic impairments. In the NHIS, impairments are coded according to a classification

U.S. Department of Education, National Institute on Disability and Rehabilitation Research (NIDRR). Number 16, September 1996.

scheme developed by the National Center for Health Statistics. Health disorders (including diseases) and injuries, however, are coded to the World Health Organization's International Classification of Diseases, Ninth Revision (ICD-9).

The classification method presents several complications. First, since many impairments are caused by ongoing disorders, both the impairment and the disorder may be coded as disabling conditions. For example, for a person who has had a leg amputated due to a bone cancer still active at the time of the interview, both the impairment (absence of limb) and the disorder (cancer) will be coded separately. A further complication results from a somewhat arbitrary distinction, in certain instances, between disorders and impairments, depending on how the condition is described. If a respondent reports "back trouble," it will be coded as an impairment, while an answer of "slipped disc" will be classified as a disorder. Thus, only by combining back-related impairments and disorders can the true number of disabling back problems be estimated.

Finally, injuries are handled in a special way. When an injury has caused an impairment, only the impairment is coded. Injuries that have not caused impairments are coded to the injuries chapter of the ICD. For example, if a person mentions last year's automobile accident as a cause of activity limitation, without specifying a particular impairment, the person's condition is coded as an injury, not an impairment.

The 37.7 million people with activity limitations report an average of 1.6 conditions per person, for a total of 61 million limiting conditions. Some 73.3 percent of these are classified as disorders and injuries, with the remainder as impairments. Among the disorders and injuries, the most prevalent are musculoskeletal disorders, which represent 17.2 percent of all limiting conditions, followed by circulatory disorders, at 16.7 percent. Respiratory conditions rank third at 7.8 percent, with nervous and sensory disorders at 7.2 percent and endocrine, nutritional, metabolic, and immunity disorders at 5.6 percent of all disabling conditions. These top five categories, each representing a chapter of the ICD, account for three-quarters (74.4 percent) of all diseases and disorders reported as causing limitation in activity, or more than half (54.3 percent) of all activity-limiting conditions.

The 16.3 million impairments reported to cause activity limitation constitute about one-quarter (26.7 percent) of all disabling conditions. More than half of these are orthopedic impairments, representing 14.1 percent of disabling conditions. A distant second is the category of learning disabilities and mental retardation, accounting for 2.6 percent.

Visual impairments rank third, at 2.1 percent, followed by hearing impairments, at 1.9 percent, and paralysis, at 1.8 percent of all disabling conditions reported. The remaining impairments—4.3 percent of all conditions causing activity limitation—include deformities, absence or loss (e.g., of a limb), and speech impairments.

Of the most common specific health conditions and impairments that cause activity limitation in the U.S. Heart disease is the most prevalent, at 7.9 million cases—13 percent of all conditions mentioned. Back problems (including those classified as impairments or disorders) are a close second at 7.7 million conditions, or 12.6 percent of all disabling conditions. Arthritis (rheumatoid arthritis plus osteoarthrosis and allied disorders) ranks third at 5.7 million, followed by orthopedic impairments of lower extremity (2.8 million), asthma (2.6 million), and diabetes (2.6 million). Mental disorders, which are mainly the mental illnesses (since learning disability and mental retardation are classified separately), rank seventh at 2.0 million conditions, followed by disorders of the eye (1.6 million, not including visual impairments), and then by learning disability and mental retardation (1.6 million). If the latter is combined with mental illnesses, the total for all mental disorders is 3.6 million, placing the category fourth overall.

Cancer ranks in tenth place (1.3 million), followed by visual impairments (1.3 million), and then orthopedic impairments of shoulder and/or upper extremity (1.2 million). The residual category of unknown and unspecified causes ranks thirteenth (1.2 million) at 1.9 percent of all conditions, followed by hearing impairments (1.2 million), also at 1.9 percent of all conditions. Cerebrovascular disease completes the list at fifteenth with slightly under 1.2 million conditions.

These data also highlight the substantial role that injury plays in causing disability. In addition to the 1.2 million injuries that limit activity but are not classified as impairments, another 7.2 million impairments have injury coded as a cause. Thus, injuries make up 13.4 percent of all disabling conditions. However, disorders clearly play the largest role as causes of disability.

—by Mitchell P. LaPlante

This abstract is based on an analysis contained in: M.P. LaPlante and D. Carlson (1996). Disability in the United States: Prevalence and Causes, 1992. Disability Statistics Report No. 6. Washington, D.C.: National Institute on Disability and Rehabilitation Research.

The Disability Statistics Abstract Series is produced by the Disability Statistics Rehabilitation Research and Training Center, Institute for Health & Aging, School of Nursing, University of California, Box 0646, Laurel Heights, 3333 California St., San Francisco, CA 94143-0646, with funding from NIDRR. Edited by Steve Kaye. Layout by Barbara L. Wenger.

Chapter 2

Understanding Rehabilitation

Rehabilitation is the science and art of enabling persons with physical, mental or sensory impairments to attain the highest degree of self-sufficiency and equality leading toward usefulness, satisfaction and full participation in community life. Rehabilitation holds promise for the estimated one out of 10 persons young or old who were born with or acquire impairments through illness, accident or disease.

Rehabilitation is a collaborative effort in which clients, parents and families play important roles. Professionals involved may include physicians, nurses, therapists, psychologists, social workers, vocational counselors, teachers, and other specialists linked through one or more agencies. Treatment and training are tailored to meet each client's physical, emotional, social, and vocational needs.

Persons receiving rehabilitation usually go through some or all of the following:

- Screening
- Assessment and diagnosis
- Goal-setting
- Medical care and treatment
- Social, psychological and other types of counseling and assistance
- Training in self-care activities
- Fitting of assistive devices
- Specialized education services

- Vocational guidance, training and placement
- Follow-up and referral

Understanding That:

Successful rehabilitation is influenced greatly by the positive belief that people can make up for the loss of one sense or ability if they focus on what they can do rather than on what they can't do. Successful rehabilitation is influenced greatly also by family and friends who:

- Participate actively in the design and arrangement of services deemed necessary for the client

- Encourage and assist the client in keeping appointments and in faithfully practicing exercises prescribed for home

- Provide support and understanding rather than pity

- Praise effort and accomplishment

- Give reassurance of being loved and useful

- Support efforts guaranteeing rights to, or opportunities for education, employment and social-cultural experiences

Rehabilitation Terms to Understand

Activities of Daily Living (ADL): The basic activities that a person with a disability can often learn to do in a routine or adapted way in order to live independently, including self-care activities such as dressing, eating, toileting, and communicating.

Advocacy: Actions by an individual or a group to ensure that the interests and the legal and human rights of persons with disabilities are safeguarded.

Assessment: A process to identify a person's competencies and limitations in order to determine services needed and ability to use services.

Assistive devices: Measures or aids, such as communication boards, artificial limbs, hearing aids, and cochlear implants intended to compensate for a loss of function or a functional limitation.

Client plan: A written program of action developed and reviewed at regular intervals with the participation of the client, the client's

8

family or representative and all agencies involved: the plan specifies objectives and goals and identifies those services planned to achieve them (also known as individual program plan).

Diagnosis: Determination of a disease or condition based on signs, symptoms and studies.

Follow-up: Support assistance for determining to what degree past and present programs have met a person's needs and for ascertaining readiness for new programs.

Medical restoration: The use of all measures needed to condition and treat a person for fullest possible recovery from disease, illness or accident.

Referral: Guidance and assistance in directing a person seeking help to select and use the most appropriate resource or service available.

Screening: Evaluation conducted prior to a person's acceptance into a program to determine the appropriateness of the program for the person.

Vocational evaluation and training: The variety of work-related experiences and services directed by specialists trained to assist the person with a disability in adjusting to suitable work.

Rehabilitation Facts

- Because no two persons with disabilities have the same needs or encounter the same barriers, basic programs of rehabilitation must be tailored to each individual.

- Even persons with severe disabilities can, to a great extent, live independently if necessary support services are provided.

- A person can make up for the loss of one sense or ability through training and practice. Even small achievements or discoveries can add meaning to life.

- The environment contributes greatly to the effect of a disability on a person's independence. Many persons with disabilities are excluded from participating in society because of doorways too narrow for wheelchairs, insurmountable steps leading to buildings and transportation systems and oral communication ignoring the needs of persons with visual disabilities.

Chapter 3

Frequently Asked Questions

Here are some answers to questions frequently asked about the specialty of physical medicine and rehabilitation:

- What is physical medicine and rehabilitation?
- What is a physiatrist?
- What kind of training do physiatrists have?
- How did the specialty develop?
- What types of conditions does a physiatrist treat?
- What is the physiatrist's role in treatment?
- How do physiatrists diagnose?
- What kinds of treatments do physiatrists offer?
- Where do physiatrists practice?
- What kinds of differences do physiatrists make?
- How can I locate a physiatrist?

What is physical medicine and rehabilitation?

Physical Medicine and Rehabilitation (PM&R), also called physiatry, (pronounced fizz ee at' tree or fizz eye' uh tree) is the branch of medicine emphasizing the prevention, diagnosis and treatment of disorders—particularly those of the musculoskeletal, cardiovascular, and pulmonary systems—that may produce temporary or permanent impairment. Physical Medicine and Rehabilitation is one of the 24 medical specialties certified by the American Board of Medical Specialties.

Physiatry provides integrated care in the treatment of all neurologic and musculoskeletal disabilities from traumatic brain injury to lower back pain. The specialty focuses on the restoration of function to people with problems ranging from simple physical mobility issues to those with complex cognitive involvement.

What is a physiatrist?

A physiatrist, (pronounced fizz ee at' trist or fizz eye' uh trist) is a physician specializing in physical medicine and rehabilitation. Physiatrists are physicians who treat a wide range of problems from sore shoulders to spinal cord injuries. They see patients in all age groups and treat problems that touch upon all the major systems in the body. These specialists focus on restoring function to people.

Physiatrists treat acute and chronic pain and musculoskeletal disorders. They may see a person who lifts a heavy object at work and experiences back pain, a basketball player who sprains an ankle and needs rehabilitation to play again, or a knitter who has carpal tunnel syndrome. Physiatrists' patients include people with arthritis, tendinitis, any kind of back pain, and work—or sports-related injuries.

Physiatrists also treat serious disorders of the musculoskeletal system that result in severe functional limitations. They would treat a baby with a birth defect, someone in a bad car accident, or an elderly person with a broken hip. Physiatrists coordinate the long term rehabilitation process for patients with spinal cord injuries, cancer, stroke or other neurological disorders, brain injuries, amputations and multiple sclerosis.

What kind of training do physiatrists have?

To become a physiatrist individuals must successfully complete four years of graduate medical education followed by four additional years of postdoctoral residency training. Residency training includes one year spent developing fundamental clinical skills and three additional years of training in the full scope of the specialty. There are currently 80 accredited residency programs in physical medicine and rehabilitation in the United States. Many physiatrists choose to pursue additional advanced degrees (MS, PhD) or complete fellowship training in a specific area of the specialty. Fellowships are available for specialized study in such areas as musculoskeletal rehabilitation, pediatrics, traumatic brain injury, spinal cord injury, and sports medicine.

To become board certified in physical medicine and rehabilitation, physiatrists are required to take both a written and oral examination administered by the American Board of Physical Medicine and Re-habilitation (ABPM&R). The ABPM&R also has agreements with each of the boards of pediatrics, internal medicine, and neurology to allow special training programs leading to certification in both specialties.

How did the specialty develop?

The field of physical medicine and rehabilitation (PM&R) began in the 1930s to address musculoskeletal and neurological problems, but broadened its scope considerably after World War II. As thousands of veterans came back to the United States with serious disabilities, the task of helping to restore them to productive lives became a new direction for the field. The Advisory Board of Medical Specialties granted PM&R its approval as a specialty of medicine in 1947.

What types of conditions does a physiatrist treat?

Physiatrists are physicians who treat a wide range of problems from sore shoulders to spinal cord injuries. The focus of the specialty is on restoring function to people. Physiatrists treat acute and chronic pain and musculoskeletal disorders. They may see a person who lifts a heavy object at work and experiences back pain, a basketball player who sprains an ankle and needs rehabilitation to play again, or a knitter who has carpal tunnel syndrome. Physiatrists' patients also include people with arthritis, tendonitis, any kind of back pain, and work and sports-related injuries. Physiatrists treat serious disorders of the musculoskeletal system that result in severe functional limi-tations as well. They would treat a baby with a birth defect, someone in a bad car accident, or an elderly person with a broken hip. Physiatrists coordinate the long-term rehabilitation process for people with spinal cord injuries, brain injuries, strokes, amputations, can-cer, and multiple sclerosis.

What is the physiatrist's role in treatment?

A physiatrist may treat patients directly, lead an interdisciplinary team, or act as a consultant. Here are some scenarios that illustrate the varied roles of a physiatrist:

A carpenter is lifting some heavy wood when he feels pain in his lower back and down his leg. He sees a physiatrist who does a thorough history and physical examination and performs all the testing needed to make the diagnosis: a herniated disc. The physiatrist develops an appropriate treatment program, monitoring and adjusting it as needed. With this treatment and rehabilitation program, the patient does not need surgery.

A woman in a diving accident has a spinal cord injury and is paralyzed below the waist. The physiatrist assesses her injury and with the patient and a team of health care professionals determines the course of her rehabilitation. The physiatrist treats the array of medical issues that occur as the result of a spinal cord injury, and also leads the interdisciplinary team to enable the woman to reach the highest level of functioning possible. The team varies in composition depending on the needs of the patient. In addition to other physicians, the team may include health care professionals such as nurses, physical therapists, occupational therapists, social workers, neuropsychologists, and vocational counselors.

A baby is born with cerebral palsy. The physiatrist is called in as the expert who advises on the correct treatment and rehabilitation that can affect the rest of the child's life.

How do physiatrists diagnose?

Physiatrists' diagnostic tools are the same as those used by other physicians, with the addition of special techniques in electrodiagnostic medicine like electromyography (EMG), nerve conduction studies, and somatosensory evoked potentials. These techniques help the physiatrist to diagnose conditions that cause pain, weakness, and numbness.

What kinds of treatments do physiatrists offer?

Physiatrists offer a broad spectrum of medical services. They do not perform surgery. Physiatrists may prescribe drugs or assistive devices, such as a brace or artificial limb. They also use diverse therapies such as heat and cold, electrotherapies, massage, biofeedback, traction, and therapeutic exercise.

Where do physiatrists practice?

Physiatrists practice in rehabilitation centers, hospitals, and in private offices. They often have broad practices, but some concentrate on one area such as pediatrics, sports medicine, geriatric medicine, brain injury, and many other special interests.

What kinds of differences do physiatrists make?

Since physiatrists focus on restoring patients to maximum function, the difference they make can be dramatic. In the case of the herniated disc, the physiatrist not only takes care of the acute problem, but also treats the patient until he or she returns to optimal functioning, usually without surgery. The physiatrist also teaches the patient how to prevent the injury in the future.

A broken hip in an elderly patient is another example. Physiatrists can provide aggressive rehabilitation so patients can walk and even exercise again. And because the physiatrist is concerned with all areas of rehabilitation—social, vocational, and medical—the quality of life is significantly increased for patients.

How can I locate a physiatrist?

There are more than 6,000 physiatrists practicing in the United States today. As a public service, the American Academy of Physical Medicine and Rehabilitation (AAPM&R) provides listings of its member physiatrists by state.

To request a list of board-certified physiatrists in your area, go the AAPM&R website at http://www.aapmr.org/paltsrch.html or contact the AAPM&R at 312-464-9700. AAPM&R provides referral listings by first class mail only at this time.

Chapter 4

Why Choose a Physiatrist?

Physiatrists are specialists in diagnosing and treating problems of the musculoskeletal system. They perform thorough histories and physical examinations to find the source of your pain, injury or disability, even when standard diagnostic tests don't reveal specific problems.

In addition, physiatrists direct your treatment team. If you need any other services, such as those of a physical therapist or athletic trainer, your physiatrist supervises, collaborates with and coordinates the other health care professionals. The result is a specially designed treatment program tailored for you.

Because physiatrists offer an aggressive, non-surgical approach to pain and injury, these physicians are the ideal choice for the treatment of a wide variety of diseases and conditions. Here's a listing of just some of the conditions that physiatrists have extensive training in diagnosing and treating:

- Low back pain
- Neck pain
- Fibromyalgia/Myofascial Pain
- Spinal cord injuries
- Brain injuries
- Acute and chronic pain
- Arthritis

- Cancer
- Burns
- Stroke and Neurological Disorders
- Multiple Sclerosis
- Cardiac Disorders
- Osteoporosis
- Musculoskeletal Disorders
- Work injuries

Most importantly, physiatrists treat the whole patient, not just the patient's symptoms. Physiatrists share their medical knowledge to help patients understand their condition and provide the tools and resources to manage it. They employ a variety of treatment methods to reduce or eliminate your problems and to decrease the possibility of a recurrence. This comprehensive approach produces not only cost-effective results, but also a high degree of patient satisfaction.

Through integrated focused care and comprehensive diagnosis and treatment, physiatrists add quality to the lives of millions of patients each year. The goal: getting you back into the game—not just back on the sidelines.

For additional information about PM&R or referral to a PM&R physician, contact Kris Rowland, marketing coordinator, by phone at (312) 464-9700 ext. 277, fax at (312) 464-0227, or e-mail at krowland@aapmr.org.

Chapter 5

How to Choose a Physical Rehabilitation Program

No one anticipates the need for physical rehabilitation services. It is an area with which most people are unfamiliar, filled with new terminology, anxiety, and uncertainty about the future.

Siskin Hospital has designed this article to help you deal with that uncertainty; helping prepare you and your family to make solid, informed decisions and to maximize available resources.

The first critical step toward achieving maximum recovery is careful selection of physical rehabilitation services that can best meet the needs of patients and their families.

The answer to each of the questions included should be "yes", and the responses are suggested to help you know what to expect about the rehabilitation provided by a particular facility.

Facilities' responses to these questions can help you choose physical rehabilitation services that satisfy the patient's needs and priorities.

The Staff of Siskin Hospital offers its best wishes during your rehabilitation journey.

Does the Facility Specialize in Physical Rehabilitation?

Facilities which are completely dedicated to physical medicine and rehabilitation devote all their time, energy, and fiscal resources to the process of rehabilitation. Because they concentrate totally on rehabilitation they offer an atmosphere which helps motivate patients to

19

concentrate their efforts and reach their goals. Facility features should include accessible bathrooms, water fountains, telephones, and oversized patient rooms.

Does the Program Provide Experienced Teams Specializing in Treatment of Specific Diseases?

Having specialized teams that treat patients with specific diagnoses such as stroke, spinal cord, brain injury, or orthopedic problems means that such patients will benefit from a higher level of knowledge and expertise. It is best if the team is headed by a physician who has specialized training or experience in the particular diagnosis. This can result in more rapid and significant progress for the patient.

Is There Adequate Staff to Provide an Intensive Physical Rehabilitation Program?

In an intensive program, the patient will participate in four to six hours of therapy per day. To achieve this, the facility must have adequate numbers of staff to work with each patient in depth. Therefore, it is important to ascertain the staff to patient ratio to insure swift and significant progress.

Can Families Observe Treatment and Are There Established Visiting Hours/Family Visitations?

In the rehabilitation setting, family support is very important. Families are encouraged to become actively involved in therapy and are trained on how to assist the patient upon their return home.

Visiting hours may be limited due to the intensity of the program in which the patient is participating. Usually, the limitations are restricted to only daytime hours, with visiting hours in the evening and on weekends.

Does the Program Have a Good Success Rate in Returning Individuals to Their Home, Work or School?

A major goal of physical rehabilitation is to help individuals return to home, work, or school. This is accomplished by helping patients meet their rehabilitation goals and by educating family members to provide whatever care may be needed. Facilities should be asked what percent of their patients are discharged to the home environment.

Is the Program Headed By Physicians Who Specialize in Physical Medicine and Rehabilitation and Are They Board Certified?

An individual will benefit most from a rehabilitation program that is headed by a physiatrist—a physician who specializes in physical medicine and rehabilitation—and is based in or supported by a hospital. The physicians should be certified by the American Board of Physical Medicine and Rehabilitation.

Are There Proper Arrangements for Medical Specialist Support in the Event of a New Illness or Major Complication?

Facilities should have a large and active medical consulting staff with all specialties represented should any new illness or complication arise. Also, facilities should be closely located to an acute care hospital to facilitate emergency transfers or more standard procedures if required.

Do Patients Have the Same Treatment Team Members Throughout the Rehabilitation Stay?

For consistency in the patient's treatment, it is valuable for the patient to have the same therapists throughout the rehabilitation stay. Communication between team members is also improved when the multi-disciplinary team remains constant. The team should be put together based on the patient's particular needs and meet regularly to evaluate the goals and progress being made by the patient.

Does the Facility Have a Variety of Rehabilitation Programs That Patients Can "Graduate Through" As They Progress?

Effective rehabilitation is based upon progressive skills development, ultimately leading to patient independence. By matching the level of care to the patient's stage of progress, effective and efficient physical rehabilitation programs result. Therefore, facilities should have a variety of programs such as inpatient, outpatient, day hospitalization and others to provide a full "continuum" of services.

Does the Facility Have Special Accreditation to Operate?

Rehabilitation facilities should have accreditation from nationally known organizations. The Commission on Accreditation of Rehabilitation Facilities (CARF) and Joint Commission on Accreditation of Healthcare Organizations (JCAHO) are independent organizations that accredit facilities and serve as "quality control intermediaries" in the rehabilitation industry. Facilities invite CARF and JCAHO to send trained teams to survey and evaluate their physical rehabilitation programs against standards of excellence for rehabilitation patient care. Facilities that meet or exceed these standards are awarded accreditation. Certificates of accreditation should be displayed in a public area in the hospital.

Chapter 6

A Guide to Choosing a Comprehensive Inpatient Medical Rehabilitation Facility

Acknowledgments

In November 1985 the Governing Council of the Section for Rehabilitation Hospitals and Programs approved the concept of developing a guide on how to identify appropriate facilities for the rehabilitation of patients requiring comprehensive inpatient rehabilitation. As a result, a survey was sent to section members to identify the "indicators of quality" that they felt were relevant in choosing a comprehensive, inpatient medical facility. Their comments and responses have been combined to form the basis of this guide and to them we extend our most sincere appreciation and gratitude. In addition to thanking the governing council, we would also like to acknowledge the following for their generous contributions:

- Francis G. Mackey, M.D., consulting medical director, Carondelet Rehabilitation Centers of America, Culver City, CA

- John L. Melvin, M.D., medical director, Curative Rehabilitation Center, Wauwatosa, Wl

- Jane Gardner Newton, R.P.T., St. Francis Medical Center, Chicago, IL

23

Purpose of the Guide

The recent proliferation of facilities providing rehabilitation services and programs has created the need for guidance in choosing a facility. This guide is intended to help individual consumers, insurance companies, and employers in selecting a rehabilitation provider to care for family members, clients, and employees.

This guide to choosing a comprehensive inpatient medical facility was developed by the American Hospital Association Section for Rehabilitation Hospitals and Programs in response to an identified need to assist consumers in selecting appropriate facilities for the rehabilitation of patients requiring comprehensive inpatient rehabilitation, and to explain to consumers how coordinated programs of comprehensive inpatient medical rehabilitation differ from individual rehabilitation services. Although consumers of rehabilitation services can include patients and their families, this guide is geared more for employers and insurers who are trying to find the right rehabilitation services to meet a patient's needs. Hospitals wishing to use the guide to promote their own services can answer the questions and make the guide, along with their own answers, available for consumers to review and compare.

This guide does not advise consumers about the degree of rehabilitation services required to meet a particular patient's needs, nor does it make available information and statistics on specific facilities. This publication simply provides a framework for consumers to enter into a dialog with rehabilitation providers for the purpose of assisting in the selection process. The questions that follow are a good starting point for dialog and, when answered, will help consumers to make informed decisions and choices about rehabilitation services.

Use of the Guide

Section 1 provides essential background on rehabilitation services. Sections 2 and 3 consist of a checklist of questions consumers can ask of facilities to determine whether a comprehensive inpatient medical rehabilitation program is provided. The checklist is arranged with the suggested questions first, followed by possible responses, and then interpretations that consumers may find helpful to evaluate the answers.

The questions on the checklist are not the only ones consumers should ask. These questions are suggested to stimulate a dialog that will help consumers know what they can expect about the rehabilitation care provided by a particular facility. Facilities' responses to these questions can help the consumer choose rehabilitation care that satisfies the patient's priorities. A consumer must weigh answers to all questions before deciding which rehabilitation programs or services best meet the patient's needs.

Facilities that are proud of their comprehensive inpatient rehabilitation programs look for ways to let consumers know about their records of performance and can readily provide answers to most of the checklist questions.

Section 1

What are Rehabilitation Services?

Rehabilitation services are measures taken to restore an ill or disabled person to the fullest degree of physical, cognitive, emotional, psychological, social, and economic usefulness, and thereafter to maintain the individual at the maximal functional level.

What Is Comprehensive Inpatient Medical Rehabilitation?

A program of comprehensive inpatient medical rehabilitation is a coordinated program of inpatient care that promotes optimum attainable levels of physical independence as well as optimum psychological, social, vocational, educational, and economic adjustment of the individual. The essential elements of a comprehensive medical rehabilitation program are as follows:

1. that the program is an organizational and physical entity;

2. that it is medically directed by a physician knowledgeable and experienced in rehabilitation medicine;

3. that 24-hour rehabilitation nursing care is provided;

4. that the services are multidisciplinary, coordinated, and integrated;

5. that the services for a patient are determined by an individual periodic assessment of basic functional ability; and

6. that the program accomplishes its rehabilitation goals within appropriate time frames.

A comprehensive inpatient medical rehabilitation program differs from individual rehabilitation services in that it meets the most frequently encountered physical, psychological, and social needs of patients, providing, at a minimum, rehabilitation medicine, rehabilitation nursing, social work, occupational therapy, physical therapy, and speech-language pathology services.

The medical care and services are provided in a rehabilitation hospital or in a unit of a hospital that is organized to provide a coordinated program of rehabilitation care. While some rehabilitative treatment can begin when a patient is in the general hospital, the patient usually is transferred to a rehabilitation hospital or a rehabilitation unit within an acute care hospital for the care needed to bring the patient to the highest level of functioning.

Rehabilitation hospitals and units offer services to patients who can benefit best from an intensive, coordinated, multidisciplinary rehabilitation program. These programs have the following features:

- Hospital licensure for geographically congregated rehabilitation beds

- Medical direction by a physician trained in rehabilitation or a related field and experienced in rehabilitation

- Nursing care provided 24 hours a day and directed by a registered nurse who is experienced in rehabilitation

- An administrator who manages the center's daily operations

- The following rehabilitation services generally provided daily, if not twice daily, when required in the rehabilitation plan of treatment:

  Physical therapy
  Occupational therapy
  Speech/hearing/language therapy
  Social work services
  Psychological services

  and, where appropriate:

  Recreation therapy
  Vocational services
  Special education services

An intensive level of physical and occupational therapy *must* be provided daily, and other services are expected to also address a wide range of problems—medical, physical, psychological, communication, social, vocational, educational, avocational, and so forth. Specialists, including dietitians, prosthetists, and orthotists are also available to provide specialized services.

For the patient's benefit, the multidisciplinary team coordinates the various rehabilitation services in conferences that are scheduled at least every two weeks. During conferences, team members discuss the patient's problems, needs, and rehabilitation goals. Team members also exchange information about the patient's care between conferences. Planning and preparing for the patient's eventual discharge and possible follow-up care also begin in early team conferences. Many teams include the family members routinely and the patient when appropriate.

The hallmark of a comprehensive inpatient medical rehabilitation program is the way health care professionals act as a team together with the family and patient. This level of communication, the exchange of information among everyone involved in the patient's care, and the setting of a "patient agenda" often are not present or needed in facilities that offer limited rehabilitation services. An effective rehabilitation team works together toward the common goal of helping the patient to achieve the highest level of function.

Who Needs Comprehensive Inpatient Medical Rehabilitation?

Not all patients need comprehensive inpatient medical rehabilitation. For instance, some patients may need just a few weeks of physical therapy from the hospital's outpatient department for treatment of an isolated knee, shoulder, or back injury to achieve their highest level of physical functioning.

Patients who need comprehensive inpatient medical rehabilitation suffer from one of many conditions that are caused by accidents or diseases and that severely impair their physical functioning or understanding—for instance, strokes, spinal-cord and head injuries, arthritis, burns, neurological conditions, birth defects, cancer, or amputations.

For example, a prime candidate for comprehensive inpatient medical rehabilitation is a person who has had a stroke that prevents him from communicating or managing his personal needs at home and whose potential for improved independence has been identified by a physician.

The patient would require intensive and daily rehabilitation, medical, and nursing care (that is, assessment, planning, intervention, and evaluation), appropriate therapies, and other services to meet the specific needs, such as social work, psychological, and vocational services.

Rehabilitation nurses would help such a patient relearn feeding, bathing, toileting, and dressing skills and would reinforce the self-care skills taught the patient by other therapists. Therapists would teach the patients these skills as well as how to regain various physical functions and communication skills. The patient can expect five to seven hours of therapy daily, as well as classes and counseling to help in relearning daily living skills and coping with any remaining disability. The patient and family can expect to meet at least every two weeks with the patient's physician and rehabilitation team to review, revise, and set treatment goals and a target discharge date and to review early discharge planning.

Patients are admitted to a rehabilitation program after they are evaluated for their potential to make gains in physical or cognitive functioning. While in the program, patients are expected to show significant practical gains within a reasonable time period. When patients no longer can make functional progress, they are discharged from the rehabilitation program, perhaps to return at a later date when they have gained more stamina and potential to tolerate more intensive therapy.

If necessary, the staff members treating the patient (the team) may coordinate family education and training sessions, as well as trial overnight stays, to help prepare the family members and the patient for the return home. Sometimes, members of the team also visit the patient's home to assess the need for and the availability of space for equipment as well as to discuss future therapy needs and to schedule follow-up home visits by hospital staff members. Often patients are taken on community recreation outings and shopping tours to assess their ability to return to social functioning.

A patient's primary care physician or family doctor can advise whether the patient needs a comprehensive inpatient medical rehabilitation program or whether individual services are appropriate. If the former is recommended, then the consumer responsible for the decision should "shop and compare" facilities to determine which one best meets the patient's needs.

Section 2

Questions to Ask Facilities about Their Comprehensive Inpatient Medical Rehabilitation Program

Consumers should ask facilities the questions provided on the following pages, being certain to record their responses for future reference. It is also recommended that the following information be recorded for easy reference:

- Name of Facility
- Location
- Contact Person
- Telephone Number
- Date

Does the Facility Meet Nationally Accepted Standards of Care?

What Special Accreditation / Certification for Rehabilitation Does the Facility Hold?

- Commission on Accreditation of Rehabilitation Facilities (CARF) Comprehensive Inpatient Rehabilitation/Hospital-Based

- How long has the facility been accredited by CARF?

- When does CARF accreditation end?

- How long has the facility been accredited by the Joint Commission?

- When does Joint Commission accreditation end?

- No special accreditation

Interpretation: The Commission on Accreditation of Rehabilitation Facilities (CARF) and Joint Commission on Accreditation of Healthcare Organizations are independent organizations that accredit facilities and serve as "quality control intermediaries" in the rehabilitation industry. CARF and Joint Commission standards are considered by the rehabilitation field to be the minimum that facilities should meet to be considered high-quality rehabilitation programs. *Facilities are not required to meet these standards; they do so on a voluntary basis.*

Facilities invite CARF and the Joint Commission to send trained teams to survey and evaluate their rehabilitation programs against standards of excellence for rehabilitation patient care. Facilities that meet or exceed these standards are awarded accreditation. *A facility need not hold both CARF and Joint Commission accreditation for inpatient medical rehabilitation to be considered a comprehensive program; however, some facilities do.*

Does the Facility Hold Additional Accreditation for Specialty Rehabilitation Programs?

- Yes
- No

Interpretation: In addition to inpatient medical rehabilitation programs, CARF accredits specialty rehabilitation programs according to separate standards for spinal cord injury, brain injury, chronic pain management, alcohol and drug abuse, and infant and early childhood developmental programs, as well as vocational rehabilitation and outpatient medical rehabilitation programs.

Who Is on the Staff?

What is the Medical Staffing of the Rehabilitation Program?

- Full-time physiatrist (a physician who specializes in physical medicine and rehabilitation) (40 hours a week)

- Full-time physician in a related specialty with rehab experience (40 hours a week)

- Part-time physiatrist (20-30 hours a week)

- Part-time physician in a related specialty with rehab experience (20-30 hours a week)

Is the Medical Director Board Certified?

- Yes
- No

If yes, specify the type of board certification

How Many Years of Rehabilitation Experience Does the Medical Director Have?

Are Other Rehabilitation Physicians Board Certified?

- Yes
- No

If yes, specify the type(s) of board certification

How Many Years of Rehabilitation Experience Do Other Rehabilitation Physicians Have?

Total years of rehabilitation experience-

Does the Facility Have Access to Consulting Physicians and Specialists (For Example, a Neurologist, an Internist, and So Forth)?

- Yes
- No

If yes, specify the types of physicians and specialists:

In Rehabilitation Programs in Acute Care Settings, are Primary Physicians on Staff Allowed to Manage the Patients' Nonrehab Problems during Their Rehabilitation Stay?

- Yes
- No

Interpretation: To appropriately perform their duties, medical directors of comprehensive inpatient medical rehabilitation programs must devote significant time to the activities of the program and must be knowledgeable about the diagnosis and treatment of conditions and diseases for which rehabilitation is likely to be needed.

Medical supervision in a comprehensive inpatient medical rehabilitation program involves active physician participation in all of the major decisions that concern a patient's admission to and treatment in such a hospital or unit. If primary physicians manage patients' nonrehabilitation problems, they are better able to participate in these decisions and provide the continuity of care that is so important in rehabilitation. These decisions include the following:

1. Recommendation for admission

2.   Identification of problems requiring treatment

3.   Selection of treatment approaches

4.   Identification of potential functional gains to be achieved during the stay

5.   Participation in the multidisciplinary team conferences

6.   Estimation of the patient's length of stay

7.   Selection of the appropriate setting for continued rehabilitation care after discharge, if necessary

8.   Rehabilitation team coordination

It is desirable that a facility have access to specialists, either on staff or on a consulting basis, to provide an appropriate level of patient care.

Does the Facility Provide the Services That Are Needed?

What Rehabilitation Therapy and Services are Available to the Patient?

- Physical therapy

  hours/day-

- Occupational therapy

  hours/day-

- Speech/hearing/language therapy

  hours/day-

- Recreation therapy

  hours/day-

total therapy hours-

- Social Work services

  hours/day-

- Psychological services

  hours/day-

- Vocational rehabilitation
  hours/day-

- Orthotic services
  hours/day-

- Prosthetic services
  hours/day-

- Biomedical engineering services
  hours/day-

total service hours-

How Many Years of Experience In Rehabilitation and Advanced Degrees do These Department Heads Have?

Do Patients Have the Same Therapists and Team Members Throughout the Rehabilitation Stay and during Team Conferences?

- Yes
- No

Are the Facility's Employees Contracted From an Outside Agency?

- Yes
- No

Interpretation: Measuring the experience levels of staff in comprehensive inpatient medical rehabilitation programs can be assessed by:

1. Appropriate special licensure

2. Number of years of rehabilitation experience

3. Staff achievement of advanced education degrees and special training/ certification (such as masters and doctoral degrees)

Continuity of staff throughout a patient's stay and during team conferences helps to facilitate communication with the patient and the family. A facility that employs its own staff rather than contracting from outside agencies helps to ensure continuity and good working relationships among familiar staff members.

What are the Arrangements for Medical Specialists Support in the Event of a New Illness or Major Complication?

- The patient's illness is managed by a multispecialty medical staff that is routinely available at the hospital on a daily basis.

- A consulting medical specialist staff is available on an "as needed" basis at varying frequencies of visits.

- The patient is transferred within 24-48 hours to an acute care facility in the event of major complications or a new illness. The time of transfer relates to the severity and complexity of the illness.

Interpretation: When a complication arises, it is important that physicians can see patients quickly and with the necessary frequency to manage the complication.

Hospitals with distinct-part rehabilitation units and freestanding rehabilitation hospitals should be able to provide daily availability of a multispecialty medical staff in the event of an illness or complication. It may be appropriate for a facility to transfer a patient with an illness or complication to another facility offering the needed level of care. However, this arrangement may be disruptive to the rehabilitation process, so great care must be given to making these kinds of decisions.

How does the Facility Respond to Life-Threatening Cardiopulmonary Situations?

Personnel certified in cardiopulmonary resuscitation are immediately available to provide basic life support to the patient until advanced life support can be provided by one or more of the following:

- An organized team with a physician who is certified in advanced cardiac life support (ACLS) or advanced life support responds with regularly checked emergency equipment and medications within three minutes.

- An organized internal emergency team with a physician without ACLS training and with team members certified in ACLS or advanced life support responds with regularly checked emergency equipment and medications within three minutes.

- An organized internal emergency team without immediate physician availability, but with team members certified in ACLS or advanced life support responds with regularly checked emergency equipment and medications within three minutes.

- External paramedics certified in advanced life support respond with regularly checked emergency equipment and medications within three minutes.

- No organized advanced life support emergency team is available within three minutes with regularly checked emergency equipment and medications.

Interpretations: Patients at risk of life-threatening complications would be better treated in a facility providing an organized method of emergency ACLS.

ACLS includes the ability to read and care for cardiac arrhythmias, give drug and intravenous therapy, defibrillate, and suction by certified physicians and personnel who have passed course requirements. Organized emergency teams with advanced cardiac life support or emergency rooms staffed with ACLS physicians that are available to the patient in three minutes are the most effective.

Emergency equipment, supplies, and medications should be checked regularly (daily or after every use) and be appropriate for the population to be served (for example, pediatric airways must be available at a pediatric facility).

What Kind of Patients are Treated?

Does the Facility Have Experience in Treating the Patient's Disability?

- Yes
- No

What Number of Cases of Each of the Following Conditions does the Facility Treat Per Year? What Percentage Is This Number of the Total Patient Population at the Facility?

- Stroke-
- Head injury-
- Spinal-cord injury-
- Other neurological disorders-
- Multiple trauma-
- Arthritis/ rheumatology-
- Hip fracture-
- Amputation-

- Burn-
- Pain-
- Cardiac-
- Pulmonary-
- Other (specify)-

Interpretation: The number of patients treated by a facility for a particular condition and the percentage of the total population of patients are usually an indicator of the facility's degree of experience in treating a particular illness or disability.

In addition to specializing in particular disorders, some comprehensive inpatient medical rehabilitation programs are organized to treat the various conditions affecting certain groups in the population, like rehabilitation programs for children or aged persons. The consumer may want to ask if other patients with similar injuries or of a similar age will be at the facility during the patient's rehabilitation stay. Peer group interaction has the potential for providing significant therapeutic benefit.

Does the Facility Offer Special Program Needed for the Patient's Condition?

- Yes
- No

If yes, which ones?

- A spinal-cord injury program (or a regionally designated spinal-cord injury center)

- A head injury program

- A chronic pain management program

- An infant and early child development program

- A vocational program for work adjustment, work hardening, occupational skill training, job placement, programs in industry, and so forth

- An outpatient medical rehabilitation program

- Patient/family support groups by disability or diagnosis

- Disabled driver education program

- Sexuality education and counseling

- Dental care for disabled patients

- Athletic programs such as wheelchair sports, swim teams, horseback riding, and so forth

- Organized clinics (brace, wheelchair, amputee, and so forth)

- Recreational therapy programs outside the facility (bowling, concerts, vacation trips, self-defense classes)

- A home health agency

- A resource library

- Urodynamics studies to help the patient and rehabilitation nurse to achieve the best bladder management outcomes

- Others (specify)

Interpretation: The ready availability of many extensive programs does not in itself ensure high-quality rehabilitation. When selecting a facility, a consumer must take care to identify those programs offered by a facility that meet the patient's and family's particular needs and goals. For example, a patient who is retired is unlikely to need a vocational rehabilitation program. Also, patients who have longer stays in the rehabilitation program may need a broader range of programs than patients who have shorter stays.

How Well Suited Is the Facility and Its Equipment?

Does the Hospital Offer the Equipment or Physical Facilities Needed for the Patient's Condition?

- Social and recreational areas outside patient rooms, including a patient dining area. A specific dining area is a requirement for licensure in many states and for accreditation by CARF.

- A facility with real, not token, access to all rehabilitation treatment areas, grounds, nursing units, patient rooms, restrooms, telephones, elevators, disabled parking areas, and so forth.

- Appropriate equipment to lend to the patient for trial use in the facility (for example, wheelchairs, training braces, canes, and walkers).

- A training area for activities of daily living that simulates a kitchen, bath, bedroom, car, and so forth.

- A driver simulator trainer.

- A therapy pool or pools.

- Treatment areas that ensure visual and auditory privacy.

- Cardiac telemetry (heart monitoring) during patient activity for persons with associated heart disease.

- Other

Interpretation: Not all patients require all or the same types of physical facilities during the rehabilitation process. For example, a child or a patient with a limited attention span might benefit from a treatment room with visual and auditory privacy, but not need a driver simulator trainer to practice driving a car. Facilities that specialize in comprehensive inpatient medical rehabilitation have removed architectural and other barriers so patients can fully use the premises. Eliminating stairs, providing ramps, widening doorways, lowering telephones and drinking fountains, and providing parking for disabled persons allows easy access to facilities by persons in wheelchairs.

Comprehensive inpatient medical rehabilitation programs provide social and recreation areas and specialized equipment to encourage patients to practice learned skills.

Where Were the Facility's Rehabilitation Beds Located?

- Beds located in a freestanding rehabilitation hospital

- Beds organized in a distinct geographic site or unit within a hospital or medical center

- Beds organized in a hospital rehabilitation unit

- Beds scattered throughout various locations in the hospital

Interpretation: Efficiency and effectiveness are usually improved when rehabilitation beds are located together. The requirement for CARF and Joint Commission accreditation and for a Medicare comprehensive rehabilitation unit or facility is that rehabilitation beds be located together in one area.

Section 3

Coordination of Care and Follow-Up

What are Team Conferences, and How Is the Family Involved?

How often are Interdisciplinary Team Conferences Held to Plan the Patient's Rehabilitation Program?

- Weekly
- Every two weeks
- Every four weeks
- Occasionally
- Never
- Other (specify)

Are Patients (When Able) and Family Members (When Available) Included in Team Conferences?

- Yes
- No

  If yes, how often?

- Routinely
- Occasionally
- Rarely
- Upon request

Interpretation: All rehabilitation programs are expected to hold a multidisciplinary team conference about every patient at least every two weeks. The team consists of the physician, rehabilitation nurse, therapists, social workers, psychologist, and other health professionals involved in the patient's rehabilitation program.

Since the team conference is when team members plan and coordinate the patient's rehabilitation treatment, most rehabilitation professionals believe the team conference is an excellent time to have the patient and family present at periodic intervals. Insurance and employer representatives are important members of the rehabilitation team and should also be consulted or invited to participate in the team conferences. Team conferences improve communication. In recent

years, team conferences, when held weekly, have been found to reduce average length of stay.

Is There Continuity of Care and Follow-up Care?

*Does the Facility Use Preadmission Criteria to Assess the Rehabilita-
tion Potential of Patient?*

- Routinely
- Occasionally
- Rarely
- Never

Interpretation: In order to have CARF and Joint Commission accreditation, comprehensive medical inpatient rehabilitation programs
generally have written criteria that define the kinds of patients believed to have the potential for improving their physical function over a
particular time to justify the money and effort spent for rehabilitation.

*Is Discharge Planning Initiated Early in the Rehabilitation Treatment
Plan?*

- Routinely
- Occasionally
- Rarely
- Never

Interpretation: Discharge planning should begin on the day of
admission. An anticipated length of stay or tentative date for discharge should be set before or at the time of admission.

*Is Home Assessment by the Rehabilitation Team, Patient, and Fam-
ily Part of the Treatment Program?*

- Routinely
- Occasionally
- Rarely
- Never

Interpretation: The rehabilitation team may need to make an on-
site visit to the patient's home to look for architectural barriers, teach
the patient and family about mobility and activities of daily living in
the home, and make any recommendations before discharge.

Does the Facility Encourage Trial Home or Community Visits for Patients?

- Routinely
- Occasionally
- Rarely
- Never

Interpretation: A trial daytime or overnight visit to the home or community is an opportunity for the patient to practice skills and achieve functional objectives in the home. Questions or problems arising during the visit can then be resolved with the help of the rehabilitation team before the patient leaves the facility. These objectives must be carefully written in the record.

Is There a Systematic Process of Referring Patients to Other Agencies (Outpatient, Home Health, Discharge and Follow-Up)?

- Routinely
- Occasionally
- Rarely
- Never

Interpretation: Comprehensive inpatient medical rehabilitation programs allow ample time for referrals to other agencies, preparation of discharge summaries, and planning follow-up visits or contacts. This coordinated activity helps the rehabilitation team to make sure that further services are provided and to determine whether a patient's rehabilitation has been successful. In many programs, up to 50 percent of all rehab patients are referred to home care at the time of discharge.

Can Families Observe Treatment?

- Yes
- No

Interpretation: Observation is important in the treatment process and helpful to all concerned. Patients and families learn techniques of coping with the conditions, and communication about treatment is easier when team members can demonstrate strategies.

What are the Facility's Objectives for Returning Patients Home?

What Percentage of Rehabilitation Inpatients Return Home Following Treatment?

- 90% - 100%
- 80% - 89%
- 70% - 79%
- below 70%

Interpretation: The percentage of rehabilitation inpatients who are discharged home or to private residences can vary somewhat depending on of the type of disability and available family support. Consumers can reasonably ask specific facilities their objectives concerning patient discharges and their performance in this area. For example, a comprehensive inpatient medical rehabilitation program may have as a stated objective:

> "To maintain an average length of stay for stroke patients at about 30 days and for 80 percent of stroke patients to be discharged to the home."

The best measure of a facility's success rate is not whether the patient was discharged home, transferred to a skilled-nursing facility, or readmitted to a general hospital; instead, the success rate can be measured by the attainment of discharge objectives that were planned for individual patients.

Note: The overall national percentage of rehabilitation inpatients who are discharged home or to private residences is approximately 80 percent.

Questions and Concerns an Employer and Insurance Company May Have:

Does the Facility Have a Track Record of Success and the Expertise Needed to Handle the Patient's Case?

- Yes
- No

Is a Coordinator Assigned to Each Patient to Help the Patient and Family During Treatment and to Answer Questions for the Insurance Company and Employer?

- Yes
- No

Are Complete Reports about the Care Provided Periodically and are Billings Itemized In detail?

- Yes
- No

Does the Rehabilitation Facility Have an Adequate Staff to Coordinate Physical and Psychological Rehabilitation with Occupational Therapy, Vocational Rehabilitation, and Job Replacement or Return-to-Work Goals?

- Yes
- No

Does a Staff Member Visit the Patient's Employer to Review the Patient's Actual Job and Worksite, if Necessary?

- Yes
- No

What Percentage of Patients with This Condition Return to Work Following Rehabilitation?

Interpretation: From the viewpoint of an employer or insurer, the objective of physical rehabilitation is to return injured persons to their regular jobs as quickly as possible or to modify jobs to accommodate any residual disability. In the case of catastrophic injuries, the objective is to make injured persons as self-sufficient as possible so they can live independently, take care of their own needs, and require less care from others.

Although the major beneficiary of successful physical rehabilitation is the injured person, employers recognize the value of a skilled employee's return to work and are generally willing to help the patient and the rehabilitation program. Insurance companies and employers have come to realize that physical rehabilitation, properly handled by experienced and qualified persons, can bring about medical results well beyond those achieved just a few years ago.

An insurer most often selects a rehabilitation program on the basis of the quality of its staff and the excellence of treatment outcomes.

However, many other factors must be considered when selecting a facility, for instance, distance from the patient's home and costs.

Does the Facility Evaluate the Success of Its Program?

Does the Facility Measure the Effectiveness of the Rehabilitation It Provides?

- Yes
- No

    If yes, how?

Does the Facility Measure Its Efficiency in Providing Rehabilitation Services?

- Yes
- No

    If yes, how?

Are Evaluation Results Used in the Facility's Decision Making?

- Yes
- No

    If yes, how?

Is There a Mechanism to Review the Adequacy of the Facility's Evaluation System?

- Yes
- No

    If yes, what is it?

Does the Facility Measure Its Rates of Hospital-Acquired Infections and Pressure Sores?

- Yes
- No

    If yes, what are these rates?

Interpretation: Program evaluation improves decision making, planning for effective programs, and the care given to patients. Facilities that provide comprehensive inpatient medical rehabilitation use a program evaluation system to measure their efficiency in providing services and to measure the effectiveness of these services. These are both measured according to specific written criteria.

Quality of care measurements are based on accurate, timely, and useful information about patients, their progress in the hospital, and how well they keep their functional skills after rehabilitation. Program evaluation records patients' functional status several times during the rehabilitation program, with a particular emphasis on the patients' admission, discharge, and follow-up status. A facility gathers various types of patient information to analyze and share with its staff. With this information, rehabilitation professionals can identify weaknesses and strengths in providing patient care.

Hospital-acquired infections include urinary, respiratory tract, bloodstream, and surgical wound infections that appear after a patient has been in the hospital for 72 hours. In high quality facilities, the rates of infections are low; for example, urinary infections are 2.3 per 100 discharges; respiratory infections are 1 per 100 discharges. Pressure sores are ulcers that appear on the skin when poor circulation occurs from the lack of proper positioning for relief from pressure.

Hospital-acquired infections or pressure sores can lengthen patients' hospital stays and add costs to their treatment. Low rates of infection are desirable, as is a system to monitor and solve problems, usually through infection control and quality assessment departments in the facility.

Chapter 7

Rehab Partners: Clients and Counselors

Rehabilitation has been an assemblage of partnerships from its inception—first between the federal government and the states, then among a broad array of professional disciplines, later between the public and private sector, and now, increasingly between those who get services and those who give them. The Fifteenth Institute on Rehabilitation Issues—sponsored by the Research and Training Center at the University of Wisconsin-Stout—resulted in a state-of-the-art monograph titled *Client Involvement: Partnerships in the Vocational Rehabilitation Process* (see Sources Corthell and Van Boskirk). This *Rehab BRIEF* presents highlights from portions of the monograph devoted to analysis of the emergent client-counselor partnership, a watershed moment in the evolution of rehabilitation.

History

The counselor-client relationship was identified in law in the Rehabilitation Act of 1973. The preceding period of social change and unrest brought on revisions in the Act designed to further the rights of people with disabilities. Affirmative action received legal support from Title V in sections 501, 503, and 504. The Architectural and Transportation Barriers Compliance Board was created and the Client

Rehab Brief Bringing Research into Focus, Vol. XIII, No. 4 (1990), ISSN: 0732-2623; National Institute on Disability and Rehabilitation Research, Office of Special Education and Rehabilitative Service, Department of Education, Washington, DC 20202.

Assistance Demonstration Projects were established. Service priority was given to people with the most severe handicaps. The Individual Written Rehabilitation Program (IWRP) was required.

The IWRP requirement represented a major shift in philosophy: clients were to be considered full partners in decisions affecting their lives. This resulted from consumer influence on the political process and caused further consumer involvement. The Rehabilitation Act Amendments of 1978 provided a legal basis for the independent living movement. The Amendments of 1986 added support for client rights provided a legal basis for supported employment, and IWRP revisions included clients' statements of rehabilitation goals.

Partnership Principles

A partnership is an interpersonal business relationship that is more successful if the partners adopt a collaborative style of mutual respect and honesty. Six building blocks—equality, shared responsibility, mutual growth opportunity, goal or task orientation, limited tenure, and contractual agreement are described.

Equality: Partners must have parity with regard to perceived worth and ability to contribute to success. In imitation of the traditional medical model, rehabilitation has tended to use an authoritarian relationship wherein a dominant, overactive service provider acts upon a passive, submissive consumer. The status differential reinforces the attitude that the expert has the answers, and it blocks development of collaboration.

The conventional casework approach is said to set the stage for frustration and disappointment on both sides. The consumer may view the counselor as a bureaucrat who deliberately withholds services. The counselor may view the consumer as uncooperative and unreasonable. Conflict can only give way when both recognize their stakes in the relationship. They must view the service process as providing critical resource tools to clients. In place of the self-defeating traditional casework model, a democratic, participatory, co-management model is suggested and its components described.

Shared Responsibility: This implies a complementary effort wherein partners doing either similar or different work make sustained, valued contributions reflecting their interests and strengths (e.g., counselors are experts on world-of-work realities; clients are experts on their own life histories and present needs). Partners must communicate what actions need to be taken by whom, with a consistent focus on increasing consumers' involvement in and responsibility for their own rehabilitation.

Mutual Growth Opportunity: Maximizing one's potential is assumed to be a primary motivating force for everyone. There are many opportunities for doing so within rehabilitation and independent living activities—for example: clients developing their economic and personal independence, and counselors renewing themselves and expanding their horizons in order to avoid burnout. They are resources to each other in these endeavors, critical reference groups with tremendous power to reward and motivate each other.

Goal or Task Orientation: The partnership is governed by a common, identified goal and a task orientation toward success. The partners should be committed to the same goals before implementing a plan.

Limited Tenure: The partners' work together knowing that when agreed upon goals are reached the business relationship will end.

Written Agreements: Unlike social relationships, the partnership is contractually agreed upon in written action plans prepared at the end of an assessment and planning period.

Personal Attributes that Enhance Partnerships

Four broad categories of desirable characteristics are identified: attitudes, communication, contracting and negotiating skills, and what is called "individualization/ flexibility."

Attitudes: The primary traits are the classics: respect and acceptance of others, empathy, genuineness, and a style of being specific and concrete in communications. Three additional traits are cited. Humor is valuable in reducing stresses and increasing bonding. Commitment or motivation is considered critical—not a romantic notion of selfless devotion, just a realistic appraisal of what is needed and a determination to do one's best.

Trust is at the core of commitment, closeness, bonding, and risk taking in relationships. When trust is high, progress is rapid, behavior is assured, and the exchange of ideas and feelings is substantive. When trust is lacking, progress is slow, behavior is tentative, and involvement is superficial. The following are signs of mutual trust and respect in a relationship: (a) information, impressions, and evaluations are promptly and openly shared; (b) collaborators can express their feelings, needs, and priorities without worrying about being labeled in a derogatory way; (c) they can ask each other for help without feeling weak or incompetent, and can say "I don't know" or "I don't understand" without fearing loss of credibility; and (d) they avoid jargon that would make the other feel like an outsider.

Communication: An essential function of human service professionals is to develop and maintain communication with consumers, colleagues, and task-significant people in the community. Verbal and nonverbal communications influence others' thoughts, feelings, and actions on external issues (jobs, salaries) and internal issues (self-esteem, acceptance of limitations). True experts in communicating, can convey attitudes and feelings, as well as ideas and information, and can adapt communication techniques to suit individual consumers.

Contracting and Negotiating Skills: These are communication skills that warrant special attention, since conflict is inevitable when emotional and economic stakes are high. When the stakes are people's lives, conflict cannot always be resolved but it can be managed through mutually developed agreements. Contracting a broad working agreement occurs following assessment. Negotiating occurs periodically, as specific changes seem needed.

Individualization/Flexibility: The ability to be flexible and present to the moment in perceptions as well as behavior allows partners to respect and facilitate expressions of each other's authentic selves instead of stereotypes they are thought (or preferred) to be.

Ecological Influences

The ecological relationship between people and their environment is one of mutual influence. By the time people meet counselors for the first time they have usually encountered many professionals who have known many clients with similar demographics. The culture inherits beliefs, attitudes, and deep-rooted ideas of stigma. The slate is written upon; both come into the relationship with preconceptions. The authors try to shape a better road map for the future based on five environmental influences: philosophy, view of time, work settings, organizational structures, and support systems.

Philosophy: This establishes a conceptual framework for action, guiding the formation of missions, goals, objectives, processes, outcomes. Differing theoretical models represent contrasting philosophies regarding, consumer-professional partnerships, and each has profound implications for rehabilitation success. Three relevant models previously encapsulated by Cunningham and Davis include the expert, consumer, and transplant models.

Expert Model: Users view themselves as having the expertise in relation to their clients; they decide what information is relevant, control the decisions, and give little importance to consumer views on relationship. The model is efficient but demands excessive time and gives disproportionate responsibility to professionals; it fails to build client self-sufficiency and may reinforce dependency.

Consumer Model: Users view clients, families, and advocates as business customers with rights to make decisions and select services. The professional provides resources, consults, and instructs in a relationship wherein negotiation is a key tool. It is not applicable to clients who wish to be dependent or passive or who don't respect organizational constraints. When suitable, its benefits to long-range skill and self-esteem building are great.

Transplant Model: Called a hybrid between the traditional-expert and new-wave-consumer models, users operate as if some of their expertise can be uprooted and transplanted into the hands of consumers. They sometimes assume the role of technical expert but often involve consumers as self-help resources. Key roles are instruction and ongoing consultation.

Time and Space: Time represents caring and worth and is important emotionally as well as pragmatically to relationships. The sense that another does not have time for you is frustrating and destructive when you feel you need it. Rehabilitation partners must contract for realistic time to avoid these problems. Can partners work efficiently in the space provided? Is the place conducive to feelings of warmth, acceptance, comfort, freedom of expression, and feelings of hope that agendas will mesh and joint efforts will lead to accomplishment? Is the place accessible, quiet, private, safe, well lighted, comfortable, convenient to reach? Does the decor encourage interaction? Are phone calls held?

Organizational Structure: Do the partners understand, respect, tolerate the formal policies, rules, regulations, eligibility criteria, budget constraints, operational procedures, informal politics, and climate of the agency? This is critical so they do not waste time blaming each other over limitations inherent in the service delivery structure.

Support System: *"Reaching one's potential to live independently is not accomplished without substantial contributions from significant others."*

John Donne recognized this need for a support system (at the turn of the 16th century) in his great poem beginning *"No man is an island..."* Rehabilitation and medicine are charged with ignoring it until recently. Now, many writers view the family as an ally that has been treated as if it were the enemy; one says the family *is* the client. The authors say. "If the primary consumer wants family involvement, then the professional should support it and find ways to help".

This broadening of the defined consumer calls for applying systems theory in a broad framework, forcing professionals to view the ecological unit (client in situ) as the proper focus of assessment and intervention. Their primary purpose, then. is teaching environmental coping skills; and environmental modification and concrete assistance are as important as face-to-face counseling. In summary, the authors believe the occupational role of "system/network consultant" should be added to those of treatment agent, teacher-counselor, service broker and advocate.

Strategies

General strategies that help establish empowering partnerships between counselors and consumers include mutual respect, honesty, awareness of preconceptions about one another, and two-way communication. Specific strategies include using nontechnical language, confirming each other's understanding, understanding each person's roles, using self-assessment techniques, accentuating the positive, involving support system members, follow along, and networking.

Awareness of Preconceptions: Preconceptions are introduced by previous service providers in written records. Counselors are urged, whenever possible, to see new clients once before reviewing files. "This is especially important because some clients have 'bought' a view of themselves based on others perceptions and behaviors." After files are reviewed, counselors are enjoined still to put some of the information aside until they can determine the accuracy of interpretations and conclusions on their own.

Two-Way Communication: Consumers say things more openly when counselors are not attached to an outcome. With a flexible counselor agenda, consumers can be more open and honest.

Nontechnical Language: When counselors use technical language, clients often misunderstand, yet nod their heads to prevent embarrassment. This very human characteristic leads to confusion, then anger and defensiveness. To say counselors must speak at the client's level does not imply phony imitation: it means using clear nonjargon language.

Confirming Understanding: Eliciting responses from clients to validate understanding and coaching them to reciprocate also draws clients into active participation in the counseling process.

Understanding Roles: In different times and situations counselors play different roles—counselor, case manager or coordinator, and advocate being three primary ones. It is important for both partners to know which hat is being worn and why because situations may arise that counselors cannot handle—for example, suicide threats—and each must be prepared for a referral to another source of help.

Self-Assessment: Both counselor and client need all the valid assessment information they can get in order to make good decisions. They may decide together what areas to assess. Although clients may have insufficient background to set the scope of the assessment, they should have a loud voice in the direction it takes. Feedback should be balanced so clients are not dejected by information about "weaknesses" not counterbalanced by good news about "strengths."

Follow Along: Provisions for post-counseling follow along should be made in advance so clients and their support people will not slip between the cracks. Unannounced visits to a person's work site may cause embarrassment: it's better to ask to be invited. You probably will not be unless a true partnership has developed. An empowered consumer should have access to the counselor when a need arises, but dependency should not be fostered.

Networking: A consumer's success in the community may depend on access to resources—vocational, personal, social, religious, medical, financial, and so forth. Counselors must establish linkages—networking—which can be used and clients must be taught to network for themselves.

Consumers must make their own vocational decisions. Counselors can only facilitate and guide, especially by focusing, on the client's decision-making capabilities. When these fall short, offer additional counseling, teaching, and assessment, etc. as needed. An instrument is recommended—the Vocational Decision.Making Interview (VDMI) described by Czerlinsky and McCray—which gives information about employment readiness and self-appraisal as well as decision-making readiness. Use of such instruments may draw clients into active participation and give them immediate feedback on their strengths and weaknesses.

Families and Communities

The family is the basic support system—a group of interdependent individuals who are in turn interdependent with the community. For individuals disabled before the age of 30, parents seem to be critical to future success—setting expectations and standards by which to facilitate adjustment and development or barring it through guilt, over-protectiveness, and so forth. An extremely high percentage of successful adults with disabilities cite their parents as primary contributors to their achievements. Consequently, professionals need to accept parents as key partners in achieving rehabilitation, teach them what they need to know in order to be better teammates, and—when relevant—help them confront any economic or emotional disincentives to promoting their child's independence. Clients lacking familial supports will be disadvantaged, and providers need to help them compensate. Families with marginal economic status may perceive loss of Social Security as a barrier. Counselors should provide information about other options, but exercise of options is not the counselor's responsibility.

Managers' and Supervisors' Roles

Management is most effective when it concentrates on obtaining resources for counselors and provides an environment conducive to good client-counselor relationships. Supervisors can provide counselors information on their experiences with individual cases in a "coaching" relationship.

Reducing Barriers to IWRP Development and VR Success

Political decisions affect who will be eligible and how services will be provided. Legal, operational, attitudinal, and socioeconomic exigencies may bar client-counselor partners from implementing a plan. A barrier exists in that the rehabilitation and consumer communities have not developed effective coalitions and networks to influence public policy. Correcting this might be a prime strategy toward resolution. The authors suggest also:

- Teach consumers to be self-advocates, from basic assertiveness training to political process techniques.

- Encourage providers, professional societies, community organizations, etc. to jump on the advocacy bandwagon.

- Involve consumers in agency budgeting processes. They learn what the problems are and gain ammunition for future self-advocacy activities. Maybe they can help get bigger appropriations.

- Involve consumers in new policy and program development through advisory committees, public hearings, surveys, and requests for feedback and comments. The powerfully enabling supportive employment initiative came about as a result of massive consumer input to the legislature.

Misunderstandings as Barriers: When clients do not understand eligibility criteria, needs tests, feasibility issues, they may question how it's "fair" for consumers to get different kinds and levels of service, and IWRP development may be blocked. Reconciliation strategies include:

- Use of agency brochures and other print handouts explaining commonly encountered misunderstandings.

- Agencies and Client Assistance Programs might jointly conduct consumer workshops covering these issues.

- Agencies might offer consumer orientations covering why diagnostic information is needed, how plans are developed, etc.

- Agencies should develop good networking relationships with referral sources and might conduct annual interagency training on commonly misunderstood issues.

- Agencies should make clear policy statements and might use the public media to clarify issues along with promotional efforts.

Failures of Courage: The ultimate barrier may be the absence of risk taking—on the parts of clients, parents, counselors, supervisors, and managers. To avoid a spiral of reinforcing self-fulfilling prophecies of under-achievement, all partners can bolster each other's courage to take risks that might lead to success for all.

Estimation Errors: Counselors and clients alike may overestimate or underestimate client potentials for success in given vocational pursuits. A major reason is lack of consumer involvement in all stages of the testing/evaluation process. Rarely chosen vocations may be discounted before discovering whether they might be valid. Emphasizing clients' roles in selecting tests and evaluation situations and providing feedback on results are suggested as prime correctives. (See *Rehab BRIEF* Vol. S. No. 5 for a model that asserts only clients can truly interpret testing findings.)

The Institute on Rehabilitation Issues

The Institute on Rehabilitation Issues began in 1947 as a workshop for state supervisors of guidance, training, and placement. They picked topics that warranted detailed study, explored them in small work groups, and presented their findings at an annual meeting.

In 1962 universities become involved as sponsors of a broadened scope of prime study groups. In 1973, the present name was selected and three vocationally oriented Research and Training Centers (RTCS) were selected as permanent, rotating sponsors—West Virginia, Arkansas, and Wisconsin-Stout.

The objectives are (a) to identify content areas and issues in vocational rehabilitation where training materials are needed. (b) to develop training resource materials in areas of priority interest, and (c) to utilize publications prepared by IRI for the training of state VR agency staff.

The call for topics goes to state VR agencies, RSA offices, NIDRR, all RTCs, the National Council of Rehabilitation Educators, and others. The Planning Committee selects one topic from those submitted by the state VR agencies (through CSAVR), one from those submitted by RSA, and a third topic from any source. Prim study group members are chosen on the basis of relevant knowledge, leadership, ability to write, and willingness to work.

Prime study groups meet twice for 3 or 4 days. Each member is given a writing assignment at the first meeting and drafts are assembled for review and editing at the second. Second drafts are assembled for the annual meeting, where input from other participants is encouraged. Following the annual meeting, final drafts are compiled and the book is printed and distributed.

Source

Corthell, D. & Van Boskirk, C. (1988). *Client involvement: Partnerships in the vocational rehabilitation process.* Fifteenth Institute on Rehabilitation Issues, Menomonie, WI: RTC, Stout Vocational Rehabilitation Institute.

Chapter 8

Culturally Sensitive Rehabilitation

If what you [the rehabilitation counselor] are going to do to a client is unacceptable in his culture, or renders him unacceptable to other members of his culture, you can't do it, even if you consider it common rehabilitation practice.

Carol Locust, Ph.D. Director of Training NARTC

Racial and ethnic minorities constitute an increasing proportion of the American population and work force. People of Asian descent are the fastest growing Minority group in the United States. A 1988 census study reported that the Hispanic population totals almost 20 million. There are more than 300 federally recognized American Indian tribes with a total population of 1.4 million. And people of African descent form the nation's largest minority.

Members of minority groups are disproportionately represented at the lower end of the economic spectrum and in the ranks of people who are unemployed. Census Bureau data document a high correlation between low socioeconomic status and disability; research corroborates the high incidence of disability among minority groups with 14.3 percent of black males and 14 percent of black females reporting a disability, compared with 9 percent of white males and 7.8 percent of white females. Data from the 1980 census indicate a rate of work-related disability for American Indians at about one and one-half

1993 *Rehab Brief*, Vol. XV, No. 8, (1993), ISSN: 0732-2623; National Institute on Disability and Rehabilitation Research.

times that of the general population, a higher rate than for other minority groups. Also, while most people think that the Asian/Pacific community is well educated and well off, in fact 12 percent of this population lives below the poverty level, and the number of Asian/Pacific persons with disabilities is disproportionate to the population.

What is the experience of members of racial and ethnic minority groups in rehabilitation? Having a disability and being a member of an ethnic minority group have often presented what many see as a "double bias." Studies show that there have been serious problems in service delivery and in success rates. Placement rates among nonwhite clients are proportionately lower than those of white clients. There is a greater tendency for cases of white clients to be closed "rehabilitated," at or above minimum wage, than for nonwhites. Of the 2.5 million Hispanics of working age who were reported disabled in 1981, only 25,000 were rehabilitated by public rehabilitation programs. Similarly, Asian-Americans, American Indians, and blacks have experienced difficulty accessing the rehabilitation system and benefiting from it; this has been manifested by low referral rates, high dropout rates, and low success rates.

Cultural Insensitivity

Many members of ethnic minorities, and those who work on their behalf, believe that part of the problem has been that of cultural insensitivity. Robert Davila, former Assistant Secretary of the U.S. Department of Education's Office of Special Education and Rehabilitative Services (OSERS), himself a Mexican-American with a disability, has said that in order to improve the quality of service delivery, rehabilitation professionals need to learn to recognize the cultural values of minority individuals and to adapt service delivery, approaches accordingly. This chapter focuses on the issue of culturally sensitive rehabilitation. It highlights recent research in the field and introduces the two Rehabilitation Research and Training Centers (RRTCS) devoted to this chapter.

Cultural Pluralism

The familiar metaphor of this nation as a "melting pot" has led to confusion and disagreement. Some people believe that immigrants and second or third generation Americans should become acculturated, that they should assimilate themselves into American society, believe and behave like Americans, and shake off characteristics of their cultural and ethnic backgrounds. Others believe that such acculturation is never fully possible, nor even desirable. The concept of cultural pluralism suggests that cultural diversity is, in itself, a mark of the "American" culture and that such diversity, in all of its manifestations, should not only be recognized but honored, celebrated, and encouraged.

Whatever one believes should be true of American society, the fact is that many different cultures do coexist here and it is impossible to separate individuals from their histories or their cultures. If rehabilitation professionals wish to serve all clients effectively, it is important to recognize culturally based beliefs, values, and behaviors. Cultural elements such as language, family roles, sex roles, and religious beliefs can play a significant role in the etiology, symptom manifestation, and rehabilitation treatment of disabilities. Culture can influence beliefs about causation of illness or disability, the conditions that qualify as "sickness," the expectations about what an affected. person should do, and the expected actions of others. When socio-cultural elements are included in the assessment and rehabilitation process, clients can be more accurately evaluated and effectively rehabilitated than when these elements are excluded.

Counselor Education

There is a growing movement among rehabilitation counselor education programs to include a focus on cultural differences in their curriculums. Rehabilitation counselors need to be trained to be sensitive not only to individual differences among clients but also to cultural differences.

While discrimination must never be tolerated, many in the field say that it is not always best to treat clients without regard to gender, race, creed, or cultural background; such differences must be acknowledged and taken into account in order for appropriate services to be provided. Rehabilitation students and all practitioners need to develop awareness, sensitivity, and respect for other cultures and offer services that reflect the belief that clients' values, although different, are equal to their own.

Focus on Mexican-Americans

Hispanic clients in rehabilitation experience low referral rates, high dropout rates, and poor overall success rates, despite the fact that they are over represented in physically demanding jobs and incur many job-related disabilities. Mexican-Americans are the dominant Hispanic group in the United States. Julie Smart, a Mary E. Switzer Merit Fellow, recently conducted a study funded by the National Institute on Disability and Rehabilitation Research (NIDRR) to find out more about Mexican-Americans in public rehabilitation programs and to suggest ways of improving outcomes.

Smart believes that Mexican-Americans with disabilities may be said to by handicapped by two conditions: the disability itself and the subordinate status that many Mexican-Americans occupy in the social and economic structure of the United States.

The state/federal rehabilitation program consists of a system of laws, regulations, knowledge, beliefs, norms, values, attitudes, techniques, and procedures. Smart describes this system as undeniably part of the dominant culture, reflecting an Anglo-centric or Eurocentric world view and value system. According to Smart, one set of cultural beliefs determines the way in which services are provided, but other—often conflicting-sets of cultural beliefs held by clients can influence how these services are utilized. If a deeper understanding of the Hispanic culture and its impact on clients with disabilities could be obtained, then rehabilitation services that are more culturally relevant could be extended.

Julie Smart's research focused on the issues of acculturation and acceptance of disability among Mexican-Americans.

Acceptance of Disability

Good health is an interest of people of all cultures. However, the ways in which various cultures view, react to, and treat disability vary. It may be said that acceptance of disability is culturally determined. Thus, attitudes and perceptions of Mexican-Americans toward disability are determined to some extent by the Mexican-American culture.

Smart points out that the degree of acceptance of disability may influence an individual in his or her decision to apply for services and may subsequently enhance or retard the success of the entire rehabilitation process. She identifies several factors that may be said to be associated with acceptance of disability among Mexican-Americans and other Hispanics:

- **Well-defined gender roles**. Many Hispanic men have been taught that it is their responsibility to provide for their families, and being strong is considered an important male attribute. Acceptance of disability may therefore be more difficult

62

for a Hispanic male than for clients who perceive their roles less stringently.

- **Stoic attitude toward life**. Acceptance of disability among Mexican-Americans may be affected by what many researchers identify as a culturally based attitude of resignation and acceptance of life problems. There may be less inclination to question, complain, or strive for change than among people of other cultural backgrounds.

- **Cohesive, protective, family-oriented society**. Researchers agree that Mexican-American families play important roles in rehabilitation outcomes. On the one hand, the reaction to disability by the tightly knit, family-oriented Hispanic culture can be described as uniquely supportive and comforting. However, some have seen this cultural characteristic as overprotective and paternalistic, making independence and self-sufficiency for the Hispanic disabled person nearly impossible to achieve.

- **Religious views**. Religion plays an important role in the definition, response, and acceptance of disability for many Hispanic clients. Smart cites research that points out that in the Hispanic world view, disability is often seen as a punishment for one's sins or for the sins of one's parents. It is important for counselors to understand that such a "theological etiology" may be ascribed to disability by many Hispanic clients.

- **Reliance on physical labor**. Mexican-American and other Hispanic people are over represented in physically demanding jobs that have a high risk of illness, disability, and fatality. They also have lower levels of education. For many Mexican-Americans who are disabled, options for employment or training may be very limited.

Acculturation

Smart's research indicates that in order to provide culturally relevant and successful rehabilitation services, some judgment or measurement of acculturation and biculturalism must be made. This is not to say that it is better for a client to be acculturated; it says that for rehabilitation efforts to be successful, they must be culturally appropriate for each client. The more acculturated a client is, the more likely it is that traditional (Anglo- or Euro-centric) assessment tools and counseling strategies will be successful. A client who is less acculturated, that is, more closely tied to his or her home culture, may benefit more from assessment techniques and interventions that take into account his or her language, value system, and beliefs.

Another telling finding of Smart's discussion concerning acculturation is this: rehabilitation practitioners tend to view acculturation as a predictor of client success. If a client retains the language and continues to embrace the cultural characteristics of his or her home country, that client may be viewed by a rehabilitation counselor as being at high risk of not reaching rehabilitation goals. Smart suggests that instead of viewing level of acculturation as a predictor of success, practitioners should view it as a tool for determining what assessment techniques and interventions might be most appropriate.

Implications

Smart's work with Mexican-Americans makes it clear that the rehabilitation process must be responsive and appropriate for each client. Cultural awareness and sensitivity can help practitioners and policymakers design and carry out programs that are best suited for clients whose world views and value systems are culturally different from their own. Smart suggests some important implications that could apply widely in rehabilitation practice:

- Level of acculturation should become a routine part of the evaluation of Mexican-American clients. Individualized Written Rehabilitation Plans (IWRPS) could be devised and implemented that take into account level of acculturation. Also, since there are so few bilingual, bicultural rehabilitation counselors, it would be possible to make better use of them by making a determination, based in part on an acculturation instrument, of who actually would profit most by working with bilingual, bicultural professionals.

- Obviously there are not enough bilingual, bicultural rehabilitation counselors in all geographic areas to serve Mexican-American clients. Therefore, more and better training about cultural sensitivity must be made available to rehabilitation counselors.

- Smart recommends that two courses be added to the curriculum for rehabilitation counselors:

    1. **Rehabilitation Counseling with Culturally Diverse Clients**. This would have both a theoretical and a clinical component. The clinical component would include a supervised

practicum in which students would work with clients of different ethnic groups. Not only would the students become sensitized to the issues and concerns of these groups but they could also learn to use culturally enhancing rehabilitation techniques.

2. **Training Course for the Use of Paraprofessional Bilingual, Bicultural Interpreters.** Smart found during the process of gathering data that many clients who consider themselves to be bilingual express different content when speaking Spanish than when speaking English. Moreover, these clients expressed more content in Spanish than in English. The use of bilingual, bicultural interpreters would help address the needs of Mexican-American clients and also the needs of monolingual English-speaking rehabilitation counselors who work with these clients. In fact, Smart proposes two courses for the rehabilitation curriculum; the first would train interpreters to work with rehabilitation counselors, and the second would train counselors in the use of interpreters in the counseling setting.

For more information about this study, contact The National Rehabilitation Information Center (NARIC), 8455 Colesville Road, Suite 935, Silver Spring, MD 20910. Ask for the NIDRR document Level of Acculturation of Physically Disabled Mexican-Americans and Acceptance of Disability, project number H133F90017.

The Native American Research and Training Center

The Native American Research and Training Center (NARTC) was established in 1983 at the University of Arizona and serves as a national resource for American Indian communities and for people working with Indian populations.

Under funding from the National Institute on Disability and Rehabilitation Research (NIDRR), NARTC investigates health and rehabilitation issues, helps determine rehabilitation and service needs, defines barriers to service, and devises innovative and culturally relevant interventions. One of the central objectives of the Center is to promote active participation and partnership of Indian communities in the Center's programs.

Each year, NARTC conducts workshops, conferences, and training programs on a number of rehabilitation and healthcare issues. In addition, as part of its mandate to disseminate the results of its research and training programs, NARTC publishes a monograph series and produces training videotapes. A few of these are highlighted here and give a flavor of this Center's commitment to culturally sensitive rehabilitation practice.

- **We Look–You Look: Perspectives**. After defining the levels of acculturation and the process of assimilation of American Indians into contemporary American society, this video discusses American Indian cultural values and philosophies. The presentation emphasizes Indian perspectives about time, death, social interaction, religion, the significance of life, child rearing and behavior.

- **Communicating With Native American Patients**. A Navajo practitioner discusses some of the communication problems that arise in the Indian client/service provider relationship as a result of cultural differences and suggests culturally appropriate solutions to these problems.

- **American Indian Concepts of Health and Unwellness**. Based on a monograph of the same title, this videotape presents 10 basic beliefs about health and handicaps common to the traditions of the majority of American Indian tribes and provides interesting comparisons between Indian and non-Indian attitudes and beliefs about health.

- **Culture and Disability**. The relationship between culture and the perception of disability is discussed in this video by Jennie R. Joe, Ph.D., director of NARTC. The presentation is particularly helpful for those wishing to understand how cultural differences impact on perception and treatment of disabilities and handicaps.

For more information about culturally sensitive rehabilitation practice and the American Indian community, or to obtain more information about NARTC's publications and videotapes, contact:

Jennie R. Joe, Ph.D., MPH
Director
NARTC
1642 E. Helen Street
Tucson, AZ 85719

Chapter 9

Rehabilitation and the Power of Attractiveness

With a disability, you look in a mirror and compare yourself to Miss America or Robert Redford and it's all over as far as sex appeal or dress-for-success is concerned. Right? WRONG. The mature person who takes stock of the situation accurately will see more than the mirror shows.

[Readers are urged to] decide what they want from others and from themselves—how they would like to appear, wish to be seen... on use of imagination to begin a process of evolving toward what you want to be within the framework of what you are.

—Excerpts from a book review Rehab Lit. *1986, 47(5-6)*

A comely lass—A winsome lad—A fox—A hunk. The words and stereotypic images they conjure may have changed, but physical appearance seems as important today as ever. Advertisers use "the beautiful people" to promote their products and services, and sometimes all they're selling is an image. (Once we only looked to see how jeans fit; now we read the label.) Traditionally the beauty business focused on attracting sex, love, and marriage partners. Now something has been added—dressing for success, attaining the proper corporate or other career-related image. The image is usually as attractive as possible—and it's useful to pay attention to that word. We shape our looks

Rehab Brief, Vol. X, No. 4, ISSN: 0732-2623; National Institute on Disability and Rehabilitation Research, undated.

and that ineffable something referred to as "presence" to attract some-one or something—bring closer to ourselves some person, job success, or perhaps money.

Along with this has come rising social science interest in the impact of attractiveness on such variables as self-esteem, marital satisfac-tion, career success, and "happiness" in general. With few exceptions, research findings over the last decade and a half have shown that the better looking and more appealing judges rate research subjects to be, the more likely the subjects are to report that they are successful in their work, social, and/or love lives and describe themselves as "happy." Elaine Hatfield, considered a pioneer psychological researcher on attractiveness, has coauthored a state-of-the-art monograph with sociologist Susan Sprecher (see sources). *Mirror, Mirror... The Impor-tance of Looks in Everyday Life* reviews what behavioral scientists have learned about the effects of physical attractiveness, supple-mented with anecdotal material from medical casebooks, classical lit-erature, and other sources.

The "Lookin Good" industry is enormous, encompassing fashions, jewelry, hair styling, cosmetics, fitness, health food, secrets of personal magnetism, and much more. An expanding array of goods and ser-vices promises to take us closer to a goal that is generally unattain-able. Most of us think this is silly or wrong, and get caught up in it anyway.

Rehabilitation Takes Notice

A possible reason why the field of rehabilitation has remained al-most silent on this subject until very recently, is that we don't like the value system that imbues looks with a great deal of power; it doesn't seem right, or fair, so we ignore the matter. However, if we believe the research reports—as well as our day-to-day, observations—looks do count. A 1981 textbook on the psychological aspects of dis-ability points out: "It doesn't help to label it shallow, irrelevant, inhumane, or undemocratic. It is a force to be reckoned with." Still, in the belief that some clients may be hurt or offended, providers of-ten avoid the topic. A little thought suggests the following questions:

- A reasonable capsule summary, of attractiveness research find-ings is: impaired attractiveness handicaps a person relative to more attractive peers in achieving success and happiness. Doesn't a person who is handicapped by a disability need more than most to avoid any additional handicapping?

- It usually feels cruel to tell people they're never going to walk, see, or hear again, but at some point, with many clients, it has to be done because postponing the confrontation with reality could be more damaging. Is this situation analogous? Is it irresponsible not to attend to a factor that may palpably affect a client's future?

Rehabilitation workers are beginning to ask such questions—and answer them with decisions to include some form of attractiveness-enhancement services among those they provide. Lacking a strong rehabilitation research base to guide them, pioneers in service settings typically start doing what seems needed and the supporting or disaffirming research comes later. On the subject at hand, there is at least a general research base, which found its way quickly into the popular press, plus a scattering of articles in the rehabilitation literature.

For example, a brief notice in the November 1986 *Psychology Today* titled "Look good, get well" states:

Two patients with similar backgrounds and symptoms are released on the same day from a psychiatric hospital. One patient is quite attractive, the other decidedly homely. Who will adjust better to community life? .... The findings do not prove conclusively that attractive patients have easier recoveries, but they do show that attractiveness is related to later adjustment .... Farina [the investigator] suggests that when mental health professionals prepare patients for discharge, "attending to topics of appearance could well be as important to the patients as fostering interpersonal skills."

Later adjustment is, of course, just what rehabilitation professionals are interested in. Before highlighting additional research reports and articles, it may be useful to provide an orienting summary of the scope of topics found that relate to attractiveness enhancement—it proved to be surprisingly broad.

The Body

Health / Fitness: diet and nutrition, exercise, health habits (e.g., rest; alcohol/drug, caffeine, tobacco use), attitudes, habitual moods and emotions.

Hygiene: sanitary practices, bathing, odor management, care of teeth.

Grooming: skin care, hair care, nail care, cosmetics usage.

Surgical Options: dental and plastic surgery.

Adornments

Fashions: adapted clothing, styles.

Accessories: functional usage.

Presence

Social Personality: poise, self-confidence, charm/wit/humor.

Interpersonal Skills: conversation, listening, negotiating.

Voice: sound, quality, speech.

The health/fitness area was covered in *Rehab BRIEF*, vol. 8, no. 12, and will be excluded here. Certain aspects of "presence" were touched upon in *Rehab BRIEF*, vol. 5, no. 9, on job clubs; however, this area is excluded here because the "social personality" and "voice" elements are too impoverished in the literature and the "interpersonal skills" element too voluminous to cover here. The following material is drawn from the other topics listed above.

Some Attitudes Reflected in the Literature

A fair amount of rehabilitation literature is available on techniques and devices for making the basic functions of bathing, grooming, and dressing easier or more independent. Usually, the aspiration is to render the person clean and presentable. There may or may not be passing references to the more dynamic concept of attractiveness. A sense of struggle to eliminate the negative—and little sense of joyful accentuation of the positive—is often conveyed. For example, one report uses the terms "appearance management" and "impression management" in lieu of the more positive attractiveness enhancement."

These attitudes—so ingrained that they are held by people with disabilities as well as people without them—are beginning to change. Dressing for success is being picked up by job placement specialists as requisite to getting their clients placed expeditiously. (See the end of this chapter, which describes one program for enhancing job-ready clients' "presentation" of themselves at job interviews and in other settings.)

The traditional personal hygiene and grooming literature does hold many useful facts and ideas, and an illustrative sampling is offered next.

Sampling of Personal Hygiene Hints

Bathing

- To prevent scalding when sensation is impaired, use a floating plastic bath thermometer.

- Use of soap suspended on a cord can reduce the danger of slipping or falling in the shower.

- People with grip problems may find bathmits with elastic bands or velcro closings easier to use than washcloths.

- Long handled sponges may help in washing and drying hard-to-reach parts of the body.

Hair Care

- A good cut and a simple style are the first steps in making hair care easier.

- A hose that attaches to a faucet in a sink or tub, or a plastic shampoo tray, may be helpful.

- No-rinse shampoos and conditioners may be useful.

- Detangler conditioners are very helpful for people with arm weakness; and battery-powered hairbrushes are available.

- Velcro-covered curlers come in differing sizes and can be managed with one hand.

Nail Care

- A suction-based nailbrush can make nail care possible for those with use of only one arm or hand.

- To file nails with one hand, tape the file or emery board to the edge of a table, or hold a long file between the knees while seated.

- Electric manicure sets are available which can be used with one hand or when grasp is weak but coordination is good.

- An inexpensive manicure at a beauty school is easy and fun!

Shaving

- Electric shavers are safer; holders are available to keep them stable.

71

- Women may prefer to use depilatory creams or to have hair removed by waxing.

Dental Care

- Handles of toothbrushes can be lengthened to compensate for limited reach or built up for easier grasping.
- A wide elastic band around the palm can compensate for lack of grip.
- Electric toothbrushes are good options for some people.
- Some communities have clinics that specialize in dental care for people with physical disabilities.

The Psychotherapeutic Value of Cosmetics

Controlled studies conducted by Jean Ann Graham, a psychologist who has worked in the cosmetics industry, have demonstrated the psychological benefits of cosmetic treatment for various groups of people, including those with disabilities. A new field, the psychology of cosmetics, is now emerging.

The social psychology literature indicates that unattractiveness can be a severe handicap, socially, while physically attractive people appear to gain many advantages in a variety of situations. According to Graham, the skillful use of cosmetics can provide an effective way to manipulate attractiveness.

Her research findings suggest that cosmetic therapy has both short- and long-range beneficial effects on appearance, socialization, self-confidence, self-esteem, and outlook on life. This has been demonstrated among elderly people; patients hospitalized for physical illness, disabilities, and mental disorders; and others who were discontented with their appearance. Two kinds of cosmetic treatment are described:

- beautifying or enhancing cosmetics
- camouflage cosmetics—heavier masking to correct disfigurement such as burns, scars, birthmarks, and skin diseases.

Facial deformities that require plastic surgery may be followed up by both camouflage and beautifying cosmetics.

Cosmetic intervention to promote psychological well-being can be particularly effective in the recovery phases of certain mental and physical disabilities, making the individual feel attractive again. It can also help break a negative cycle that develops frequently: feelings of lowered self-esteem lead to neglected appearance, leading in turn to negative responses from others, which further lower self-esteem and confidence.

Cosmetic Surgery and Down Syndrome

Robert Brent, while chairing a 1983 conference on the subject, characterized the congenital malformations of the facial features of a person with Down syndrome as "stigmata which make the individual a recognizable entity with a negative connotation." He went on to say that judicious use of plastic surgery, by improving appearance, might increase ability by giving the person a better chance to develop in society. Although no broad-based research has been done, considerable anecdotal data from families as well as data from research reports have been accumulated by the National Down Syndrome Congress on the practices and potential of cosmetic surgery. Executive Director Diane Crutcher states:

> The National Down Syndrome Congress does not have an official position regarding plastic surgery and the person with Down syndrome but does encourage thoughtful investigation to find the most appropriate team to assist you in the investigation and (if deemed so) the implementation of the techniques. The team would ideally include not only the plastic surgeon (who has previous experience in working with people with Down syndrome) but also a psychologist and a speech therapist. Obviously, the speech therapist could help analyze whether tongue reduction surgery would be of use with the child being considered; the psychologist could assist in the emotional question faced by the family and child.

Most surgery is done early, when the child is between four and eight. In addition to tongue reduction, other correctives sometimes include raising the bridge of the nose with a silicone implant, changing the axis of the eyelids, correcting crossed eyes, augmenting small receding chins, bringing ears closer to the head, and reducing the size of lower lips.

Adapted and Stylish Clothing

Clothing can affect our moods, self-esteem, and the impressions we make on others. What we wear provides information about these

73

to others, as well as information about our social-occupational standing, sex-role identification, values, temperament, aesthetic priorities, and so forth. Most people take for granted the availability of clothing they can wear that will "say" what they want it to say about them. Not so for many people with disabilities.

There are, however, a growing number of companies manufacturing special clothing for people with disabilities. These firms supply ready-made adapted clothing or kits for customers to complete. Some will construct garments on receiving measurements. Patterns for adapted designs are also available. The following suggestions were offered in various articles and pamphlets vis-a-vis particular needs or problems.

For crutch users: Some clothing has protective padding in the underarm area to resist abrasion. Fasteners and other devices are available to keep blouses/shirts inside skirts or pants. Action pleats in the back armhole and shoulder areas may prove helpful.

For wheelchair users: Larger size clothing in soft, lightweight, stretchable, absorbent, smooth fabrics may be preferable. Garments shorter in back are less bulky. Heavy coat sleeve bulk can be avoided by wearing ponchos. Raglan sleeves, tops with sleeve emphasis (eye-catching), and bias cut skirts with minimal waistline gathering work well for women who remain seated a great deal. Special hosiery and stylish boots are available for easily chilled feet.

Clothing should pay attention to lines and view point of others. Short skirts can be indecent. Wide brim hats cut facial view from those standing and the seated person.

A Program to Enhance Presentation at Job Interviews

My awareness of the importance of how people with disabilities present themselves to others stemmed from working in a transition program for young adults in London. It became apparent during mock job interviews that many clients lacked interviewing skills, interpersonal skills, and in many cases basic hygiene and grooming skills revealing low levels of self-esteem.

From this evolved the Self Enhancement Employment Key (SEEK), designed to encourage self-help, self-esteem, and successful transition from school or unemployment to work. I'd read research reports on a vicious cycle-low self-esteem leading to negative responses from others leading to further lowering of self-esteem and neglect of appearance and interpersonal skills. Stopping such a cycle was an integral purpose of SEEK.

Many young people leave school ill-equipped to compete in the marketplace because they lack basic self-care and social skills: basic hygiene, grooming, clothing, assertiveness, and interpersonal—especially interviewing skills. I was confident that a remedial program in these areas could only enhance my clients' job competitiveness. Research reports had convinced me that appearance is a major source of information to interviewers in first-impression situations. Individuals are judged on the basis of their appearance before any verbal interaction takes place.

The British Red Cross had a program called Beauty-care and Cosmetic-service, and I relied heavily on their expertise. A cosmetic company provided free cosmetics and a trained beautician. A local hair-dressing salon (happily, barrier-free) offered low-cost styling and advice. A counselor supplied assertiveness and interpersonal skills training. And I—having worked both in personnel and the fashion industry—developed the interviewing skills and adapted clothing elements of the program.

SEEK enjoyed a high placement rate; and when I came to the United States, on encountering similar problems, I instituted the program in Michigan with funding from State vocational rehabilitation programs and local school districts.

Many practical problems arise. For example, major adaptations needed are often unavailable or at a cost that is unacceptable, or devices which might solve problems cannot be located because they are not widely advertised. Here, ABLEDATA provides some help. The outlook is improving, though. The last 5 years have seen a striking growth in the number of adapted clothing companies; cosmetics are now available that are easier to open, hold, and apply; consumer-oriented magazines provide helpful hints; and so forth.

Client Exemplar

A very attractive woman with cerebral palsy had a continual drool and severe spasticity. A college-educated writer, she was shy and withdrawn and anxious about meeting people. With help from local resources, I designed some attractive clothes in the Victorian style—with matching handkerchiefs attached to each outfit, high on the shoulder, with brooches. This allowed her to control the saliva without making her movements obvious. A short hairstyle that needed minimal

75

daily care and the attachment of grooming tools/sponges to oversize handles let her groom herself without help.

— by Jan Galvin

Information Specialist National Rehabilitation Information Center

Sources and Suggested Readings

Additional tips of use to clients can be found in the base documents for this *Rehab BRIEF* and still more in other publications. Additional information is available for those interested in the research aspects, too. Thus, a somewhat expanded reading list is offered to ease the problems of finding information in the still scattered area. (It is interesting to note that the majority of rehabilitation-related references found were in cosmetic and home economics journals, not in rehabilitation publications.)

All dated source documents with identifiable authors are listed. Copies of product brochures/pamphlets and new titles can be obtained by contacting Jan Galvin at the National Rehabilitation Information Center (NARIC), 4407 Eighth Street, N.E., Washington, DC 20017.

Caldwell, Robert, D.D.S. 1982. Dentistry for the homebound. *Journal of the Michigan Dental Association* 64 (Nov. / Dec.):453454.

Counselors create special programs for SCI women. *Movin on*. Craig Hospital. Summer 1986.

Graham, Jean Ann. 1983. The psychotherapeutic value of cosmetics. *Cosmetic Technology*. January, 25-26.

Graham, Jean Ann, and A.J. Jouhar. 1980. Cosmetics considered in the context of physical attractiveness: a review. *International Journal of Cosmetic Science* 2:77-101.

Graham, J.A., and A.M. Klingman, M.D. 1984. The psychological benefits of cosmetics in health care: dermatologic perspectives. *J. Appl Cosmetol* 2:7-18.

Hall, Holly. 1986. Crosstalk. *Psychology Today*, November, 15. (Miss Hall reported on Dr. Amerigo Farina's research that was reported in the *Journal of Abnormal Psychology* 95(2).)

Hatfield, Elaine, and Susan Sprecher. *Mirror, Mirror... The Importance of Looks in Everyday Life*. State University of New York. ($39.50; paperback, $12.95).

Hutchinson, Marcia Germaine. 1985. *Transforming Body Image.* The Crossing Press, Box 640, Trumanburg, NY 14886. ($8.95 paperback).

Kaiser, Susan et al. 1987. Acceptance of physical disability and attitudes toward personal appearance. *Rehab Psych* 32(1).

Kennedy, Evelyn S. 1981. *Dressing With Pride.* Groton, Connecticut: P.R.I.D.E. Foundation, Inc.

Mead, Marjorie. 1980. *Clothing for People with Physical Handicaps.* North Central Regional Extension Publication 101, Illinois Circular 1177.

Review of Transforming Body Image by Marcia Germaine Hutchinson. *Rehabilitation Literature.* 1986. 47(5-6):144-145.

Solomon, Michael R. 1986. Dress for effect. *Psychology Today.* April, 20-28.

Vash, Carolyn. 1981. *The Psychology of Disability.* New York: Springer.

Part Two

Types of Rehabilitation Therapy

Chapter 10

Understanding Physical Therapy

Physical therapy is often an important part of medical treatment provided to people following illness, accident or surgery. The chief aims of physical therapy are to:

- Prevent disability and pain
- Restore function and relieve pain
- Promote healing

Physical therapy treatment may involve the use of therapeutic exercise, exercise equipment, heat, cold, electrical stimulation, ultrasound, and other procedures suitable for a specific person and condition. A new area of emphasis for physical therapy is in preventive medicine. People of all ages, from children to the elderly, receive physical therapy.

Who Needs Physical Therapy?

Physical therapy is often necessary:

- After operations—to restore function to affected muscles and to keep unaffected muscles strong and useful
- Following stroke—to restore movement and independent living
- After birth—to evaluate infants suspected of having disabling conditions and to recommend corrective action
- Before illness to design programs of preventive health care

© 1992 National Easter Seal Society, reprinted with permission.

81

Physical therapy helps people with spinal cord injuries, sports injuries, broken bones, and amputations learn to use crutches, braces, wheelchairs, and artificial limbs.

Physical Therapy is Used to:

- Ease the pain of sprains and strains and prevent future injuries

- Plan treatment programs, including physical education, for children who have neurological, orthopedic and other disorders

- Reduce pain and improve motion in arthritic joints

- Test for exercise stress and to design exercise programs for individuals who have coronary artery disease or are at risk for coronary artery disease

- Evaluate low-back pain and eliminate functional causes

- Rebuild self-confidence and interest in returning to an independent active life

The Physical Therapist

The physical therapist (or P.T.) who provides the treatment is a professionally trained specialist—a graduate of a college program that includes medical, physical, biological, and social science courses and clinical education. This program is accredited by the American Physical Therapy Association.

Some therapists hold master's and doctoral degrees and concentrate on teaching, clinical practice or administration. Others may choose to specialize in a specific area of physical therapy, such as pediatrics or orthopedics, and bring this expertise to the clinic. Therapists must be licensed by the state in which they practice. They use the initials "P.T." after their name.

Physical therapist assistants are sometimes employed to work tinder a physical therapist's supervision following two years of college education in a physical therapist assistant program accredited by the American Physical Therapy Association.

The Client's Program

In planning each client's program of therapy, the physical therapist reviews the person's medical records, evaluates the person and identifies the person's problem(s).

The physical therapist performs tests and evaluations that provide information about joint motion, condition of muscles and reflexes, appearance and stability of walking, need for and use of braces and artificial limbs, function of the heart and lungs, integrity of sensation and perception, and performance of activities required in daily living.

The physical therapist consults and works closely with the individual's physician, other health care practitioners and the client in setting treatment objectives that are realistic and consistent with the individual's needs.

Chapter 11

Who Are Physical Therapists and What Do They Do?

Physical therapists are professionally educated at the college or university level and are required to be licensed in the state or states in which they practice. Graduates from 1960 to the present have successfully completed professional physical therapist education programs accredited by the Commission on Accreditation in Physical Therapy Education (CAPTE). Graduates from 1926 to 1959 completed physical therapy curricula approved by appropriate accreditation bodies. The CAPTE will limit its scope in 2002 to accredit only those professional programs that award the postbaccalaureate degree.

Physical therapists also may obtain clinical specialist certification through the American Board of Physical Therapy Specialties (ABPTS).

Practice Settings

Physical therapists practice in a broad range of inpatient, outpatient, and community-based settings, including the following, in order of most common setting:

- Hospitals (e.g. critical care, intensive care, acute care, and subacute care settings)
- Outpatient clinics or offices
- Rehabilitation facilities
- Skilled nursing, extended care, or subacute facilities

- Homes
- Education or research centers
- Schools and playgrounds (preschool, primary, and secondary)
- Hospices
- Corporate or industrial health centers
- Industrial, workplace, or other occupational environments
- Athletic facilities (collegiate, amateur, and professional)
- Fitness centers and sports training facilities

Patients and Clients

Physical therapists are committed to providing necessary, appropriate, and high-quality health care services to both patients and clients. Patients are individuals who are the recipients of physical therapy care and direct intervention. Clients are individuals who are not necessarily sick or injured but who can benefit from a physical therapist's consultation, professional advice, or prevention services. Clients also are businesses, school systems, and others to whom physical therapists provide services. The generally accepted elements of patient/client management typically apply to both patients and clients.

Scope of Practice

Physical therapy is the care and services provided by or under the direction and supervision of a physical therapist. APTA emphasizes that an examination, evaluation, or intervention—unless provided by a physical therapist or under the direction and supervision of a physical therapist—is not physical therapy, nor should it be represented or reimbursed as such.

Physical therapy, which is the care and services provided by or under the direction and supervision of a physical therapist includes:

1. Examining (history, systems review, and tests and measures) individuals with impairment, functional limitation, and disability or other health-related conditions in order to determine a diagnosis, prognosis, and intervention; tests and measures may include the following:

   - Aerobic capacity and endurance
   - Anthropometric characteristics
   - Arousal, mentation, and cognition
   - Assistive and adaptive devices

- Community and work (job/school/play) integration or reintegration
- Cranial nerve integrity
- Environmental, home, and work (job/school/play) barriers
- Ergonomics and body mechanics
- Gait locomotion, and balance
- Integumentary integrity
- Joint integrity and mobility
- Motor function
- Muscle performance
- Neuromotor development and sensory integration
- Orthotic, protective, and supportive devices
- Pain
- Posture
- Prosthetic requirements
- Range of motion
- Reflex integrity
- Self-care and home management
- Sensory integrity
- Ventilation, respiration, and circulation

2. Alleviating impairment and functional limitation by designing, implementing, and modifying therapeutic interventions that may include, but are not limited to:

- Coordination, communication, and documentation

- Patient/client-related instruction

- Therapeutic exercise (including aerobic conditioning)

- Functional training in self-care and home management (including activities of daily living and instrumental activities of daily living)

- Functional training in community and work (job/school/play) integration or reintegration activities (including instrumental activities of daily living, work hardening, and work conditioning)

- Manual therapy techniques (including mobilization and manipulation) Prescription application, and, as appropriate, fabrication of assistive, adaptive, orthotic, protective, supportive, and prosthetic devices and equipment

- Airway clearance techniques

- Wound management
- Electrotherapeutic modalities
- Physical agents and mechanical modalities

3. Preventing injury, impairment, functional limitation, and disability, including the promotion and maintenance of fitness, health, and quality of life in all age populations

4. Engaging in consultation, education, and research

  - Direct interventions, which begin with "Therapeutic exercise," are listed in order of preferred usage.

  - This category of tests and measures is referred to as "arousal, attention, and cognition" in the Guide.

Physical Therapists:

- Provide services to patients/clients who have impairments, functional limitations, disabilities, or changes in physical function and health status resulting from injury, disease, or other causes. In the context of the model of disablement [1,2] on which this Guide is based, impairment is defined as loss or abnormality of physiological, psychological, or anatomical structure or function; functional limitation, as restriction of the ability to perform—at the level of the whole person—a physical action, activity, or task in an efficient, typically expected, or competent manner; and disability, as the inability to engage in age-specific, gender-specific, or sex-specific roles in a particular social context and physical environment.

- Interact and practice in collaboration with a variety of professionals, including physicians, dentists, nurses, educators, social workers, occupational therapists, speech-language pathologists, and audiologists. Physical therapists acknowledge the need to educate and inform other professionals, government agencies, third-party payers, and other health care consumers about the cost-efficient and clinically effective services that physical therapists render.

- Provide prevention and wellness services, including screening and health promotion. Physical therapists are involved in wellness initiatives, including health promotion and education, that stimulate the public to engage in healthy behaviors. They provide preventive care that forestalls or prevents functional decline and the need for more intense care. Through timely and appropriate screening, examination, evaluation, and intervention, they frequently reduce or eliminate the need for costlier forms of care, such as surgery, and also may shorten or even eliminate institutional stays.

- Consult, educate, engage in critical inquiry, and administrate.

- Direct and supervise physical therapy services, including support personnel.

Roles in Primary Care

Physical therapists have a major role to play in the provision of primary care, which has been defined as the provision of integrated, accessible health care services by clinicians who are accountable for addressing a large majority of personal health care needs, developing a sustained partnership with patients, and practicing within the context of family and community.[3]

APTA has endorsed the concepts of primary care set forth by the Institute of Medicine's Committee on the Future of Primary Care[3], including the following:

- Primary care can encompass a myriad of needs that go well beyond the capabilities and competencies of individual caregivers and that require the involvement and interaction of varied practitioners.

- The "gatekeeper" concept is rejected because of the pejorative connotation that the primary care practitioner's role is to manage costs and, for the most part, keep the "gate" closed.

- Primary care is not limited to the "first contact" or point of entry into the health care system.

- The primary care program is a comprehensive one.

- The role of family and community in the provision of primary care is an important one, and caregivers and care-receivers function in the context of, and are dependent on, a wide range of societal and environmental factors.

As clinicians involved in examination and in the evaluation, diagnosis, prognosis, intervention, and prevention of musculoskeletal and neuromuscular disorders, physical therapists are well positioned to provide those services as members of primary care teams. On a daily basis, physical therapists practicing at acute, chronic, rehabilitative, and preventive stages of care assist patients/clients in the following: restoring health; alleviating pain; and preventing the onset of impairments, functional limitations, disabilities, or changes in physical function and health status resulting from injury, disease, or other causes. Prevention and wellness activities, including health promotion, are a vital part of physical therapy.

For acute musculoskeletal and neuromuscular conditions, triage and initial examination are appropriate physical therapist responsibilities. The primary care team may function more efficiently when it includes physical therapists, who can recognize musculoskeletal and neuromuscular disorders, perform examinations and evaluations, and intervene without delay. For patients/clients with low back pain, for example, physical therapists can provide immediate pain reduction and programs for strengthening, flexibility, endurance, postural alignment, instruction in activities of daily living, and work modification. Physical therapist intervention may result not only in more efficient and effective patient care but also in more appropriate utilization of other members of the primary care team. With physical therapists functioning in a primary care role and delivering early intervention for work-related musculoskeletal injuries, time and productivity lost due to injuries may be dramatically reduced.

For certain chronic conditions, physical therapists should be recognized as the principal providers of care within the collaborative primary care team. Physical therapists are well prepared to coordinate care related to loss of physical function as a result of musculoskeletal, neuromuscular, cardiopulmonary, or integumentary disorders. Through community-based agencies, physical therapists coordinate and integrate provision of services to patients/clients with chronic neuromuscular and musculoskeletal disorders.

Physical therapists also provide primary care in industrial or workplace settings, in which they manage the occupational health services provided to employees and prevent injury by designing or redesigning the work environment. These services focus both on the individual and on the environment to ensure comprehensive and appropriate intervention.

Roles in Secondary and Tertiary Care

Physical therapists play major roles in secondary and tertiary care. Patients with musculoskeletal, neuromuscular, cardiopulmonary, or integumentary conditions frequently are treated initially by another health care practitioner and then are referred to physical therapists for secondary care. Physical therapists provide secondary care in a wide range of settings, from hospitals to preschools.

Tertiary care is provided by physical therapists in highly specialized, complex, and technology-based settings (e.g., heart and lung transplant services, burn units) or when supplying specialized services (e.g., to patients with spinal cord lesions or closed head trauma) in response to requests for consultation that are made by other health care practitioners.

Roles in Prevention and Wellness (Including Screening Programs and Health Promotion)

Physical therapists are involved in prevention and wellness activities, screening, and the promotion of positive health behavior. These initiatives decrease costs by helping patients/clients (1) achieve and restore optimal functional capacity, (2) minimize impairments, functional limitations, and disabilities related to congenital and acquired conditions, (3) maintain health (thereby preventing further deterioration or future illness), and (4) create appropriate environmental adaptations to enhance independent function. There are three types of prevention:

- Primary prevention—Preventing disease in a susceptible or potentially susceptible population through such specific measures as general health promotion efforts

- Secondary prevention—Decreasing duration of illness, severity of disease, and sequelae through early diagnosis and prompt intervention

- Tertiary prevention—Limiting the degree of disability and promoting rehabilitation and restoration of function in patients with chronic and irreversible diseases

Physical therapists conduct screenings to determine the need for primary, secondary, or tertiary prevention services; for further examination, intervention, or consultation by a physical therapist; or for referral to another health care practitioner. Candidates for screening generally not patients/clients currently receiving physical therapy services. Screening is based on a problem-focused, systematic collection and analysis of data. Examples of screening activities in which physical therapists engage include:

- Identifying lifestyle factors (e.g., amount of exercise, stress, and weight) that may lead to increased risk for serious health problems

- Identifying children who may need an examination for idiopathic scoliosis

- Identifying elderly individuals in a community center or nursing home who are at high risk for slipping, tripping, or falling

- Identifying risk factors in the workplace

- Pre-performance testing of individuals who are active in sports

- Conducting prework screening programs

Examples of prevention and wellness activities in which physical therapists engage include:

- Back schools, workplace redesign, strengthening, stretching, endurance exercise programs, and postural training to prevent and treat low back pain, a condition afflicting millions of Americans

- Workplace redesign, strengthening, stretching, endurance exercise, and postural training to prevent job-related disabilities, including trauma and repetitive stress injuries

- Exercise programs, including weight bearing and weight training, to increase bone mass and bone density (especially important in older adults with osteoporosis)

- Exercise programs, gait training, and balance and coordination activities to reduce the risk of falls and fractures from falls in older adults

- Exercise programs and instruction in activities of daily living (ADL) (self-care, communication, and mobility skills required for independence in daily living) and instrumental activities of daily living (IADL) (activities that are important components of maintaining independent living, such as shopping and cooking) to decrease utilization of health care services and enhance function in patients with cardiopulmonary disorders

- Exercise programs, cardiovascular conditioning, postural training, and instruction in ADL and IADL to prevent disability and dysfunction in women who are pregnant

- Broad-based consumer education and advocacy programs to prevent problems (eg., prevent head injury by promoting the use of helmets, prevent pulmonary disease by encouraging smoking cessation)

The Five Elements of Patient/Client Management

The physical therapist integrates five elements of patient/client management—examination, evaluation, diagnosis, prognosis, and intervention—in a manner designed to maximize outcomes. Examination, evaluation, and establishment of a diagnosis and a prognosis are all part of the process that guides the therapist in determining the most appropriate intervention.

Examination

Examination is required prior to any intervention and is performed for all patients/clients. The initial examination, which is an investigation, has three components: the patient/client history, relevant Systems reviews, and tests and measures.

History. The history is an account of past and current health status. It includes identification of complaints, provides the initial source of information about the patient/client, and also suggests the individual's ability to benefit from physical therapy. While taking the history, the physical therapist identifies health-risk factors, health restoration and prevention needs, and coexisting health problems that have implications for intervention. This history commonly is obtained through the gathering of data from the patient/client, family, significant others, caregivers, and other interested persons (e.g., rehabilitation counselor, Workers' Compensation claims manager, employer), through consultation with other members of the health care team; and through review of the medical record.

Systems Review. The systems review is a brief or limited examination that provides additional information about the general health of the patient/client to help the physical therapist formulate a diagnosis, a prognosis, and a plan of care and select direct interventions. The systems review also assists the physical therapist in identifying possible health problems that require consultation with or referral to another health care provide.

Data generated from a systems review that may affect subsequent examination and interventions include: (1) physiologic and anatomic status (cardiopulmonary, integumentary, musculoskeletal, and neuromuscular) and (2) communication ability, affect, cognition, language, and learning style.

Tests and Measures. After analyzing all relevant information gathered from the history and systems review, the physical therapist examines the patient/client more closely, selecting tests and measures to elicit additional information. Before, during, and after administering the tests and measures, physical therapists frequently apply their hands to the patient/client to gauge responses, assess physical status, and obtain a more specific understanding of the condition and the diagnostic and therapeutic requirements.

The physical therapist may decide to use one, more than one, or portions of several specific tests and measures as part of the examination, based on the purpose of the visit, the complexity of the condition, and the directions taken in the clinical decision-making process.

As the examination progresses, the physical therapist may identify additional problems that were not uncovered by the history and systems review and may conclude that other specific tests and measures or portions of other specific tests and measures are required to obtain sufficient data to make an evaluation, establish a diagnosis and a prognosis, and select direct interventions. The examination therefore may be as brief or as lengthy as necessary. For instance, the physical therapist may conclude from the history and systems review that further examination and management are not required, that the patient/client should be referred to another health care practitioner, or both. Conversely, the physical therapist may decide that a full examination is necessary and then select appropriate tests and measures. Physical therapists frequently perform one or more reexaminations, which are examinations that take place after the initial examination is completed. Because physical therapy is most often an ongoing process delivered over a period of weeks for a single episode of care—rather than one service delivered during a single visit—physical therapists rely on reexaminations to modify or redirect intervention and to evaluate progress toward the anticipated goals and desired outcomes. If a reexamination is indicated (e.g., because of new clinical indications or failure to respond to intervention), the physical therapist selects and administers additional specific tests and measures. The reexamination has an important quality assurance component, as it allows the physical therapist to focus on the relationship between the elements of patient/client management and the outcomes.

Note: In the course of examining and establishing the diagnosis and the prognosis, the physical therapist may find evidence of physical abuse or domestic violence. In such cases, the physical therapist is bound by ethical principles—and may be bound by state law or regulation—to report such findings to the appropriate agencies.

Evaluation

Physical therapists perform evaluations (make clinical judgments) based on the data gathered from the examination. Factors that influence the complexity of the examination and the evaluation process include the clinical findings, extent of loss of function, social considerations, and the patient's/client's overall physical function and health status. Thus, the evaluation reflects the chronicity or severity of the current problem, the possibility of multisite or multisystem involvement, the presence of preexisting systemic conditions or diseases, and the stability of the condition. Physical therapists also consider the level of the current impairments and the probability of prolonged impairment, functional limitation, and disability; the living environment; potential discharge destinations; and the social supports.

Diagnosis

A diagnosis is a label encompassing a cluster of signs and symptoms, syndromes, or categories. It is the decision reached as a result of the diagnostic process, which includes evaluating the information obtained during the examination; organizing it into clusters, syndromes, or categories; and interpreting it.

The purpose of the diagnosis is to guide the physical therapist in determining the most appropriate intervention strategy for each patient/client. In the event that the diagnostic process does not yield an identifiable cluster, syndrome, or category, intervention may be guided by the alleviation of symptoms and remediation of deficits. Alternatively, the physical therapist may determine that a reexamination is in order and proceed accordingly. In carrying out the diagnostic process, physical therapists may need to obtain additional information (including diagnostic labels) from other professionals. In addition, as the diagnostic process continues, physical therapists may identify findings that should be shared with other professionals, including referral sources, to ensure optimal care. If the diagnostic process reveals findings that are outside the scope of the physical therapist's knowledge, experience, or expertise, the physical therapist refers the patient/client to an appropriate practitioner.

Prognosis

The prognosis includes the predicted optimal level of improvement in function and amount of time needed to reach that level; it also may include a prediction of levels of improvement that may be reached at various intervals during the course of therapy.

At this point in patient/client management, the physical therapist establishes plan of care. In designing the plan of care, the physical therapist integrates all of the previous data, incorporates all of the prognostic predictions, and determines the degree to which interventions are likely to achieve anticipated goals and desired outcomes. Goals generally relate to the remediation (to the extent possible) of impairments, whereas outcomes relate to minimization of functional limitation, optimization of health status, prevention of disability, and optimization of patient/client satisfaction. Thus, the plan of care specifies long-term and short-term goals and outcomes, the specific interventions to be used, the duration and frequency of intervention required to reach the goals and outcomes, and criteria for discharge.

Intervention

Intervention is the purposeful and skilled interaction of the physical therapist with the patient/client and, when appropriate, with other individuals involved in patient/client care, using various physical therapy procedures and techniques to produce changes in the condition consistent with the diagnosis and prognosis. Decisions about interventions are contingent on the timely monitoring of patient/client response and the progress made toward achieving the anticipated goals and the desired outcomes. Physical therapist intervention has three components: coordination, communication, and documentation; patient/client-related instruction; and direct interventions.

Coordination, Communication, and Documentation. These services, which are provided for all patients/clients, may include case management; communication (direct or indirect); coordination of care with the patient/client, family, significant others, caregivers, other professionals, and other interested persons; discharge planning; documentation of all elements of patient/client management; education plans; patient care conferences; record reviews; and referrals to other professionals or resources. Through these services, the physical therapist ensures appropriate, coordinated, comprehensive, and cost-effective services between admission and discharge and cost-effective and efficient integration or reintegration to home, community, and work (job/school/play), and leisure environments. Documentation should follow APTA's Guidelines for Physical Therapy Documentation.

Patient/Client-Related Instruction. These services, which are provided to all patients/clients, may include computer-assisted instruction, demonstration by patient/client or caregivers in the appropriate environment, periodic reexamination and reassessment of the home program, use of audiovisual aids for both teaching and home reference, use of demonstration and modeling for teaching, verbal instruction, and written or pictorial instruction. The physical therapist uses these services to educate the patient/client—and also the family, significant others, caregivers, or other professionals—about the current condition, plan of care, and future transition to home, work, or community roles. The physical therapist may include information and training in activities for maintenance of function and primary and secondary prevention. The educational backgrounds, needs, and learning styles of individuals must be taken into account during this process.

Direct Interventions. The physical therapist selects, applies, or modifies direct interventions based on examination and evaluation data, the diagnosis and the prognosis, and the anticipated goals and desired outcomes for a particular patient in a specific patient/client diagnostic group. Based on the results of the interventions, the physical therapist may decide that reexamination is necessary, a decision that may lead to the use of different interventions or, alternatively, the discontinuation of care.

Forming the core of most physical therapy plans of care: therapeutic exercise, including aerobic conditioning; functional training in self-care and home management activities, including activities of daily living (ADL) and instrumental activities of daily living (IADL); and functional training in community and work (job/school/play) integration or reintegration, including IADL, work hardening, and work conditioning.

Factors that influence the complexity, frequency, and duration of the intervention and the decision-making process may include the following: anatomic and physiologic changes related to growth and development; chronicity or severity of the current condition; cognitive status; level of impairment; living environment; multisite or multisystem involvement; overall physical function and health status; potential discharge destinations; preexisting systemic conditions or diseases; probability of prolonged impairment, functional limitation, or disability; social supports; and stability of the condition.

Outcomes

At each step of patient/client management, the physical therapist considers the possible outcomes (remediation of functional limitation and disability, optimization of patient/client satisfaction, and primary or secondary prevention).

Beginning with the history, the physical therapist identifies patient/client expectations for therapeutic interventions, perceptions about the clinical situation, and desired outcomes. The physical therapist then considers whether these expectations and outcomes are realistic in the context of the examination and evaluation data. In establishing a diagnosis and a prognosis and selecting direct interventions, the physical therapist asks the question, "What outcome is likely, given the diagnosis?" The physical therapist may use reexamination to determine whether predicted outcomes are reasonable and then modify them as necessary.

The physical therapist engages in outcomes data collection and analysis—that is, the systematic review of outcomes of care in relation to selected variables (e.g., age, sex, diagnosis, interventions performed)—and develops statistical reports for internal or external use.

Discharge Planning

Discharge—the process of discontinuing interventions in a single episode of care—occurs based on the physical therapist's analysis of the dynamic interplay between the achievement of anticipated goals and the achievement of desired outcomes. Other indications for discharge include the following:

- The patient/client declines to continue treatment.
- The patient/client is unable to continue to progress toward goals because of medical or psychosocial complications.
- The physical therapist determines that the patient/client will no longer benefit from physical therapy services.

In consultation with appropriate individuals, and in consideration of the goals and outcomes, the physical therapist plans for discharge and provides for appropriate follow-up or referral. If the physical therapist determines, through examination and evaluation, that intervention is unlikely to be beneficial, the physical therapist discusses those findings and conclusions with the individuals concerned, and there is no further physical therapist intervention. When a patient/client is discharged prior to achievement of desired outcomes, patient/client status and the rationale for discontinuation are documented.

A physical therapy episode of care consists of all patient/client management activities conducted by a physical therapist from initial contact through discharge. A single episode of care should not be confused with multiple episodes of care that may be required by certain individuals in particular patient/client diagnostic groups. For these patients/clients, periodic follow-up is needed over a lifetime to ensure safety and effective adaptation following changes in physical status, caregivers, the environment, or task demands.

Other Professional Roles

Consultation—Physical therapist consultants render professional or expert opinion or advice, applying highly specialized knowledge and skills to identify problems, recommend solutions, or produce a specified outcome or product in a given amount of time on behalf of a patient/client.

Patient-related consultation is a service provided by a physical therapist at the request of a patient, health care practitioner, or health care organization either to recommend physical therapy services that are needed or to evaluate the quality of physical therapy services being provided. Such consultation usually does not involve actual treatment. Client-related consultation is a service provided by a physical therapist at the request of an individual, business, school, government agency, or other organization.

Examples of consultation activities in which physical therapists engage include:

- Advising a referring practitioner about the indications for intervention

- Advising employers about the requirements of the Americans With Disabilities Act (ADA)

- Conducting a program to determine the suitability of employees for specific job assignments

- Developing programs that evaluate the effectiveness of an intervention plan in reducing work-related injuries

- Educating other health care practitioners (e.g., in injury prevention)

- Examining school environments and recommending changes to improve accessibility for students with disabilities

- Instructing employers about job preplacement in accordance with provisions of the ADA

- Participating at the local, state, and federal levels in policymaking for physical therapy services

- Performing environmental assessments to minimize the risk of falls

- Providing peer review and utilization review services

- Responding to a request for a second opinion

- Serving as an expert witness in legal proceedings

- Working with employees, labor unions, and government agencies to develop injury reduction and safety programs

Education

Education is the process of imparting information or skills and instructing by precept, example, and experience so that individuals acquire knowledge, master skills, or develop competence. In addition to instructing patients/clients as an element of intervention, physical therapists may engage in education activities such as the following:

- Planning and conducting academic education, clinical education, and continuing education programs for physical therapists, other health care providers, and students

- Planning and conducting education programs for local, state, and federal health agencies

- Planning and conducting programs for the public to increase awareness of issues in which physical therapists have expertise

Critical Inquiry

Critical inquiry is the process of applying the principles of scientific methods to read and interpret professional literature; participate in, plan, and conduct research; evaluate outcomes; and assess new concepts and technologies.

Examples of critical inquiry activities in which physical therapists engage include:

- Analyzing and applying research findings to physical therapy practice and education

- Disseminating the results of research

- Evaluating the efficacy and effectiveness of both new and established interventions and technologies

- Participating in, planning, and conducting clinical, basic, or applied research

Administration

Administration is the skilled process of planning, directing, organizing, and managing human, technical, environmental, and financial resources effectively and efficiently. Administration includes the management, by individual physical therapists, of resources for patient/client management and for organizational operations.

Examples of administration activities in which physical therapists engage include:

- Ensuring fiscally sound reimbursement for services rendered

- Budgeting for physical therapy services

- Managing staff resources, including the acquisition and development of clinical expertise and leadership abilities

- Monitoring quality of care and clinical productivity

- Negotiating and managing contracts

- Supervising physical therapist assistants, physical therapy aides, and other support personnel

The Physical Therapy Service

Direction and Supervision of Personnel Direction and supervision are essential to the provision of high-quality physical therapy. The degree of direction and supervision necessary for ensuring high-quality physical therapy depends on many factors, including the education, experience, and responsibilities of the parties involved; the organizational structure in which the physical therapy is provided; and applicable state law. In any case, supervision should be readily available to the individual being supervised.

The director of a physical therapy service is a physical therapist who has demonstrated qualifications based on education and experience in the field of physical therapy and who has accepted the inherent responsibilities of the role. The director of a physical therapy service must:

- Establish guidelines and procedures that will delineate the functions and responsibilities of all levels of physical therapy personnel in the service and the supervisory relationships inherent to the functions of the service and the organization

- Ensure that the objectives of the service are efficiently and effectively achieved within the framework of the stated purpose of the organization and in accordance with safe physical therapist practice

- Interpret administrative policies

- Act as a liaison between line staff and administration

- Foster the professional growth of the staff

Written practice and performance criteria should be available for all levels of physical therapy personnel in a physical therapy service. Regularly scheduled performance appraisals should be conducted by the supervisor based on applicable standards of practice and performance criteria.

Delegated responsibilities should be commensurate with the qualifications—including experience, education, and training—of the individuals to whom the responsibilities are being assigned. When the physical therapist of record delegates patient care responsibilities to physical therapist assistants or other support personnel, that physical therapist holds responsibility for supervision of the plan of care. Regardless of the setting in which the services are given, the following responsibilities must be held solely by the physical therapist:

- Interpretation of referrals when available. Initial examination, evaluation, problem identification, diagnosis, and prognosis

- Development or modification of a plan of care that is based on the initial examination and that includes anticipated goals and desired outcomes

- Administration of intervention and, as appropriate, determination of (1) tasks that require the expertise and decision-making capacity of the physical therapist and that must be personally rendered by the physical therapist and (2) tasks that may be delegated. Prior to delegating any procedure, the physical therapist should determine that the consequences of the procedure are predictable, the situation is stable, and the basic indicators are not ambiguous and do not require ongoing observation by the physical therapist.

- Delegation of the tasks to be rendered by the physical therapist assistant or other support personnel, including, but not limited to, specific treatments, precautions, special problems, and contraindicated procedures

- Timely review of treatment documentation, reexamination of the patient/client and the anticipated goals and desired outcomes, and revision of the plan of care when indicated

- Establishment of the discharge plan and documentation of discharge summary or status

References

1. Physical Disability. Special issue. *Phys Ther.* 1994;74:375-506.

2. Verbrugge L, Jette A. The Disablement Process. *Soc Sci Med.* 1994;38:1-14,

3. *Defining Primary Care: An Interim Report.* Washington, DC: Institute of Medicine, National Academy Press; 1995.

Physical Therapist Assistants

The physical therapist assistant is an educated health care provider who assists the physical therapist in the provision of physical therapy. The physical therapist assistant is a graduate of a physical therapist assistant associate degree program accredited by an agency recognized by the Commission on Accreditation in Physical Therapy Education (CAPTE).

The physical therapist of record is the person who is directly responsible for the actions of the physical therapist assistant. The physical therapist assistant may perform physical therapy procedures and related tasks that have been selected and delegated by the supervising physical therapist. Where permitted by law, the physical therapist also may carry out routine operational functions, including supervision of the physical aide and documentation of progress. The ability of the physical therapist assistant to perform the selected and delegated tasks should be assessed on an ongoing basis by the supervising physical therapist. The physical therapist assistant may modify a specific intervention procedure in accordance with changes in patient/client status and within the scope of the establish plan of care.

Physical Therapist Aides

The physical therapy aide is a non-licensed worker who is specifically trained under the direction of a physical therapist. The physical therapy aide performs designated routine tasks related to the operation of a physical therapy service delegated by the physical therapist or in accordance with the law, by a physical therapist assistant.

The physical therapist of record is the person who is directly responsible for the actions of the physical therapy aide. The physical therapy aide provides support that may include patient-related and non-patient-related duties. The physical therapy aide functions only with the continuous on-site supervision of the physical therapist or, where allowable by law or regulation, the physical therapist assistant. Continuous on-site supervision requires the presence of the physical therapist or physical therapist assistant in the immediate area.

Other Support Personnel

When other personnel (e.g., exercise physiologists, athletic trainers, massage therapists) work within the supervision of a physical therapy service, they should be employed under their appropriate title. Any involvement in patient/client care activities should be within the limits of their education, in accordance with applicable laws and regulations, and at the discretion of the physical therapist. If such personnel function as an extension of the physical therapist's license, however, their title and all services that they provide must be in accordance with state and federal laws and regulations.

Chapter 12

What Is Occupational Therapy?

Occupational therapists evaluate and treat individuals with injuries, illnesses, cognitive impairments, psychosocial dysfunctions, mental illness, developmental or learning disabilities, physical disabilities, or other disorders or conditions. Evaluation and intervention focuses on an individual's level of function and involves assessment of performance areas, performance components, and performance contexts. Intervention involves the use of purposeful activity for developing, improving, sustaining or restoring function in performance areas including, but not limited to, daily living skills, work performance, educational performance skills, and leisure capacities. The performance components (sensorimotor, cognitive, psychosocial, and psychological) are the elements of performance in which occupational therapists intervene for the purpose of attaining an individual's highest level of functional independence. Services of an occupational therapist also include: the design, development, adaptation, application or training in the use of assistive technology devices; the design, fabrication or application of orthotic devices; training in the use of orthotic or prosthetic devices; application of physical agent modalities; and the adaptation of environments and processes to enhance functional performance.

Certified occupational therapy assistants (COTAS) assist with the evaluation and treatment of individuals with injuries, illnesses, cognitive impairments, psychosocial dysfunctions, mental illness, developmental or learning disabilities, physical disabilities, or other disorders or conditions. Under the supervision of occupational therapists (OTs), COTAS:

1. Contribute to the evaluation process through the administration of assessments (standardized and non-standardized) for which they have established competency; and

2. Implement therapeutic interventions which use purposeful activity for developing, improving, sustaining or restoring function in performance areas including, but not limited to, daily living skills, work performance, educational performance skills, and leisure capacities.

The performance components (sensorimotor, cognitive, psychosocial, and psychological) are the elements of performance in which COTAs intervene for the purpose of attaining an individual's highest level of functional independence within the appropriate environmental context. Under the supervision of an OT, COTAs also assist in the design, development, adaptation, application or training in the use of assistive technology devices; the design, fabrication or application of orthotic devices; training in the use of orthotic or prosthetic devices; application of physical agent modalities; and the adaptation of environments and processes to enhance functional performance.

There are many definitions of occupational therapy. Here are a few of them:

"Occupational therapy is the therapeutic use of self-care, work, and play activities to increase independent function, enhance development, and prevent disability; may include adaptation of task or environment to achieve maximum independence and to enhance quality of life."

—Dictionary definition of occupational therapy, adopted and approved by the Representative Assembly in April 1986

"Occupational therapy is the art and science of directing man's participation in selected tasks to restore, reinforce, and enhance performance; facility learning of those skills and functions essential for adaptation and productivity; diminish or correct pathology; and to promote and maintain health. Its fundamental concern is the capacity, throughout the life span, to perform with satisfaction to self and others those tasks and roles essential to productive living and to the mastery of self and the environment."

—Willard and Spackman's Occupational Therapy, H.L. Hopkins and H.D. Smith (Eds.), 1993

"Occupational therapy is the use of purposeful activity or interventions designed to achieve functional outcomes which promote health, prevent injury or disability, and which develop, improve, sustain or restore the highest possible level of independence of any individual who has an injury, illness, cognitive impairment, psychosocial dysfunction, mental illness, developmental or learning disability, physical disability, or other disorder or condition. It includes assessment by means of skilled observation or evaluation through the administration and interpretation of standardized or nonstandardized tests and measurements."

—Definition of Occupational Therapy Practice forState Regulation by the American Occupational Therapy Association, 1994

Occupational therapy involves the "therapeutic use of work, self-care, and play activities to increase independent function, enhance development, and prevent disability. It may include adaptation of task or environment to achieve maximum independence and to enhance the quality of life."

—Official definition of occupational therapy as passed by the AOTA Executive Board, 1976

Occupational therapy is a vital health care service whose practitioners help to restore and sustain the highest quality of productive life to persons recovering from illnesses or injuries or coping with developmental disabilities or changes resulting from the aging process.

Occupational therapy is a health care profession that uses occupation, meaning purposeful activity, as a means of preventing, reducing or overcoming physical, social, and emotional disabilities in people of all ages.

"Occupational therapists and occupational therapy assistants work with people of all ages who, because of physical, developmental, social or emotional problems, need specialized assistance to lead independent, productive and satisfying lives."

—AOTA brochure, "What is Occupational Therapy?"

"Formerly associated only with the use of arts and crafts for the rehabilitation of the mentally ill or the psychological well-being of the elderly, occupational therapy is now an indispensable aspect of the team approach to patients who have to learn new ways of coping with the mechanics and logistics of daily living as a result of temporary or permanent impairment."

—Every Woman's Health, *D.S. Thompson, M.D.,*
Consulting Editor

Occupational therapy is helping people with physical and brain challenges achieve their highest level of performance. We help people to become as independent in their life roles as they can be. Occupational therapy translates mobility into function.

—*Administration and Management*
Special Interest Section

Occupational therapy helps children and young adults with disabilities from birth to 21 years of age to benefit from their educational programs. We focus on the student's performance in the areas of hand skills, eating, self-care, social skills and play/leisure skills. Services may include assessment to determine strength/needs; collaborating with teachers, families, students and others on environmental and material adaptations; developing strategies and activities to enhance performance; and providing student-specific interventions.

— *School System Special Interest Section*

Occupational therapy in education prepares OT practitioners to use occupations and daily life tasks to promote health and quality of life. It prepares OT practitioners to enhance role performance and adaptations necessary to specific environmental demands throughout one's life. It prepares therapist-scholars to study the effectiveness of occupations in role performance competence and promoting response to environmental demands. It prepares therapist-scholars to investigate the effectiveness of occupational therapy services and to investigate the fundamentals of occupations throughout the life span.

—*Education Special Interest Section*

The elements of occupational therapy practice in a home health setting are: to restore, compensate, and/or adapt the patient's skills and/or their environment to achieve a higher degree of functioning in his/her home and community; to promote the principles of wellness and safety appropriate to the patient's needs and goals in his/her home and community; and to address the physical, cognitive and psychosocial, cultural needs of the client.

—Home and Community Health Special Interest Section

Occupational therapists use meaningful activities of every day living to enhance and restore health. When natural environments for daily occupations are not available, occupational therapy practitioners use simulated environments to teach and have persons with disabilities practice their skills. Occupational therapy involves a collaborative relationship between the practitioner and the client, family or group accessing OT services.

—Mental Health Special Interest Section

Occupational therapists teach people how to live and function in their work environment. Occupational therapy helps people prevent injuries and promote safety. Employees know the work; occupational therapists teach employees how to do the work safely for the long term. Occupational therapy teaches individuals how to understand their abilities related to work, giving them control of themselves and ownership for their job. Occupational therapy is keeping people at work.

—Work Programs Special Interest Section

"Occupational therapy is a health profession which uses therapeutic purposeful activities to help children and adults function better physically, emotionally, academically and socially in their daily activities."

—Occupational Therapy and the School-Aged Child.
A reference guide for parents and teachers by
the Easter Seal RehabilitationCenter of
Will-Grundy Counties, Joliet, IL.

109

Chapter 13

Industrial Rehabilitation— A Natural Environment for Occupational Therapy

The trend in developing return-to-work services and/or injury-prevention education programs has become a focus in many hospital-based rehabilitation programs and physical therapy private practices during the past decade. Occupational therapy practitioners are well prepared for contributing to these programs. One of the three areas of occupational performance defined in the occupational therapy literature is "work." Facilitating maximum independence, preventing further disability, and promoting health are areas occupational therapy practitioners always consider, regardless of the injury or illness. This article discusses industrial rehabilitation programs and the role of occupational therapy practitioners participating in such programs.

Industrial rehabilitation programs continue to grow in number and recognition. Occupational therapy practitioners are formally educated and clinically trained to provide many of the services/products offered by these programs. Work hardening, injury-prevention education, job-site analysis, ergonomic analysis, treating acutely injured workers, and making recommendations for modified duty/activity adaptation are some of those services.

Industrial rehabilitation is a natural practice area for occupational therapy practitioners. Documented within the profession's roots are work programs that go back several decades (Briggs, 1949; Bunnell,

1950; Wegg, 1957). There are several basic assumptions of work programs:

1. As adults we have a drive to be "productive."

2. There are physical and psychological considerations underlying the philosophy and necessity of work.

3. There is a fear of reinjury on the part of the injured worker.

These assumptions blend well with beliefs of the occupational therapy profession.

Occupation, as defined by occupational therapy practitioners, means engagement in "purposeful activity" (Schwartzberg, 1988). The occupational therapy profession identifies three areas of occupational performance: 1) work; 2) play/leisure; and 3) self-care (Cynkin and Robinson, 1990). A basic belief of occupational therapists is that humans desire to be productive. There is a natural drive for humans to "work," and thus occupational therapy practitioners assist persons with injuries or illnesses to develop or retain their capacities for work. In a 1993 position paper of the American Occupational Therapy Association (AOTA), the Commission on Practice stated that occupational therapy education—in the nature of "purposeful activities," in activity analysis and synthesis, in behavioral and biological sciences—provides the necessary background to use activities as therapeutic modalities. These activities are considered purposeful because they are designed to assist in developing an individual's unique abilities, thus leading to the achievement of personal satisfaction and self-reliance.

American industry is driven by the need for productivity and "profits," but theirs is a different kind of productivity. Because of this, workers are frequently expected to be productive without taking into consideration health-related issues.

Education and Training

Occupational therapy practitioners assess, consult with, and treat injured workers. The knowledge and skills of occupational therapy practitioners prepares them to talk effectively with employers about an injured worker's unique issues/concerns. Their academic preparation through biological, psychological, and social sciences studies provides occupational therapy practitioners with a basic foundation that prepares them to work with this population (American Occupational Therapy Association 1991).

Activity analysis, activity adaptation, and performance of work-history interviews are part of the preparation of occupational therapy practitioners, who are trained and educated to consider the occupational performance area of "work." Practitioners have demonstrated knowledge in this area by publishing in the work rehabilitation literature. One particular journal, *Occupational Therapy Practice*, dedicated an entire issue to "work." Some of its articles included topics of supported employment and programming for brain-injured adults (Perosig and Haase, 1990; Spencer, 1990). Occupational therapy practitioners must continue to contribute to the literature in order to demonstrate their education and expertise.

The challenge facing occupational therapy practitioners in industrial rehabilitation is to become proficient in their activity-analysis skills. The complaint heard most frequently while doing presentations to students and therapists is that practitioners are frustrated in their attempts to develop appropriate "work circuits" in their industrial rehabilitation programs.

Roles in Injured-Worker and Return-to-Work Programs

A successful return-to-work program typically takes an inter-disciplinary team approach. Interdisciplinary collaboration provides an opportunity for all staff to learn about the supportive services provided to the individual and the total program plan (Muhlenhaupt, 1991). All aspects of the clients performance are thoroughly addressed.

Work hardening is a systematic and comprehensive therapeutic approach to assist clients to return to work after an injury or illness. A set of circuits are developed to address areas of weakness.

Specific circuit training is defined as "exercise that incorporates aerobic and anaerobic activity for a specified time, using different activities and muscle groups" (Altug, Hoffman, Slone, et al., 1990). This may involve the use of multiple exercise stations that vary between activities for the upper body and the lower body. The practitioner can grade the resistance and/or the static/dynamic components of each activity. The essence to designing work-specific circuits is consideration of the client's work environment, the condition of the client, the status of the injury, functional goals, and the critical demand factors of the specific job to which the client will return. Altug and co-authors (1990) described a work circuit training for a fire fighter. Occupational therapy practitioners who contributed to their article demonstrated the knowledge and skill of activity analysis.

113

Occupational therapy practitioners should address work issues with every client they serve but especially with those clients in industrial rehabilitation programs. Simulating necessary job tasks can always be a part of the treatment program. Developing a treatment plan that helps build the skills necessary for success in the three occupational performance areas (work, play/leisure, and self-care) should be a routine occupational therapy treatment goal.

Occupational therapy practitioners have the skill and knowledge to treat mental health disorders. A worker's return to the job is often impeded by psychological maladjustments or other mental health problems. Chronic-pain management clients may have psychological needs that occupational therapy practitioners are trained to address, while also addressing the physical impairments/functional restrictions of persons with mental health problems. Currently, a supervised psychosocial fieldwork experience is required by AOTA curriculum essentials (American Occupational Therapy Association, 1991).

Early work-related therapy for injured employees reduces return-to-work barriers. Tramposh (1988) stated that work-related therapy causes the patient to face many of the work issues and to discover whether he or she is capable of performing their job tasks/duties. Tramposh emphasized the need for comprehensive work-hardening programs to operate on the concept that the injured worker take responsibility for managing his or her injuries and returning to the job quickly and safely.

Injury-Prevention Education

Occupational therapy practitioners are familiar with the requirements of injury-prevention education. For a long time practitioners have recommended home programs for either maintaining or improving one's upper-extremity flexibility and hand function, for energy conservation principles, and for work-simplification techniques for many diagnoses. Within the last decade the medical community has recognized specialty areas of "occupational and environmental medicine" and "preventive medicine." The adage "an ounce of prevention is worth a pound of cure" is appropriate as occupational therapy practitioners begin the new decade.

Practitioners must take an active role in the U.S. industrial "occupational" health care era and the prevention of work-related injuries, working in collaboration with physicians and occupational health nurses. For example, a job that could result in the development of a specific injury, such as cumulative trauma disorder (CTD), should be identified and the issues should be addressed. Repetitive use of a specific group of muscles over an extended period of time with maximum force and joint torque potentially leads to dysfunction. Repetitive-motion injuries have received much attention in the current literature. Educating employers and insurance case managers about recognizing and controlling CTD is a role an occupational therapy practitioner assumes.

Job-Site Analysis and Ergonomic Analysis

Another occupational therapy practitioner role in industrial rehabilitation is performing job-site analyses as part of the rehabilitation process. The practitioner may identify the need for adaptive equipment and assistive devices, or auxiliary aids, as they are referred to in the Americans With Disabilities Act (ADA). Examples of areas of concern include workstation and/or tool redesign, environmental considerations, and so on.

Providing ergonomic analysis and recommendations to industry is a service occupational therapy practitioners may also provide. Rodgers (1992) referred to occupational therapists as "ergonomists." Ergonomics is defined as a body of knowledge about human abilities, human limitations, and other human characteristics that are relevant to design. Ergonomic design is the application of this body of knowledge to the design of tools, machines, systems, tasks, jobs, and environments for safe, comfortable, and effective human use (Board of Certification in Professional Ergonomics, 1990). Ergonomics is sometimes synonymous with human factors, according to the Board of Certification of Professional Ergonomics (BCPE). Job rotations, modified job duties, or categorizing different jobs to allow productivity benefit the employer while promoting an employee's feeling of productivity (occupation) and "being productive." Ergonomics looks at these issues and addresses problems. Joyce (1991) reported that the evidence is overwhelming, both nationally and internationally, that government agencies, corporations, and labor organizations are directing greater effort toward ergonomics.

Activity Adaptation

What is modified duty? As practitioners continue to study and share industrial rehabilitation knowledge, industry continues to talk about limited duty, light duty, modified duty, restricted duty, and alternative productive work. Modified duty is the preferred terminology for the purposes of this article. Basically, they all have the same meaning and outcome. Much of industry has learned that the 100% rule (only allowing a worker to return when he or she is 100% better) is both ineffective and expensive; therefore, industry has begun to support programs that allow employees to return to work at an earlier stage during their recovery. Unfortunately, in some cases this is not possible because of the healing process, because of labor organizations, or because performance demands are such that the job may be difficult to modify. During occupational therapy education and training, determining modified duty involves grading the activity and adapting it through the activity-analysis process (this sometimes is referred to as therapeutic grading and adaptation). Hinojosa and the Commission on Practice (1993) stated that "purposeful activities are adapted by modifying the sequence or procedures of the task," the position of the individual, the position of the materials, the size, shape, weight, or texture of materials, and nature/degree of physical handling by the employee. Employers, physicians, and occupational therapy practitioners must decide together the tasks a worker can productively perform on the job for a couple of hours, for half of the day, or for a specific time frame based on the injury. Job modification is any change in the duties, hours, or expectations of a job. Randolph and Dalton (1989) advocated that a limited-duty program at the acute-care hospital was cost effective and most significant. Bringing employees in for modified duty allows for work behaviors to continue and assists the other employees with some tasks and duties.

Summary

Occuptional therapy practitioner's recognize that much of the push for industrial rehabilitation services has been driven by federal mandates and by state workers' compensation laws. The need for programs that encourage employee independence and early return to work following injury or illness is increasing. Occupational therapy practitioners must be aware of workers' compensation programs in their states; they must determine whether a particular program has a rehabilitation and/or vocational focus. Returning a worker to some work as quickly as possible, even if it is modified duty, should typically be a goal in a treatment plan. Occupational therapy practitioners must be proactive during this decade; they must anticipate better public awareness of a great profession. As Jacobs (1992) reported, "Work has been at the heart of the philosophy and practice of occupational therapy since its inception." The area of work rehabilitation programs is truly a natural environment for occupational therapy practitioners.

—by Thomas F. Fisher

References

Altug, A., Hoffman, J., Slone, S., Tinschel, D., and Bemesderfer, L. (1990). Work circuit training. *Clin Manage*, 10(5), 41-48.

American Occupational Therapy Association. (1991). Essentials of occupational therapy education. Rockville, MD: American Occupational Therapy Association.

Board of Certification in Professional Ergonomics. (1990). Certification for ergonomists and human factors professionals. Brochure. Bellingham, WA.

Briggs, C. (1949). Graded exercise and work tolerance. *Am J Occup Ther.*, 3(2), 78-81.

Bunnell, S. 1950, *Am J Occup Ther*, 4(4), 145-177.

Cynkin, S., and Robinson, A. (1990). Occupational therapy and activities health: Toward health through activities. Boston, MA: Little, Brown.

Hinojosa, J., and the Commission on Practice. (1993). Purposeful activity: A Position paper. Rockville, MD: American Occupational Therapy Association, Commission on Practice.

Jacobs, K. (1992). Work practice for the new millennium. *Rehab Manage*, 5(2), 71-72.

Joyce, M. (1991). Ergonomics will take center stage during '90s and into new century. *Occup Health Safety*, 10(1), 31-37.

Muhlenhaupt, M. (1990). Components of program planning process. In W. Dunn (Ed.), *Pediatric occupational therapy: Facilitating effective service delivery* (pp. 125-127). Thorofare, NJ: Slack.

Perosig, A., and Haase, B. (1990). Bridging the rehabilitation gap. *Occup Ther Prac*, 1(2), 44-52.

Randolph, S., and Dalton, P. (1989). Limited duty work: An innovative approach to early return to work. *AAOHN J*, 37(11), 446-453.

Rodgers, S. (1992). Ergonomics: View from the top. *Visions*, 2(4), 2-4.

Schwartzberg, S. (1988). Generic tools: Purposeful activity, *occupational therapy*. Philadelphia, PA: Willard and Spackman, J. B. Lippincott.

Spencer, K. (1990). Supported employment: The role of occupational therapy at the job site. *Occup Ther Prac*, 1(2), 74-83.

Tramposh, A. K. (1988). Work-related therapy for the injured reduces return-to-work barriers. *Occup Health Safety*, 8(4), 55-82.

Wegg, L. (195 7). The role of the occupational therapist in vocational rehabilitation. *Am J Occup Ther*, 11(2), 252-254.

Chapter 14

Massage Therapy

Whether seeking relief for a medical condition, searching for a method to help deal with the stresses of daily life or wanting to maintain good health, more and more Americans are turning to therapeutic massage.

Massage doesn't just feel good. Research shows it reduces the heart rate, lowers blood pressure, increases blood circulation and lymph flow, relaxes muscles, improves range of motion, and increases endorphins, the body's natural painkillers. Therapeutic massage enhances medical treatment and helps people feel less anxious and stressed, relaxed yet more alert.

A writer for the Chicago Tribune stated, "Massage is to the human body what a tune-up is for a car." Therapeutic massage can be part of your regular healthcare maintenance.

The consumer demand for massage therapy is fed by the health and fitness movement as well as America's growing emphasis on wellness and alternative care. Both the demand and the healthcare profession's response are overwhelming:

- Consumers spend $2 billion to $4 billion a year on visits to massage therapists, according to an American Massage Therapy Association (AMTA) analysis of a study by Beth Israel Deaconess Medical Center and Harvard Medical School published in the *New England Journal of Medicine* in 1993.

- Current research shows people are getting more massages, and that therapeutic massage is becoming more mainstream,

119

appealing to everyone from young adults to seniors. People are experiencing the therapeutic benefits of massage and report getting massages mostly to relax, relieve aches and pains, and help reduce stress.

- A national survey conducted by the State University of New York at Syracuse found 54 percent of primary care physicians and family practitioners said they would encourage their patients to pursue massage therapy as a treatment, and a third of those said they are willing to refer patients to a massage therapist.

- The American Massage Therapy Association's membership has increased nearly four-fold in the past decade, to more than 28,000.

There also is a growing trend of offering therapeutic massage in the workplace. Your employer may be among those who have learned that massage therapy isn't just a perk, but actually increases employee productivity and morale.

According to a 1996 survey of employees who regularly receive therapeutic massage on-site at Reebok International Ltd., 98 percent said it helped them reduce work-related stress; 92 percent said it increased alertness, motivation and productivity; 83 percent said it had in some cases sufficiently addressed a problem so medical attention was not necessary; and 66 percent said it had enabled them to stay at work when they would have otherwise gone home sick.

Health insurance companies and HMOs, realizing the cost savings of therapeutic massage, are increasingly covering or reimbursing massage when it is prescribed or provided by authorized professionals.

What is Therapeutic Massage?

"Massage therapy has clearly been shown to me to be very beneficial, particularly in areas where conventional medicine has not been as successful, including chronic arthritis, musculoskeletal syndromes and chronic headache, among others."

—by Renslow Sherer, M.D.

Director of the Cook County Hospital, HIV Primary Care Center, Chicago

Therapeutic massage involves the manipulation of the soft tissue structures of the body to prevent and alleviate pain, discomfort, muscle spasm, and stress; and, to promote health and wellness. AMTA defines massage therapy as a profession in which the practitioner applies manual techniques, and may apply adjunctive therapies, with the intention of positively affecting the health and well-being of the client.

Massage therapy improves functioning of the circulatory, lymphatic, muscular, skeletal, and nervous systems and may improve the rate at which the body recovers from injury and illness. Massage involves holding, causing movement of soft tissue, and/or applying pressure to the body. It comes in many forms, including:

- Swedish a gentle, relaxing massage;
- Pressure point therapy for certain conditions or injuries; and
- Sports massage which focuses on muscle groups relevant to the particular sport.

How Can Massage Be Medically Beneficial?

"Massage therapy is a complementary therapy, not alternative anymore. It's of tremendous benefit."

— by Brad Stuart, M.D.

Hospice medical Director for the Visiting Nurse Association & Hospice of Northern California

People find that therapeutic massage can help with a wide range of medical conditions, including:

- allergies
- anxiety
- arthritis (both osteoarthritis and rheumatoid arthritis)
- asthma and bronchitis
- carpal tunnel syndrome
- chronic and temporary pain
- circulatory problems
- depression
- digestive disorders, including spastic colon, constipation and diarrhea
- headache, especially when due to muscle tension

- insomnia
- myofascial pain (a condition of the tissue connecting the muscles)
- reduced range of motion
- sinusitis
- sports injuries, including pulled or strained muscles and sprained ligaments
- stress
- temporomandibular joint dysfunction (TMJ)

Although massage therapy does not increase muscle strength, it can stimulate weak, inactive muscles and, thus, partially compensate for the lack of exercise and inactivity resulting from illness or injury. It also can hasten and lead to a more complete recovery from exercise or injury.

Therapeutic massage can be inappropriate in some cases, such as in people with:

- inflammation of the veins (phlebitis)
- infectious diseases
- certain forms of cancer
- some skin conditions
- some cardiac problems

If you have one of these or some other diagnosed medical condition, always check with your doctor before seeking a massage.

What Does Research Show About Massage Therapy?

"Massage therapy is beneficial for almost all diseases. Eighty percent of disease is stress-related, an massage reduces stress."

— by Sandra McLanahan, M.D.

family practitioner, Buckingham, Va.

Research on the effects of massage therapy has been ongoing for more than 120 years. A surge in research over the past 20 years has resulted in more than 100 published studies.

At the University of Miami School of Medicine's Touch Research Institute, 55 studies on touch, the majority on massage therapy, have been published or are under way. And, the National Institutes of Health (NIH), the government agency that oversees and conducts medical research in the United States, opened an Office of Alternative Medicine in 1992, which has funded several studies on the benefits of massage. More research is under way.

Among research findings so far:

- Office workers massaged regularly were more alert, performed better and were less stressed than those who weren't massaged.

- Massage therapy decreased the effects of anxiety, tension, depression, pain, and itching in burn patients.

- Abdominal surgery patients recovered more quickly after massage.

- Premature infants who were massaged gained more weight and fared better than those who weren't.

- Autistic children showed less erratic behavior after massage therapy.

The NIH has awarded $10 million in grants to establish 10 centers in the United States to study alternative therapies, including massage, for a variety of ailments. All are affiliated with major institutions, from Harvard Medical School in Boston, Massachusetts, to Stanford University in Palo Alto, California.

AMTA, the international 28,000-member professional association for massage therapists, supports research through the AMTA Foundation. Currently, AMTA and the AMTA Foundation are helping to fund and collaborating closely with the Center for Alternative Medicine Research at Boston's Beth Israel Deaconess Medical Center, which is conducting a study on the use of alternative treatments, including massage therapy, for lower back pain.

What Is the Cost of Massage Therapy and Will My Insurance Cover It?

"Massage is to the human body what a tune-up is to a car. It provides a physical and mental boost to the weary, sore, and stressed..."

—Chicago Tribune, April 6, 1995

While cost depends on the locality, type and length of the massage and the experience of the therapist, fees generally start from $45 an hour.

Insurance providers continue to recognize the advantages of massage therapy and coverage is increasing, particularly in the 25 states and the District of Columbia where massage therapists are licensed by state regulatory bodies. Generally, therapeutic massage is covered or reimbursable when it is given by an authorized healthcare provider. Some states are considering legislation, which would require insurance companies to cover "treatments" by licensed, alternative medicine providers, including massage therapists.

Several health and managed-care plans in the country, including Oxford Health Plans Inc., PREMERA (formerly Blue Cross of Washington and Alaska, and Medical Services Corp.), Prudential Insurance Company of America, Great-West Life & Annuity, Group Health Cooperative of Puget Sound and Alternative Health Insurance Services, cover prescribed massage therapy in many cases.

Check with your healthcare insurance provider. Once massage therapy is prescribed, you or your doctor may need to seek authorization from the insurer if coverage is not clearly spelled out in your policy or plan.

What Can You Expect?

The first appointment generally begins with the massage therapist asking what prompted you to get a massage, your current physical condition, medical history, lifestyle, stress level, and painful areas. The massage therapist may ask you about your health goals and what you hope the massage will do to help you achieve those goals.

Some massages, such as those on-site at your place of business, are done while you are fully clothed. For a full-body massage you will be asked to remove clothing to your level of comfort. Undressing takes place in private, and a sheet, towel or gown is provided for draping. The therapist will undrape only the part of your body being massaged, insuring that modesty is respected at all times. Your massage will take place in a comfortable atmosphere and on a padded table. You should expect a peaceful, relaxing experience.

How Can You Find a Qualified Massage Therapist?

"I had neck problems that limited my activities. Massage therapy cleared up the stiffness and pain in my neck—now I am playing golf and tennis, even biking. Thanks to massage therapy, I feel I have a more pain-free life."

—by Paula Marcotte
Silver Spring, MD

The American Massage Therapy Association has over 30,000 members in more than 20 countries. Approximately 22,000 members have demonstrated a high level of skill and expertise through testing and/ or education. Another 6,000 associate members are working toward such qualifications. Founded in 1943, AMTA provides a massage therapist locator service for consumers and healthcare professionals, and it offers consumer education materials about therapeutic massage.

AMTA also has a code of ethics and practice standards that promote the highest quality assurance in the profession and has a certification program for event sports massage therapists.

New AMTA Professional Active Members must be graduates of training programs accredited or approved by the Commission on Massage Training Accreditation (COMTA); have a current AMTA accepted city, state or provincial license; or be National Certification Board for Therapeutic Massage & Bodywork (NCTMB).COMTA-accredited programs require a stringent course of study including at least 500 hours of classroom instruction in anatomy, physiology, massage therapy techniques, first aid, and CPR.

Certification by the National Certification Board for Therapeutic Massage & Bodywork (NCTMB) is an indication that a massage therapist has attained the highest professional credential in the field. The certification process incorporates testing in competency, ethics and practice standards; also, it requires periodic evidence that the massage therapist participates in continuing education to keep current and competent in the field.

To find a qualified massage therapist, contact:

American Massage Therapy Association
820 Davis Street
Suite 100
Evanston, Illinois 60201-4444
phone: (847) 864-0123
fax: (847) 864-1178
email: info@inet.amtamassage.org
http://www.amtamassage.org

AMTA Mission

The mission of the American Massage Therapy Association is to develop and advance the art, science and practice of massage therapy in a caring, professional and ethical manner in order to promote the health and welfare of humanity.

Massage Therapy is a profession in which the practitioner applies manual techniques, and may apply adjunctive therapies, with the intention of positively affecting the health and well being of the client.

Glossary of Terms

Cranio-Sacral is a technique for finding and correcting cerebral and spinal imbalances or blockages that may cause sensory, motor or intellectual dysfunction.

Deep Tissue, releases the chronic patterns of tension in the body through slow strokes and deep finger pressure on the contracted areas, either following or going across the grain of muscles, tendons and fascia. It is called deep tissue, because it also focuses on the deeper layers of muscle tissue.

Reflexology (zone therapy) is organized around a system of points on the hands and feet that are thought to correspond, or "reflex," to all areas of the body. Though the massage is specific to an area, it is intended to affect the whole body.

Shiatsu and Acupressure are systems of finger-pressure massage, based on Oriental healing concepts, which treat special points along "meridians," the invisible channels of energy flow in the body. Energy blocked along these meridians can cause physical discomfort, so the aim is to release the blockage and re-balance the energy flow. They can be used for the full body or for specific areas of the body.

Sports Massage Therapy is classified into three main categories: maintenance, event and rehabilitation. Maintenance massage is a regular program of massage to help the athlete reach optimal performance through injury-free training. Event massage takes place before, during and/or after competition to supplement an athlete's warm-up, readying the athlete for top performance, and/or to reduce the muscle spasms and metabolic build-up that occurs with vigorous exercise. Such techniques enhance the body's recovery process, improving the athletes return to high-level training and competition, and reducing the risk of injury. Rehabilitation massage techniques are effective in the management of both acute and chronic injuries.

Swedish Massage uses a system of long strokes, kneading, and friction percussive and vibration techniques on the more superficial layers of muscles, combined with active and passive movements of the joints. It is used primarily for full-body sessions and promotes general relaxation, improves blood circulation and range of motion, and relieves muscle tension. Swedish is the most common type of massage.

Trigger Point Therapy (a.k.a. Myotherapy or Neuromuscular Therapy) applies concentrated finger pressure to "trigger points" (painful irritated areas in muscles) to break cycles of spasm and pain.

Physical Benefits of Therapeutic Massage

- Helps relieve stress and aids relaxation
- Helps relieve muscle tension and stiffness
- Fosters faster healing of strained muscles and sprained ligaments; reduces
- pain and swelling; reduces formation of excessive scar tissue
- Reduces muscle spasms
- Provides greater joint flexibility and range of motion
- Enhances athletic performance
- Promotes deeper and easier breathing
- Improves circulation of blood and movement of lymph fluids
- Reduces blood pressure
- Helps relieve tension-related headaches and effects of eyestrain
- Enhances the health and nourishment of skin
- Improves posture
- Strengthens the immune system

Massage Therapy and Well-Being: Mental Benefits

- Fosters peace of mind
- Promotes a relaxed state of mental alertness
- Helps relieve mental stress
- Improves ability to monitor stress signals and respond appropriately
- Enhances capacity for calm thinking and creativity
- Emotional Benefits
- Satisfies needs for caring nurturing touch
- Fosters a feeling of well being
- Reduces levels of anxiety
- Increases awareness of mind-body connection

To locate a qualified massage therapist in your area, contact:

American Massage Therapy Association
820 Davis Street, Suite 100
Evanston, Illinois 60201-4444
phone: (847) 864-0123
fax: (847) 864-1178
e-mail: info@inet.amtamassage.org
http://www.amtamassage.org

Chapter 15

Research Shows Massage Therapy Works

Massage not only feels wonderful, research has proved it has myriad health benefits, from controlling pain, to decreasing stress, to reducing heart rate and blood pressure.

"It's been indisputably shown that massage moves blood and lymph through the body," said E. Houston LeBrun, president-elect of the American Massage Therapy Association (AMTA). "Increasingly, there are research studies being done on the benefits of massage therapy—especially on massage for people with low-back pain and for AIDS patients."

Research in massage therapy has been ongoing for more than 120 years. A recent resurgence in research over the last 30 years has resulted in more than 100 studies being published.

AMTA, the international 28,000-member professional association for massage therapists, supports research through the AMTA Foundation. Since 1993, the AMTA and the Foundation have awarded more than $82,000 in grants for researchers to study the effects of massage. Among the findings of the studies:

- Medical school students at the University of Medicine and Dentistry of New Jersey-New Jersey Medical School who were massaged before an exam showed a significant decrease in anxiety and respiratory rates, as well as a significant increase in white blood cells and natural killer cell activity, suggesting a benefit to the immune system.

- Preliminary results suggested cancer patients had less pain and anxiety after receiving therapeutic massage at the James Cancer Hospital and Research Institute in Columbus, Ohio.

- Women who had experienced the recent death of a child were less depressed after receiving therapeutic massage, according to preliminary results of a study at the University of South Carolina.

Studies funded by the National Institutes of Health (NIH) have found massage beneficial in improving weight gain in HIV-exposed infants and facilitating recovery in patients who underwent abdominal surgery. And at the University of Miami School of Medicine's Touch Research Institute, studies have found massage helpful in decreasing blood pressure in people with hypertension, alleviating pain in migraine sufferers and improving alertness and performance in office workers.

Because of Congressional pressure and public insistence, the NIH, the government agency that oversees and conducts medical research in the United States, founded the Office of Alternative Medicine in 1992. As part of the effort to further study therapeutic massage and other alternative treatments, the NIH awarded $10 million in grants to establish 10 centers in the United States to study alternative therapies for a variety of ailments. All are affiliated with major institutions.

Researchers at the Center for the Study of Complementary and Alternative Therapies at the University of Virginia, Charlottesville, will study the effects of massage therapy on pain with their NIH grant. A study at Stanford University, Palo Alto, California, will focus on massage after removal of lymph glands during surgery for breast or uterine cancer. Massage therapists will be working with people with HIV and AIDS in a study at Bastyr University AIDS Research Center, Seattle.

AMTA and the AMTA Foundation are helping to fund and collaborating closely with another NIH site. The Center for Alternative Medicine Research at Boston's Beth Israel Deaconess Medical Center is conducting a study on the use of alternative treatments, including massage therapy, for lower back pain.

AMTA provides free informational brochures to consumers and helps consumers or health professionals locate qualified massage therapists in their area. Contact AMTA at 820 Davis St., Suite 100, Evanston, IL 60201-4444; phone (847) 864-0123; fax (847) 864-1178; or via the Web at www.amtamassage.org.

Chapter 16

Massage Therapy Is Effective for Many Childhood Conditions

Massage therapy is proving to be an effective therapy for children and adolescents with medical and psychological problems. In our studies with children, we use parents as the massage therapists; the children can be massaged daily at no cost; and the parents can feel less helpless and more involved in the child's treatment. Parents' involvement in their children's treatment is often negative because they must give shots or monitor dietary compliance, as with diabetic children. Being involved in a more positive treatment such as massage therapy can be very helpful to these parents.

Asthmatic Children

Asthmatic massages at bedtime by their parents for a one-month period. At the end of the study the parents' anxiety decreased, and the children's anxiety and stress hormone levels decreased. Most importantly, over the one-month period. At the end of the study the parents' anxiety decreased, and the children had fewer asthma attacks and were able to breathe better based on daily peak air-flow readings.

Autistic Children

In this study, we wanted to determine whether massage therapy improved the classroom behavior of preschool autistic children. Data analyses revealed that after one month of massage therapy, the autistic children a) were less touch-aversive; b) were less distracted by sounds; c) were more attentive in class; d) showed better relationships with their teachers; e) received better scores on the Autism Behavior Checklist (sensory, relating and total scale scores); and f) scored better on the Early Social Communications Scales (joint attention, behavior regulation, social and initiating behaviors). These were very surprising findings because we expected, based on anecdotal reports, that autistic children would find massage—as with other forms of touch—aversive. Instead, they enjoyed massage. Massage may be less aversive than other kinds of touch because it is predictable. Autistic children may find unpredictable stimulation too arousing.

Children with Severe Burns

This study was designed to reduce anxiety levels prior to the very painful skin-brushing procedure that burn patients experience, and thereby reduce pain during this procedure. Since massage therapy is noted to decrease levels of anxiety and stress hormones in children, we used this therapy prior to the anxiety-provoking, painful skin brushings. After one week, the children had lower anxiety levels and lower levels of stress hormones.

Cancer

In this study, the children were massaged prior to chemotherapy sessions to reduce anticipation anxiety/nausea (short-term effects). The parents also massaged their children prior to bedtime to help them sleep and to give parents an active positive role in their children's treatment. Other benefits included decreased touch aversion (sometimes noted in children with cancer) and improved immune function. In turn, massage could reduce opportunist infections such as pneumonia in children with cancer.

Dermatitis in Children

In this study, stress levels were reduced (stress levels are known to contribute to skin allergic conditions), and having the parents give the massage helped the parents' treatment compliance and reduced their aversive reaction to touching the dermatitis area (and the child's sense that others have an aversive reaction). Finally, measures of the children's skin condition suggested clinical improvement.

Diabetes

Parents' typical involvement in treatment of this condition, as with monitoring dietary compliance and taking blood samples and giving insulin shots, is negative. We gave parents a more positive role in their children's treatment by having them massage their child daily before bedtime. Immediately after the massage sessions, the parents' and children's anxiety and depressed mood levels decreased. At the end of one month, blood glucose levels had decreased to a low value within the normal range.

Eating Disorders (Bulimia)

Adolescents with eating disorders such as bulimia or anorexia are typically depressed. In this study, we hoped to decrease depression and anxiety and to improve the body images of adolescents who were hospitalized for bulimia. The adolescent girls were massaged twice weekly for a five-week period. Data analyses revealed the following significant effects: the massaged adolescents had a) fewer depressive symptoms; b) lower anxiety levels; c) a less distorted body image; and d) lower urinary cortisol levels.

Juvenile Rheumatoid Arthritis

Children with this disease experience chronic pain because anti-inflammatory agents have ceiling effects and narcotic drugs cannot be used due to the addiction risk. Thus, other pain-relieving therapies are being explored. In a massage therapy study in which parents gave daily massages to their children, preliminary data analyses comparing massage and progressive muscle relaxation revealed that the massage therapy group showed several advantages: a) a greater decrease in anxiety and stress hormone levels (cortisol) after the first and last sessions; and b) a greater reduction in pain over the one-month period.

Posttraumatic Stress Disorder (PTSD)

This study was conducted with children who were traumatized by Hurricane Andrew and displayed behavior problems in the classroom. The children were massaged at their school two times weekly for one month. A control group watched relaxing videotapes during their sessions. The results showed that the massaged children had less depression, lower anxiety levels and lower levels of stress hormones, and their drawings had fewer depressive and disorganized features.

Psychiatric Problems

In this study, we gave a 30-minute back massage to 52 hospitalized depressed and conduct-disordered adolescents every day for a five-day period. The following significant differences were found between the control group, who watched relaxing videotapes, and the massage therapy group: Massaged children a) were less depressed; b) were less anxious; and c) had lower saliva cortisol levels after the massage therapy sessions. After five days, nurses rated the adolescents as being less anxious and more cooperative; nighttime (time-lapse videotaped) quiet sleep increased; and urinary cortisol and norepinephrine levels decreased.

Summary

Massage therapy has generally resulted in lower anxiety levels (both self-reported and observed), lower levels of stress hormones (cortisol and norepinephrine), better mood (less depression) and improved clinical course. Other findings were unique to specific conditions.

Massage therapy may work by increasing vagal activity, slowing down the nervous system to a more alert, relaxed state in which people characteristically feel better, perform better, are able to sleep and are less likely to get sick. Enhanced attentiveness or decreased off-task behavior in our studies on autistic and attention-deficit disorder children may relate to increased vagal activity. Lower heart rate and greater heart rate variability generally accompany attentiveness. Increased quiet sleep, which we have noted in our studies on child and adolescent psychiatric patients and infants of depressed mothers, may derive from increases in vagal tone and parasympathetic dominance. Enhanced quiet sleep might also relate to the reduction in anxiety and depression levels noted across most of our studies.

The reduction in pain noted during our studies on children with burns and juvenile rheumatoid arthritis could relate to the "gate theory" of pain. The theory posits that, because touch or tactile nerve fibers are longer than pain fibers and because they are more myelinated, their transit time to the central nervous system is shorter and they "close the gate" to the slower moving pain signals. A similar phenomenon has been noted by Elliott Blass and his colleagues at Cornell University, who report both an opiate-mediated, pain-alleviating mechanism (for example, using sucrose to reduce pain in preemies as they receive heelsticks) and a non-opiate-mediated, pain-alleviating mechanism that needs to be further explored as a potential explanation for pain reduction following non-nutritive sucking (intraoral stimulation) in preemies.

An increase in serotonin also may contribute to these effects (serotonin being the base of many pain medications and antidepressants).

Continuing multimethod/multivariable research is needed on the effects of massage therapy with infants and children.

— by Tiffany M. Field.

Tiffany M. Field is director of the Touch Research Institute at the University of Miami School of Medicine's department of pediatrics. For more information, contact her at PO Box 016820 (D-820), 1601 N.W. 12th Ave., Miami, FL 33101.

Chapter 17

Dance/Movement Therapy— Frequently Asked Questions

Purpose of the American Dance Therapy Association

Since its founding in 1966, ADTA has worked to establish and maintain high standards of professional education and competence in the field.

ADTA stimulates communication among dance/movement therapists and members of allied professions through publication of the *ADTA Newsletter*, the *American Journal of Dance Therapy*, monographs, bibliographies, and conference proceedings.

ADTA holds an annual conference and supports formation of regional groups, conferences, seminars, workshops and meetings throughout the year.

What Is "Dance/Movement Therapy"?

Dance/movement therapists use movement and the body as a whole as the medium for effecting change, growth and healing in the individual. In our official definition, Dance/Movement Therapy is defined as "the psychotherapeutic use of movement as a process which furthers the emotional, cognitive and physical integration of the individual."

Where Do Dance/Movement Therapists Work?

Dance/Movement Therapists work with individuals who have social, emotional, cognitive and/or physical concerns or problems. They are employed in general and psychiatric hospitals, clinics, adult day care, community mental health centers, infant developmental centers, correctional facilities, schools and rehabilitation facilities as well as in private practice. Therapists work with people of all ages in groups and individually. They also act as consultants and engage in research.

How are Dance/Movement Therapists Trained?

Professional training occurs on the graduate level. Studies include courses such as dance/movement therapy theory and practice, psychopathology, psychotherapeutic theory, human development, observation and research skills, and a supervised internship in a clinical setting. There are two levels of certification: DTR, Dance Therapist Registered, received after completing a Masters level program; and ADTR, Academy of Dance Therapists Registered, which one can apply for after a requisite number of supervised hours of employment in the field.

Currently there are 5 Masters level programs approved by the ADTA:

- Antioch New England, contact: Susan Loman, Director of Dance Movement Therapy Program, sloman@antiochne.edu
- Columbia College, Chicago
- Allegheny University
- Naropa Institute, (303) 444-0202
- Also Naropa Institute Report (on charm.net)
- UCLA

Approval of Graduate Programs:

The Association has established an Approval Procedure based on "Guidelines for Graduate Degree Programs." Any Graduate Program may apply for ADTA Approval after graduating two classes.

Undergraduate Training Is Preparation for Graduate Study in Dance/movement Therapy

The following is recommended:

- A broad liberal arts background with an emphasis in psychology; extensive training in a variety of dance forms with courses in theory, improvisation, choreography and kinesiology; experience in teaching dance in normal children and adults.

- Introductory or survey courses in dance/movement therapy can help students evaluate their interests and aptitudes before entering a graduate program.

Credentials

The Association has always distinguished between dance/movement therapist prepared to work in professional settings within a team or under supervision, and those prepared for the responsibilities of working independently in private practice, or providing supervision.

DTR—Dance Therapist Registered

Therapists with this title have a Masters Degree and are fully qualified to work in a professional treatment system.

ADTR—Academy of Dance Therapists Registered

Therapists with this title have met additional requirements and are fully qualified to teach, provide supervision, and engage in private practice.

Membership In A.D.T.A.

Professional Membership: Open to any person prepared through dance therapy training and professionally involved in the field of dance/movement therapy.

Associate Membership: Open to those individuals interested in and supporting the objectives of the profession.

Contributing Membership: Open to institutions, schools, organizations, foundation, and associationist interested in the profession.

Student Membership: Open to all students verified by a student I.D. Card.

For more information

If you're interested in more information about dance/movement therapy, please send a note to Kathy Wallens, ADTA Newsletter Editor at: KWallens@Slip.net

Or you can write or call the national office of the ADTA at:

American Dance Therapy Association
10632 Little Patuxent Parkway
2000 Century Plaza
Columbia, MD 21044-3263
410-997-4040 (Voice)
410-997-4048 (FAX)
E-Mail: info@adta.org
http://www.adta.org

The American Dance Therapy Association is the national professional support organization for Dance/Movement Therapists. For a description of Dance/Movement Therapy, see either of these two excellent Web pages:

- Denny Balish-LaSaine

- Maria Brignola Lee

ADTA ListServe

The ADTA also has a ListServe. If you're interested in finding out about it, you can write to either:

Kathy at: KWallens@Slip.net or at: ADTA@Capital.citi.net or,
ADTA ListServe at: listproc@list.ab.umd.edu

To subscribe, send "SUB ADTA, first name, last name" to listproc@list.ab.umd.edu

Chapter 18

Dance and Drama Therapies Stimulate Creativity, Enhance Patient Well-Being

An elderly man in a wheelchair feels invigorated, swaying his arms and kicking his legs to the rhythm of his favorite music. Originally stiff and withdrawn, his movements have helped him to feel better, develop increased self-esteem, and feel more comfortable communicating with others.

A group of residents leave a room singing, feeling a sense of accomplishment and an awakened sense of creativity. The same residents, only a week before had been withdrawn and isolated from each other, having little energy or desire to try new things.

What has Caused the Changes in These Residents?

Alternative therapeutic techniques—dance and movement therapy and drama therapy, although fairly new to long-term care settings, have proven very effective in achieving a wide variety of therapeutic goals. These types of therapy help participants to activate their bodies, use their imaginations, release tension, become more coordinated, and develop better self-images.

Group movement and drama therapy can help residents to learn how to interact with each other better. These sessions also are effective in helping residents discover and confront emotions that may not be accessible to them through traditional verbal therapies.

© 1995 Manisses Communications Group, Inc., *Council Close-Up*, Feb.25, 1994, and Dec. 10, 1993, *The Brown University Long-Term Care Quality Letter*, July 24, 1995; reprinted with permission.

Movement activities for the elderly should involve both relaxation and vitalization techniques. The therapist should lead residents through breathing and stretching exercises that revitalize and motivate.

You can use movement therapy to inspire reminiscence. Reminiscence encourages cognitive reorganization in confused residents and increases self-esteem and social interaction. Certain movements often are linked to past events, and the memories that are triggered can bring back pleasurable emotions. For example, for some residents, swaying the arms may bring back the memory of dancing with a spouse or loved one.

By participating in movement session, the residents can have physical contact with others. They also can share memories and emotions. Susan Schaefer, a dance/movement therapist says, "I try to keep the session very playful, so that the participants will feel comfortable in expressing themselves. Through this sharing and contact, they develop a greater comfort level in the group and feel less inhibited."

Using Drama as Therapy

Drama therapy is a progressive group technique designed to increase self-awareness and enhance self-expression. It has been shown to strengthen self-esteem, improve interpersonal relationships, enhance coping skills, reduce stress, and stimulate spontaneity. David R. Johnson, clinical instructor of psychology at Yale University, defines drama therapy as "the intentional use of creative drama toward psychotherapeutic goals of symptoms relief, emotional and physical integration, and personal growth."

Drama therapy provides integration between the residents' internal and external worlds. By encouraging self-expression, drama therapy helps residents to develop better coping mechanisms and improve their adaptation skills.

Drama therapy brings a sense of renewal. It helps residents to forget about their pains and troubles and become creative and productive. As Marilyn Richman, drama therapist with the Institute of Therapy through the Arts (ITA) says, "the loss of role that often accompanies old age and retirement can lead to feelings of isolation and worthlessness. But by belonging to a lively, relaxed drama group, participants take on creative roles and recover a feeling of being vibrant, connected, and effective."

Getting Residents to Improvise

In both forms of therapy, participants need not follow any set routine. Instead, group leaders provide a loose structure for improvisation. In dance and movement therapy, leaders play music and encourage residents to move their bodies in response to the rhythm. For drama therapy, the starting point might be a particular setting or situation—"waiting at a bus stop," or "at the grocery store." Then, encourage participants to use their imaginations, and work with each other to allow a scene to unfold.

When planning movement or drama therapy sessions, it is important to take physical or mental impairments into account. Assess all residents before involvement, and make sure that all movement techniques—in either type of therapy—fall within residents' capacity to experience and perform without pain or discomfort.

Follow-Up With Discussion

After sessions, therapists can facilitate discussion among the group members. They can address themes and ideas raised through the session, and participants can discuss their own responses to the activity—how it felt to take on certain roles, or what emotions were evoked, and why.

Residents reap many benefits from these kinds of sessions and discussions. One patient with residual stroke said after one of the sessions, "I feel like a surge of life." Another woman commented that the movement therapy "makes me feel beautiful." "When you finish a class," says another resident, "you're raring to go. It's really a lift."

—by Kevin Kavanaugh

Mr. Kavanaugh is editor of *The Council Close-Up*, a news-letter dedicated to residents and employees of nursing homes, published by the Illinois Council on Long-Term Care.

For more information on educational programs for movement and drama therapy, contact the American Art Therapy Association, Inc., at (847) 566-4580, and the American Music Therapy Association, at (301) 589-3300.

Chapter 19

Frequently Asked Questions about Art Therapy

Art therapists work with individuals of all ages, races, and ethnic backgrounds who have developmental, medical, or psychological impairments.

What Is Art Therapy?

Art therapy is a human service profession which utilizes art media, images, the creative art process and patient/client responses to the created art productions as reflections of an individual's development, abilities, personality, interests, concerns, and conflicts. Art therapy practice is based on knowledge of human developmental and psychological theories which are implemented in the full spectrum of models of assessment and treatment including educational, psychodynamic, cognitive, transpersonal, and other therapeutic means of reconciling emotional conflicts, fostering self-awareness, developing social skills, managing behavior, solving problems, reducing anxiety, aiding reality orientation, and increasing self-esteem.

Art therapy is an effective treatment for the developmentally, medically, educationally, socially or psychologically impaired; and is practiced in mental health, rehabilitation, medical, educational, and forensic institutions. Populations of all ages, races, and ethnic backgrounds are served by art therapists in individual, couples, family, and group therapy formats.

Educational, professional, and ethical standards for art therapists are regulated by the American Art Therapy Association, Inc. (AATA). The Art Therapy Credentials Board, Inc. (ATCB), an independent organization, grants post-graduate registration (ATR) after reviewing documentation of completion of graduate education and post-graduate supervised experience. The Registered Art Therapist who successfully completes the written examination administered by the ATCB is qualified as Board Certified (ATR-BC), a credential requiring maintenance through continuing education credits.

How Did Art Therapy Begin?

Although visual expressions have been basic to humanity throughout history, art therapy did not emerge as a distinct profession until the 1930's. At the beginning of the 20th century, psychiatrists became interested in the art work done by patients, and studied it to see if there was a link between the art and the illness of their patients. At this same time, art educators were discovering that the free and spontaneous art expression of children represented both emotional and symbolic communications. Since then, the profession of art therapy has grown into an effective and important method of communication, assessment, and treatment with many populations.

Where Do Art Therapists Work?

Art therapists work in private offices, art rooms, or meeting rooms in facilities such as:

- hospitals—both medical and psychiatric
- out-patient facilities
- clinics
- residential treatment centers
- halfway houses
- shelters
- schools
- correctional facilities
- elder care facilities
- pain clinics
- universities
- art studios

The art therapist may work as part of a team which includes physicians, psychologists, nurses, rehabilitation counselors, social workers, and teachers. Together, they determine and implement a client's therapeutic, school, or mental health program. Art therapists also work as primary therapists in private practice.

What are the Requirements to Become an Art Therapist?

Personal Qualifications: An art therapist must have sensitivity to human needs and expressions, emotional stability, patience, a capacity for insight into psychological processes, and an understanding of art media. An art therapist must also be an attentive listener, a keen observer, and be able to develop a rapport with people. Flexibility and a sense of humor are important in adapting to changing circumstances, frustration, and disappointment.

Educational Requirements: One must complete the required core curriculum as outlined in the AATA Education Standards to qualify as a professional art therapist. Entry into the profession of art therapy is at the master's level. Avenues of completion offered by graduate level art therapy programs include:

- a master's degree in art therapy
- a master's degree with an emphasis in art therapy
- twenty-one (21) semester units in art therapy with a master's degree in a related field

Contact the AATA National Office for more information concerning educational requirements and programs.

Registration and Board Certification Requirements: The ATR and ATR-BC are the recognized standards for the field of art therapy, and are conferred by the ATCB. In order to qualify as a registered art therapist (ATR), in addition to the educational requirements, an individual must complete a minimum of 1,000 direct client contact hours. One hour of supervision is required for every ten hours of client contact.

What Is the Employment Outlook for the Profession of Art Therapy?

Art therapy is a growing field. Employment continues to increase as it becomes recognized by professionals and clients. Graduates of art therapy programs are successful at finding employment in both full and part-time positions. Those with ATR and ATR-BC have a distinct advantage as it is the recognized credential of the profession.

Earning for art therapists vary geographically depending on the type of practice and job responsibilities. Entry level income is approximately $25,000, median income between $28,000 and $38,000, and top earning potential for salaried administrators ranges between $40,000 and $60,000. Art therapists with doctoral degrees, state licensure, or who qualify in their state to conduct private practice, have an earning potential of $75.00 to $90.00 per hour in private practice.

State requirements for private practice vary across the country. Practice rules and regulations are available from state licensing boards.

How Do I Find a Job as an Art Therapist?

There are several sources available to an art therapist seeking employment, including college placement offices, contacts formed during internship placements, and through state affiliation chapter memberships. Memberships in AATA and AATA affiliate chapters, newsletters and job information hotlines are resources for employment opportunities. Those desiring work in federal or state agencies may write or call the local branch of the Office of Personnel Management for details on the application process. Letters and resumes sent to the facilities listed above often bring invitations for an interview. Professional journals and local newspapers may list positions available.

Chapter 20

Therapeutic Recreation

What Is Therapeutic Recreation?

Therapeutic recreation consists of leisure activities specifically designed to help people get the most out of their lives. People with physical or developmental disabilities, the mentally ill, and older adults with activity limitations can benefit from therapeutic recreation.

Recreational therapists plan activities to promote physical, mental, emotional and/or social wellness. A program of therapeutic recreation is made up of many types of education, therapy, and recreational activities.

Why Is Therapeutic Recreation Important?

Therapeutic recreation can help people of all ages to get well, live well, and stay well so that they can enjoy life more. Goals are developed to help people learn and practice the new skills needed to care for themselves and to be independent. As people become more self-reliant and independent, therapeutic recreation can help relieve tension and promote a sense of accomplishment. Activities are designed to provide opportunities to be with other people, to gain self-confidence, and to learn to cope in different situations outside the home.

After an evaluation of the person's abilities, interests, needs, and desires, goals for a therapy program are set. A written plan is developed against which progress toward the goals is measured. Some activities that may be included are:

- shopping
- swimming
- group sports
- cooking
- exercises
- games
- arts and crafts
- woodworking
- painting.

The therapist may draw upon the skills of other professionals to achieve the goals outlined in the recreational plan. Those professionals may include doctors, nurses, psychologists, physical therapists, occupational therapists, vocational counselors, speech/language pathologists, social workers, prosthetists, and orthotists.

How Can Recreation Therapy Help?

Recreation therapy helps people get involved in a variety of activities needed to improve everyday living. Examples of activities and possible benefits include:

- improved balance, muscle strength, and coordination through exercise activities
- increased flexibility and movement through sports
- increased self-esteem, self-confidence, and interpersonal skills through group participation and discussions
- enhanced opportunity for the development of social relationships through parties, community arts programs, and community relations activities.
- participation in activities, such as swimming or hiking, that relax both mind and body and help manage stress.

Who Provides Therapeutic Recreation?

Recreational therapists, also called specialists, have completed an accepted program of study at a college or university. An associate's degree is needed to be a recreational therapist assistant and a bachelor's degree is needed to be a recreational therapist/specialist. The National Council for Therapeutic Recreation Certification, Inc., certifies therapists and assistants. In many cases, therapists are also licensed by the state.

Where Can I Find a Recreation Therapist?

Therapeutic recreation specialists can be associated with your doctor's office, senior center, health club, or city recreation department. They can also practice independently. Ask your doctor to recommend specialists available in your community.

Where Does Recreation Therapy Take Place?

Activities take place in many different settings depending upon the needs of the client. Those settings may include the home, hospitals, senior centers, swimming pools, city parks, health clubs, schools, and shopping malls.

Does Insurance Cover Recreation Therapy?

Many health insurance policies cover recreation therapy, as does Medicare. Check with your insurance company and doctor to determine the requirements for a therapy referral.

Where Can I Get More Information About Therapeutic Recreation?

Write or call:

National Therapeutic Recreation Society NRPA 12th Floor 3101 Park Center Drive Alexandria, VA 22302 Phone: (703) 820-4940

American Therapeutic Recreation Association P.O. Box 15125 Hattiesburg, MI 39402-5215 Phone: 1-800-553-0304

— by Carolyn Norrgard, RN-C, BA, MEd. and
Carol Matheis-Kraft, Ph.D., RN-C, NHA,
for Clinical Reference Systems, Ltd.

Part Three

Assistive and Adaptive Devices Used during Rehabilitation

Chapter 21

What Is an Assistive Device?

An assistive device is an aid used to help a person with an activity, a tool used to make life easier. Assistive devices are used to make changes in the physical environment or to serve as an extension of the person's body. Assistive devices are used for many types of activities of daily living (ADLs). ADLs include bathing, dressing, eating, grooming, transferring (moving in and out of bed, chairs, or cars), and walking.

Some examples of assistive devices are:

- braces and prostheses such as artificial limbs
- wheelchairs, walkers, and canes
- reachers
- knives, forks, and spoons with larger blades or handles
- cooking or eating utensils that can be used with one hand
- bath chairs
- large print books or magnifiers
- computers that are voice activated.

Why Are Assistive Devices Used?

When an assistive device is used, tasks are easier to perform. For example, eating is easier for the person with arthritis when a fork or spoon with an enlarged handle is used.

Clinical Reference Systems, December 1997, page 1998; ā 1997; reprinted with permission.

An assistive device can provide a feeling of security. For example, a walker gives the person better balance and is more comfortable than using crutches to walk.

With assistive devices the person has better function and more independence. For example, assistive devices used for walking enhance the ability to get around.

Why Don't Some People Use Assistive Devices?

There are a variety of reasons why people never start using an assistive device or abandon the use of it. The best reason for not using a device is that it is no longer needed because function has been regained. Other reasons include not having proper instruction in its use, loss of the device, failure of the device to accomplish the desired task, feelings of embarrassment at using an aid, or a poor fit leading to discomfort.

How Do I Find Someone to Help Me Decide Which Device I Should Use?

Local hospitals, home health care agencies, long-term care facilities, and assisted living facilities can refer you to physical and occupational therapists and to orthotists, who specialize in making the devices to best meet an individual's needs. Your doctor can tell you how to locate professionals in your community who sell or rent assistive devices.

How Do I Get an Assistive Device?

Assistive devices for walking, bathing, dressing, and grooming can be purchased at medical equipment stores, rented from community agencies, or supplied by an agency providing home care. Some pharmacies provide assistive devices for rent or sale. Medicare Part B will generally cover 80% of the cost of these devices if they are ordered by a physician. Braces and prostheses are constructed by orthotists skilled in following your doctor's directions. Devices to use for moving in and out of bed, chairs, or cares can be developed with the assistance of therapists.

Physical and occupational therapists:

* can identify the best devices to use
* are skilled in adapting equipment and supplies

- can teach people how to use and care for the assistive device prescribed.

—by Carolyn Norrgard, RN-C, BA, MEd. and Carol Matheis-Kraft, Ph.D., RN-C, NHA, for Clinical Reference Systems, Ltd.

Chapter 22

Understanding Assistive Technology Services

The Rehabilitation Act Amendments of 1986 directed the National Institute on Disability and Rehabilitation Research (NIDRR) to establish Rehabilitation Engineering Centers (RECS) in Connecticut and South Carolina. The mission of the two Rehabilitation Engineering Centers was as follows:

1. Develop, demonstrate, and disseminate innovative models for the delivery of cost-effective assistive technology services to individuals with disabilities.

2. Promote the use of rehabilitation and other technological developments to assist in meeting the employment, education, and independent living needs of individuals with severe disabilities.

3. Assist in identifying and removing barriers confronting individuals with disabilities and the agencies providing the services to them.

4. Coordinate information dissemination and other activities with consumers and providers as well as with relevant NIDRR-sponsored programs.

The purpose of this *Rehab BRIEF* is to report on the work done by these two Rehabilitation Engineering Centers and to look at implications for professionals in the field of rehabilitation.

1993 National Institute on Disability and Rehabilitation Research from *Rehab Brief*, Vol., XV, No. 9, 1993; Issn: 0732-2623.

Connecticut REC

The Connecticut REC performed a search of technology services models already available. Consumers and experts in various areas were consulted throughout the project and participated on advisory boards. After reviewing the state of technology service delivery in Connecticut, the REC concluded that it was most appropriate to assist and augment existing service delivery mechanisms. To accomplish its goals, the REC developed the products summarized below.

"How To" Manuals

The REC developed a series of "how to" manuals for implementing technology services in various settings:

- a preschool day care center
- an independent living center (ILC)
- a post-secondary academic setting
- a public school setting

Each of these handbooks pertains to delivering technology services in a specific environment, and each addresses both philosophical and day-to-day planning issues unique to each environment.

For example, the guidebook *Accessible Day Care Centers* is part of a total training program available for individuals wanting to insure accessibility in children's day care centers. This guide deals with physical accessibility and functional aspects of the environment, such as light/color, scale and proportion of equipment, play areas, how to select and fund adaptive equipment, and toys. The training program gives ideas regarding selection and arrangement of equipment and is a logical and inclusive approach to the adaptation of environments for children with disabilities.

The manual *Establishing Assistive Technology Services in a Center for Independent Living* examines different types of technology services and how they could be integrated into an ILC. Technology services discussed include information and referral, evaluation and recommendation, individual and systems advocacy for technology, technology demonstration center, loan service, funding, sales, repair and maintenance, fabrication and modification, training in the use and maintenance of technology, consumer satisfaction follow-up, and community access consultation. Specific suggestions for how to develop and implement each of the above-listed types of technology programs, through an ILC ensuring integration within the ILC philosophical structure, are included.

Establishing an Adaptive Computer Lab in a Post-Secondary Setting: Ideas and Resources contains developmental suggestions beginning with whom to recruit for a planning committee, how to perform a needs assessment, proposal writing, ideas regarding space selection, and choice and funding of equipment-including borrowing equipment from other departments. Day-to-day operations are outlined, beginning with program development, recruitment, publicizing, the lab, staffing, ongoing funding, program follow-up, and long-range planning. A review of three established computer labs is included along with accessibility guidelines, resources, and sample service delivery forms.

Developing Technology Teams in a Public School Setting, How to Get Started is an excellent "how to" manual. Challenges for the educational system as identified by the REC are "keeping abreast of changing computer technology, successfully matching computer technology with the individual needs of students, integrating the technology into the curriculum and the student's individualized education plan, and providing these services within a limited budget. A technology team can meet these challenges within the school system." The manual defines a technology team, names potential members, discusses the benefits of developing such a team, and indicates how a team might function in a public school setting. Information on getting started and training the team is included.

Software Library

Another goal was to develop a model for statewide databases and electronic networks. The REC determined that a cost-effective method of obtaining software was through the use of adapted public domain software; therefore, a library focusing on adaptive software was developed. The REC has published an excellent catalog of public domain software for the Apple computer. The Apple computer was emphasized because REC research concluded that there is more adapted software available for the Apple than for IBM and compatibles. Over 200 public domain software programs are identified and can be ordered from the National Rehabilitation Information Center (NARIC). In addition, the REC has developed short resource directory for public domain and shareware software. This resource directory is not meant to be all inclusive. Throughout its materials, the REC has included resources, many of them computerized databases on rehabilitation products.

161

Training

As part of its research, the Connecticut REC identified a major gap "between the possibilities offered by technology and the realities of their application or use, based largely on lack of adequate, available information about technology targeted to those who could benefit from such knowledge. Methods of information dissemination continue to be a problem. Typically, information regarding technology is disseminated through a labor-intensive, process oriented, highly idiosyncratic 'apprentice' model not directed to those most affected by technology— the consumer." To bridge this gap, the Connecticut REC developed curriculum guides, train-the-trainer manuals, participant workshops, and graphics/slide displays with the following titles:

- *Rehabilitation Technology: What is It? How Can It Help?*
- *Ecological Assessment*
- *Adaptive Computer Systems*
- *Technology Informational Resources*
- *Accessible Day Care Centers*
- *Activities of Daily Living*
- *Accessible and Adaptable Environments*
- *Communication Aids*
- *Environmental Controls*
- *Switch Selection*
- *Home and Worksite Modifications*
- *Americans With Disabilities Act and Its Impact on the Workplace*

These training materials are meant for volunteers, professionals in the field of rehabilitation, consumers, and others who need training in technology services. They are self-paced for individual use or for use by a group.

South Carolina REC

The Rehabilitation Engineering Center in South Carolina has been named the Center for Rehabilitation Technology Services (CRTS) and is located within the South Carolina Vocational Rehabilitation Department. The CRTS explored various methods of planning statewide assistive technology service delivery, and staff decided that, "in

162

identifying resources needed for the delivery of comprehensive assistive technology services, it has become evident that a single technology services network designed to support the existing delivery programs and agencies would be most desirable." It was determined that the model technology service delivery system would be implemented in stages and would be based on a "hub and node" multilevel service provider network. First, the system would initiate a centralized resource center on rehabilitation technology. Then it would develop regional technology service areas providing clinical services in geographic regions across the state. Finally, it would implement a statewide network of user assistance centers. In these, trained technology resource specialists would help match the needs of individuals with disabilities with appropriate technology solutions and services.

The centralized resource center operated a technology demonstration project for consumers and professionals to learn about and try out assistive aids and devices. This central center also concentrated upon increasing general awareness about assistive technology services and promoted cooperative programming among the various agencies and service delivery programs in the state. It acted as the organizational and administrative hub of the project.

For the second stage of implementation, the state was divided into four regional service areas, which provided information and referral and specialized technology services. Each regional service area was located in a facility that already provided specialized technology services, such as a hospital or rehabilitation agency. Assessment and evaluation were performed through the regional service area. Referrals were made, as necessary, to local vendors for purchase, fabrication, and modification of equipment.

The last aspect of the service delivery system was the implementation of user assistance centers located in nine areas throughout the state. These centers were to form a statewide network of trained resource specialists who would respond to requests from consumers about technology applications and who would recommend potential solutions to selected assistive technology problems. It was decided that the user assistance centers could most appropriately operate within the South Carolina Vocational Rehabilitation Department because offices were already established in geographical areas, which would allow access by most individuals in the state needing services.

In addition to implementing the above described "hub and node" service delivery system, the CRTS developed training and dissemination mechanisms.

Training

The CRTS identified a need for more trained assistive technology specialists. It developed a proposal and curriculum to add assistive technology courses within long-term training programs such as those for occupational and physical therapists and vocational counselors and evaluators at local colleges and universities. In addition, the CRTS developed a curriculum for a telecommunications training program designed for consumers and professionals in order to increase awareness of assistive technology and its applications. Rationale for the telecommunications training was that South Carolina has many individuals who could benefit from the training but who could not attend training in a central area due to travel difficulties and cost.

The CRTS also explored the use of consumer volunteers as trainers and demonstrators of assistive technology. It was suggested that with proper training, consumer volunteers could provide excellent information to others who are considering assistive technology, and would be an asset to the overall system.

Information Dissemination

The CRTS developed a catalog of resource materials for consumers and professionals regarding assistive technology. These materials include reference materials such as symposium reports, a national directory of organizations related to assistive technology, assistive technology planning guides, information support packets about adaptive driving, battery-powered scooters and three-wheelers, and recommendations for the design of a barrier-free home; information resource center listings, including *Home / Worksite Accommodations* and *Barrier-free Design, Computer Applications, Video Tapes on Assistive Technology*; Quick Reference Guides on assistive technology available at the Technology Demonstration Center, such as South Carolina Durable Medical Equipment Dealers, Augmentative Communication Devices, Recreational Aids, Switches, and guides on Apple, Macintosh and IBM-compatible assistive devices and software; Issues and Applications in Assistive Technology, including *Critical Issues Impacting on the Use of Assistive Technology, Who is a Rehabilitation Engineer?*; survey forms; audiovisual materials; and back issues of the newsletter, *Spectrum*.

The project developed a systematic method to integrate assistive technology into the planning process at any point along the continuum of services provided by schools, rehabilitation agencies, or hospitals.

This project also studied the problem of providing assistive technology services to individuals who live in rural areas. Service provision was accomplished by development of the user assistance centers, which are located so that potential clients would be within 60 miles of service. Mobile outreach capabilities were explored, and an 800 telephone number was established for information and referral services.

Throughout this project, great care was taken to utilize existing resources and much time was spent forging alliances, cooperative agreements, and collaborative relationships among already existing service providers.

Funding

Funding was addressed through a symposium on various types of service delivery providers. From this symposium was published *A Guide to Funding Resources for Assistive Technology in South Carolina*, which walks an individual through the process to develop a funding proposal.

Implications

For Consumers: Most people who use technology will be users for life, and the decision of what types of assistive technology will be most useful is an important one. Assistive devices are very personal; what works well for one person may not work for another. Therefore, each potential device needs to be investigated and, if possible, tried before purchase. The programs established by the Connecticut and South Carolina RECs offer organized methods for disseminating information and try-out opportunities for consumers with disabilities in those states. Consumers may wish to advocate for similar programs in other states.

For Rehabilitation Engineers: Identifying, selecting, and funding appropriate assistive technology can be an overwhelming task for a consumer or professional. It is important that information in this area be standardized so that users of the information can make intelligent comparative decisions. Currently, there does not appear to be widespread standardization of information, although a major effort was made by the Connecticut and the South Carolina RECS. Also, quality assurance standards need to be developed for design of devices and production of devices. In addition, performance standards for individuals who recommend devices are needed.

For Practitioners: Practitioners need to have trustworthy referral sources available who have overall knowledge of the field and employ technical specialists to help consumers make appropriate adaptive technology decisions to adequately meet their needs. Both RECs have evaluated needs within their respective states and have produced products that can be replicated. These include training programs, resource libraries, information and referral models, and model programs—located in various settings, allowing consumers to try equipment before purchase.

In addition, system changes are needed by which individuals may obtain technology to enhance activities of daily living, learning, and employment, and to improve access to all aspects of life. System changes can occur only if practitioners document the needs and applicability of assistive technology and submit such information to payors on a regular basis.

For Insurers: Insurers can work together with practitioners to re-evaluate decision-making and paperwork processes so that suitable assistive technology is provided to individuals who can benefit from it. In the past, insurance providers have refused to provide assistive technology on the basis that it is "experimental" when, in fact, it has been successfully used many times and will assist the individual in being productive.

For Educators: These two RECs have demonstrated the need for staff of assistive technology centers to be well trained and qualified. Ensuring quality among personnel may entail certification for assistive technology specialists. A need for standardized training and continuing education to upgrade skills as technology advances is also indicated. The use of well-trained volunteers in conjunction with assistive technology specialists was explored by the RECs and could be further evaluated along with training programs for volunteers.

For Information Brokers: There is a need to manage, update, and disseminate continually the large volume of information available to consumers and people in the field of rehabilitation. The RECs have made starts in this area, but it remains to be determined whether information should be maintained on a state, regional, or national basis or all three.

For VR Agency Administrators: The program in South Carolina shows the apparent importance of developing alliances and cooperative relationships among existing service delivery programs in each state. Most VR agencies already have such relationships with other agencies, service delivery programs and vendors; but reviewing current alliances and developing new cooperative relationships could further ensure efficient and effective delivery of assistive technology services. As part of this process, VR agency administrators can work closely with payors to streamline the funding process and ensure that required technology is provided.

Sources

The following sources are from Connecticut Rehabilitation Engineering Center for Technology Resources, Institute for Human Resource Development:

Cema, R.G. (1990, January). *Rehabilitation technology: What is it? How can it help?*

Cema, R.G. (1990, February). *Ecological assessment.*

Cema, R.G. (1990. May). *Accessible day care centers.*

Cema, R.G. (1991, November). *American With Disabilities Act of 1990: Making it work for you.*

Follow the rainbow, to a golden opportunity: Public domain and shareware software, resource directory. (1991, September).

Follow the rainbow to a golden opportunity: Public domain software catalog, Apple.

Hartmann, K.D., & Navickis, R.M. *Developing technology teams in a public school setting: How to get started.*

McGarvey, D.L. (1992). *Establishing an adaptive computer lab in a post-secondary setting: Ideas and resources.*

Program overview.

Project report, October 1, 1990-September 1991. (Grant No. H133E80500 from the National Institute on Disability and Rehabilitation Research, Office of Special Education and Rehabilitative Services, U.S. Department of Education).

Shreve, M., & Weston, D. (1992). *Establishing assistive technology services in a center for independent living.*

The following sources are from Center for Rehabilitation Technology Services, South Carolina Vocational Rehabilitation Department:

Accessible public transportation in South Carolina. (A report on research and symposium proceedings).

Anderson, S.L., Stevens, J.H., & Trachtman, L.H. (1990, January; updated 1992, April). (Revised and updated by C. Flynn, L. Gaster, & T. Poland). *A guide to funding resources for assistive technology in South Carolina.*

Capilouto, G.J. (1991, October). *Alternative and augmentative communication.* Information Support Packet. No. 4.

Capilouto, G.J. (1991, October). *Manual communication.* Information Support Packet. No. 5.

Capilouto, G.J. (1992, January). *Electronic communication devices.* Information Support Packet. No. 5.

Counselor handbook for the South Carolina Handicapped Services Information System Assistive Technology Information and Referral Network.

D'Andrea, S. (1989, September). *An annotated bibliography on assistive technology service delivery models.*

Gaster, L.S., & Gaster, J.C. (1992, March). *Acceptance of rehabilitation engineering: A survey of healthcare administrators.* Issues and Applications in Assistive Technology.

Gaster, L.S. *Continuous quality improvement in assistive technology.*

Lake, L.D., Trachtman, L.H., Parker, R.W., & Stevens, J.H. (1992, August). *Development of an assistive technology information resource center: A final report.*

Langton, A.J. (1991, July). *Critical issues impacting on the use of assistive technology.* Issues and Applications in Assistive Technology.

Langton, A.J. (1991, July). *Making more effective use of assistive technology in the vocational evaluation process.* Issues and Applications in Assistive Technology.

Langton, A.J. (1991, July). *Utilizing technology in the vocational rehabilitation process.* Issues and Applications in Assistive Technology.

Langton, A.J., Parker, R.W., & Reagin, D.J. (1990, September). *Assistive technology service provider directory.*

Langton, A.J., & Trachtman, L.H. (1989, April). *Assessing the availability of program resources within a state.*

Quick Reference Guides: *Adaptive toys, Aids for daily living, Adaptive office environment, Apple IIGS assistive devices, Apple IIGS software, Augmentative communication devices. Environmental control units, IBM compatible assistive devices, IBM software, Listening aids, Macintosh assistive devices, Macintosh software, Mobility aids, Recreational aids, Rehabilitation Engineering Centers, Seating and positioning. South Carolina durable medical equipment dealers, Switches, and Vision aids.*

South Carolina Assistive Technology Project: Executive summary. (Funding for this project is supported by the National Institute on Disability and Rehabilitation Research, U.S. Department of Education, Grant No. H224AI0031).

Southeast Regional Symposium on Assistive Technology. Proceedings, February 26-28, 1990.

Spectrum. (Newsletter published by the Center for Rehabilitation Technology Services).

Stevens, J.H. (1991, October). *Adaptive Driving Equipment.* Information Support Packet No. 1.

Stevens, J.H. (1991, December). *A barrier-free home.* Information Support Packet No. 3.

Trachtman, L.H. *A review of practices among assistive technology information resource programs.*

Trachtman, L.H. *Who is a rehabilitation engineer?*

Trachtman, L.H., & Brown, J.G., Jr. (1990, September). *Technology resources nationally.* Second Edition.

Trachtman, L.H., & Wiles, D.L. (1990, April). *Access technology: Statewide information and referral for assistive technology services.* Six-month Progress Report.

169

Chapter 23

Adaptive Equipment and Techniques for Home and Family Management Activities

There are four types of intervention strategies that can be used with clients demonstrating deficits in home management or caregiving:

1. Remediating performance areas and performance component deficits.

2. Teaching new methods of task performance to compensate for performance area or performance component deficits.

3. Suggesting environmental modifications to make task performance easier.

4. Educating clients and families to support the above approaches or as a means of preventing future problems.

Each of these approaches will be summarized below.

Remediation

The focus of remediation is to improve or restore the client's performance and performance components to pretreatment levels. This approach is appropriate when a client's condition or diagnosis (e.g., generalized weakness or deconditioning, acute arthritis) or performance component deficits are likely to improve enough to allow pretreatment levels of task proficiency. For example, a practitioner may teach a client with arthritis exercises to improve the client's shoulder ROM so that he or she could perform ideal preparation tasks such as reaching into a cabinet for cooking supplies or dishes. Various parameters need to be considered when grading activities and measuring the effectiveness of treatment using a remediation approach. These parameters include the following:

1. *Physical assistance.* There should be an inverse correlation between the amount of ability demonstrated by the client and the amount of assistance provided by the practitioner or caregiver. That is, as a client displays increased skill in completing a task, the practitioner or caregiver should intervene less frequently.

2. *Supervision and cuing.* Supervision and cuing can include the number of cues given, in addition to the types (written materials, tactile, and verbal) of cues used. Written materials (booklets, handouts, written home programs with illustrations or pictures) can be used to reinforce teaching that has occurred during occupational therapy treatment. Tactile cues can be used effectively to modify or guide client performance (e.g., guiding a stroke client's involved arm to reach for a glass in a cabinet). Lastly, the type of verbal cue can affect client performance. While on a community outing to the grocery store, a direct cue provides the client with a specific instruction, such as: "The spaghetti is here," as the practitioner points to the aisle where spaghetti is located. An indirect cue provides assistance to the client in a less directive manner, such as: "Can you find the foods listed on your grocery list?"

3. *Task demands.* Task demands (i.e., the amount of cognitive and physical skill required to perform the task) affect quality of client performance. in selecting the type of task, consider the complexity of performance skills demanded by the task. As a general rule, with neurologically involved clients, it is better to select a task with low motor and high cognitive demands or with high motor and low cognitive demands (Chapparo, 1979), and then progress to increasing levels of both. As an example, for a client with stroke, participating in a community outing is an activity that requires high cognitive demand. In addition, the client's mobility may become compromised. Thus, the client may ambulate for a short amount of time, but as the quality of the client's gait decreases, the

client may need to complete the community outing in a wheel-chair (high cognitive, low motor demand).

4. *Amount of task.* Increasing the number of steps or tasks that a client needs to complete can be indicative of increased proficiency. During a community outing, a client may be able to progress from completing one errand in 1 hour to completing three errands in 1 hour.

5. *Type of task.* Cognitive tasks can be graded from routine and familiar to unfamiliar or new. As an example, it is less demanding for a client to cook a familiar recipe from memory than to follow a new recipe from a cookbook. A task organized by the client without assistance from the practitioner is a high level of performance.

6. *Environment.* Environment plays a role in task performance. A familiar environment (e.g., kitchen at home) is less demanding than a new environment (e.g., clinic kitchen). In addition, the type of stimulation can vary from a quiet, nondistracting environment, such as a room with no noise or other people, to a distracting, busy environment, such as the community. For clients in wheelchairs, lack of wheelchair accessibility can prohibit the client's ability to access services (banks, restaurant, stores) in the community.

By altering the various parameters in treatment, an activity can be upgraded or downgraded to provide a difficult, but not overwhelming, challenge that results in a successful experience for the client.

Compensation

The compensation approach focuses on using remaining abilities to achieve the highest level of functioning possible in the areas of home and family management. If the client cannot perform these tasks in the usual manner, then adapted techniques or equipment are used to maximize client abilities. This strategy can be used (1) when a client's condition is temporary, such as for hip replacement; (2) when precautions need to be taken; (3) when the condition is not amenable to remediation; or (4) when task speed and proficiency are greatly improved by use of adaptive equipment or adaptive techniques. Use of adaptive techniques is preferable to use of equipment because techniques allow the client more flexibility. Use of adaptive equipment is less preferable because of the cost incurred for equipment purchase and maintenance and the inconvenience of having to transport the equipment for task performance. Table 23.1 outlines specific adaptive equipment and techniques that can be used for various impairments (Hopkins & Smith, 1993; Klinger, 1978; Pedretti, 1996; Trombly, 1989).

Energy conservation and work simplification techniques can help clients perform home management and caregiving tasks in spite of the mobility and endurance problems imposed by many disabilities (American Heart Association, date unknown; Hopkins & Smith, 1993; Pedretti, 1996; Rehabilitation Institute of Chicago (RIC), 1988; Trombly, 1989). These techniques require that the practitioner and client address the following points:

1. Determine what tasks need to be improved; that is, according to the client, what tasks take too long, cause fatigue, or take too much energy.

2. List all the steps of the task, including setup, performance, and cleanup.

3. Analyze the task.

    a. Why is the task necessary?
    b. What is the purpose of the task?
    c. When and where should it be done?
    d. What is the best way for the client to accomplish it?

4. Develop a new method of performing the task. Consider eliminating unnecessary steps, combining motions and activities, rearranging the sequence of the steps, and simplifying the details of the task by taking the following steps:

    a. Use correct work height to reduce fatigue and promote good posture. Correct work height in standing should be 2 inches below the bent elbow; in sitting, client should avoid positions that require lifting the shoulders or "winging out" the elbows.

    b. Preposition supplies and equipment in work areas. Clear area of unnecessary items. As an example, to pay bills, obtain needed supplies, such as calculator, bills, and stamps, before beginning task.

    c. Organize the work center. Having necessary supplies and equipment increases productivity with less effort. In the kitchen, place the can opener near the canned goods. Place the most frequently used items within easy reach on counters or shelves immediately above or below counter height.

d. Use laborsaving devices. This includes using wheels for transport; in the kitchen, using electric appliances, such as an electric mixer and food processor; for outdoors, using an electric garage door opener and motorized lawn mower. Transport heavy objects using wheels.

e. Fatigue can result in poor body mechanics and reduced safety awareness. Regular rest breaks should be incorporated into the client's schedule. The client should alternate light and heavy tasks throughout the day and week. Heavy work tasks, such as cleaning the oven, stripping and waxing floors, or doing yard work, should be delegated to another family member or done by a professional cleaning service.

f. Use proper body mechanics. This includes use of a wide base of support, using both sides of the body and keeping objects close to the body, facing objects when reaching or lifting to avoid twisting, pushing rather than pulling objects, and alternating positions and motions to avoid fatigue.

5. Implement new methods.

Environmental Modifications

Environmental modifications are considered a compensatory strategy. Compared with remediation and compensation, in which the practitioner directly influences client functioning, environmental modification is a means of indirectly maximizing client function. Modifications can range from extensive home modifications to make a home wheelchair accessible, to low-cost strategies, such as removing obstacles to make a household safer for an older person who has impaired vision and mobility.

Education of Client and Family Members

The final type of occupational therapy intervention strategy is client and family education. This is a key component to the occupational therapy treatment plan because the approaches of remediation, compensation, and prevention involve learning new strategies and, more importantly, incorporating these strategies into client and family habits and lifestyles. In some circumstances, the practitioner may provide education to the family in addition to client education or in place of client education. The following issues are central to effective client and family education (Bowling, 1981; Kautzman, 1991):

1. *Have a clear plan about the purpose of the teaching session.* An observable goal for teaching can assist both the practitioner and client regarding expectations and anticipated outcome. Based on client and family motivation, cognitive status, and skill level that need to be achieved, and time availability for the teaching and learning process, the expected outcomes or goals may vary. The three levels of goals include knowledge, application, and problem solving. At the level of knowledge, a client is asked to recall basic facts presented by the practitioner. For example, the practitioner may ask a client to name the five techniques used for good body mechanics. At the application level, the client and family are shown ways of incorporating this information into home management. The practitioner may demonstrate how to use body mechanics when retrieving food from the oven during performance of meal preparation and then ask the client to incorporate the same strategy while performing the task. At the level of problem solving, the client is asked to use information in new situations that have not been demonstrated by the practitioner. For example, the practitioner may ask the client to demonstrate how to use good body mechanics when shoveling snow.

2. *The presentation of information needs to be appropriate to the clients' educational and emotional levels.* The choice of terminology used with a client who has had a few years of formal education should vary from that used with a client who has a college education. Client readiness to receive information will vary. The client may be overwhelmed with life changes caused by the disability and unable to concentrate on issues that the practitioner feels needs to be addressed. Therefore, for a task that a client may not be concerned with, but that will be needed at home, the inpatient practitioner may try to increase client awareness by introducing appropriate adaptive equipment. Once the client has returned home, the motivation to perform in this area may increase. Then the outpatient practitioner

can promote client application and problem solving in the outpatient occupational therapy program.

3. *Instructions must be clear.* Clear instructions increase the possibility of client carryover. For example, instead of telling a client to use proper body mechanics for all activities, it is preferable and more realistic to begin with having the client identify one or two activities that require these techniques. The client may need assistance to do this. Another strategy to increase carryover is to explain the rationale for the therapy recommendations.

4. *Ask open-ended questions to ensure client understanding.* For example: Why is it important for you to incorporate proper body mechanics into your day-to-day activities?

5. *Use client response to determine the amount of information presented during a session.* If the client's attention is waning or if the client's learning ability is decreased, termination of the teaching session is recommended. If the amount of information is extensive, it may be preferable to present it over several sessions. Taking the added time to ensure client competence in performance is time well spent.

6. *Promote the highest level of learning possible, preferably the problem-solving level.* Involve the clients by asking questions about how information presented might affect their lifestyles. For example, a practitioner may ask of an arthritic client: "Which joint protection techniques do you think you would use at home? How could you use these techniques while cooking?" It is preferable to follow this up with client demonstration to ensure that the client has integrated the information into pertinent tasks.

7. *Illustrate or demonstrate the points being taught.* Use of such aids as demonstration, pictures, videotapes, and handouts reinforces teaching and helps the client and family remember the information presented. A study of client doctor visits found that only half of the information covered was remembered by the client (Ley, 1972). Some of the ways of reinforcing teaching include repeating information throughout the session and allowing adequate time for practice by the client or family members to ensure that they are comfortable with and capable of using the information outside the therapy situation.

If the client or family member cannot gain adequate competency or perform the task in a safe manner, then other options such as a paid caregiver or identifying community support (e.g., home health aide) need to be considered.

Table 23.1. Adaptive Equipment and Techniques for Home and Family Management Activities

Impairment:
One upper-extremity or body side impairment

Common Diagnoses Resulting in This Impairment:
Hemiplegia (cerebrovascular accident (CVA) or head injury), unilateral trauma or amputation, temporary conditions such as burns and peripheral neuropathy.

Rationale for Using Compensatory Strategies:
To allow for safe, one-handed performance; to stabilize objects for task completion; with hemiplegia, to compensate for loss of balance and mobility.

ADL Area: Meal Preparation and Cleanup

Adaptive Equipment

To stabilize objects consider use of:

- Adapted cutting board with stainless steel or aluminum nails for cutting or peeling. Raised comers on the board can stabilize broad to spread ingredients or make a sandwich.
- Sponge dishes Dycem™ or suction devices to stabilize bowls or dishes during food preparation.
- Pot stabilizer.

To allow for safe, one-handed performance:

- Adapted jar openers.
- Electric appliances such as food processor and hand mixer save time and energy. Note: client safety and judgment need to be considered when electrical appliances are considered.
- Rocker knife.
- Whisk to mix food.

To compensate for decreased standing tolerance and mobility, consider use of:

- Utility cart to transport objects.
- If cooking is done at wheelchair level or seated, use angled mirror over the stove to watch food on the stove.

For cleanup, consider use of:

- Handhold spray for rinsing dishes.
- Rubber mat at bottom of sink to reduce breakage.
- Suction-type brush to clean glassware.

Adaptive Techniques

If balance is affected, it is recommended that the task be done in a seated position.

- Objects can be stabilized by using the knees.
- Pots and pans can be slid across counters, rather than lifted.
- To open a jar, place it in a drawer, then lean against it to stabilize it before opening.
- Scissors can be used to open plastic bags.
- Milk cartons can be opened by using the prolonged portion of a fork.
- An egg can be cracked by holding it in the palm of the hand, hitting the egg against the edge of the bowl, and separating the egg shell with the index and middle fingers.

For clean-up:

- Soak and air-dry dishes for easier clean-up.

ADL Area: Clothing management (laundry, Ironing, clothing repair)

Adaptive Equipment

Laundry can be transported to and from and dryer using a wheeled cart

ADL Area: Housecleaning

Adaptive Equipment

- A tank-type vacuum permits the client to sit and reach areas to be cleaned up.
- Long-reach duster.
- Long-handled dustpan and brush.
- Self-wringing mop.

Adaptive Techniques

- Incorporate energy conservation by making bed completely at each comer before progressing to the next comer. No-wax floors are easier to care for.
- If balance and ambulation problems are present, some floor care can be managed from a seated position.

ADL Area: Child Care

Adaptive Equipment

For feeding use:
- High chairs with one-handed tray release mechanism.
- Electric baby dish keeps food warm during the meal.
- Tongs can be used to remove baby food from heated water.
- Use screw top, rather than plastic liner bottles.
- If breastfeeding, pillows or commercially available carriers can be used to position baby.

For bathing.
- Strap the baby into a suction-based bath seat.

For dressing:
- Use Velcro strap on dressing table to reduce squirming.
- Use disposable diapers with tab closures for cloth diapers, use diaper covers with Velcro covers.

For transporting child:
- Try various child carriers (front, side, and back types available).
- Use a bassinet on wheels, a stroller, or a wagon to transport child from room to room.

Adaptive Techniques

For feeding:

- Prop the infant on pillows, in an infant seat, or against arm or an upholstered chair. If breastfeeding, try various positions to accommodate affected side (sidelying).
- Premixed formula can eliminate the need for measuring.
- Stabilize the bottle inside a coffee cup and use funnel to pour into bottle.

Impairment:
Reduced upper-extremity range of motion and strength

Common Diagnoses Resulting in This Impairment:
Quadriplegia, burns, arthritis, upper-extremity amputation, multiple sclerosis, amyotrophic lateral sclerosis, orthopedic and other traumatic injuries.

Rationale for Using Compensatory Strategies:
To compensate for lack of reach or hand grip; to compensate for lack of strength or tolerance for prolonged activity; to allow gravity to assist; to compensate for decreased balance.

ADL Area: Meal preparation and cleanup

Adaptive Equipment

Consider the use of:
- Adapted jar opener.
- Foam or built-up handles on utensils.
- Universal cuff to hold utensils to compensate for reduced grip.
- Long-handled reacher to obtain right-weight objects from overhead or low places.
- Wheeled cart to transport objects.
- Adapted cutting board.
- Loop handles can be added to utensils to substitute for reduced grasp.
- If using a walker, a walker basket can help transport objects.

For marketing:

- Marketing by phone or mail is recommended because many objects may be out of reach in store.

Adaptive Techniques

- joint protective measures for rheumatoid arthritis.
- Position electrical appliances within easy reach. This helps to conserve energy.
- To conserve energy, work at a seated position.
- Use teeth to open containers.
- Purchase convenience foods to eliminate food preparation.
- Tenodesis action (wrist extension and finger flexion; wrist flexion and finger extension) can be used to pick up lightweight objects.
- Use a fork to open milk cartons.
- Use lightweight pots, pans, and utensils.

ADL Area: Housecleaning

Adaptive Equipment

- Long-handled reacher allows objects be picked up from the floor.
- Long-handled sponge to clean bath tub.
- Self-wringing mop.
- Use lightweight tools such as sponge mops and brooms for floor care.

Adaptive Techniques

- Use aerosol cleaners to dissolve dirt before cleaning surfaces.
- When making the bed, do not tuck sheets in.

ADL Area: Laundry

Adaptive Equipment

- If client is ambulatory, the preference is for a top-loading washer to avoid the need to bend.
- Push-button controls on the washer and dryer are easier to use than knobs. If knobs are present. they may need to be adapted.

- If client chooses to iron, set iron at a low temperature setting. An asbestos pad can be placed at the end of the ironing board to eliminate the need to stand iron up after each ironing stroke.

Adaptive Techniques

- Use premeasured packages of soap or bleach to avoid handling large containers. It may be more economical to buy larger containers and have someone else measure soap or bleach into single packets.

Use energy conservation:

- Place hangers near dryer to hang permanent press items as they come out of the dryer. Remain seated to do ironing.

ADL Area: Child Care

Adaptive Equipment

- If client lacks mobility to get up and down from the floor, then a crib with a swing open side allows the parent in a wheelchair to wheel close to the baby.

For feeding.

- Feeding can be done with a child in an infant seat or propped up on pillows.
- An electric baby dish can be placed in a convenient area to keep food warm throughout the meal.
- Formula can be prepared by another family member and placed in bottles for use during the day.

For dressing:

- Clothing should be large with closures that are easily handled.
- Disposable diapers with tabs are easily manipulated.

Adaptive Techniques

Use energy conservation:

- Have client do the more enjoyable tasks, delegate other tasks to a helper.

The safest place to handle an infant is on the floor. All tasks, including sponge bathing, feeding and playing, can be done on the floor.

- A method to obtain assistance in an emergency needs to be determined.
- Dressing and diapering can be done on a table or desk that allows for wheelchair access.

Impairment:
Incoordination of upper extremities

Common Diagnoses Resulting in This Impairment:
Head injury, cerebral palsy, CVA, multiple sclerosis, tumors, other neurological conditions

Rationale for Using Compensatory Strategies:
To stabilize proximal portion of limbs; to reduce movements distally by using weight; to stabilize objects for task completion; to provide an environment in which client is safe and proficient; to avoid breakage or accidents with sharp utensils or hot food or equipment.

ADL Area: Meal Preparation and Cleanup

Adaptive Equipment

- Use heavy cookware, ironstone dishes to aid with distal stabilization.
- Use pots and casseroles with double handles to provide greater stability.
- Weighted wrist cuffs may reduce tremors.
- Use nonslip materials such as Dycem™ to provide stability.
- Use adapted cutting board to stabilize food while cutting.
- A serrated knife is less likely to slip than a straight-edged knife.
- Using a frying basket to cook foods, such as vegetables, makes for safe removal and reduces the chance of burns.
- Free-standing appliances, electric skillet, and countertop mixer, are safer than transferring objects out of oven or using handheld mixer.
- Use a milk carton holder with handles to pour milk.

- A stove with front controls is preferred so the client does not need to reach over hot pots to the back of the stove.
- A wheeled cart that is weighted is one alternative for transporting food.
- Place a rubber mat or sponge cloth at the bottom of the sink to cushion fall of dishes.

Adaptive Technique

- During food preparation, such as cutting and peeling, stabilize arms proximally to reduce tremors.
- Start the stove after the food has been placed on the burner.
- Sliding food and dishes over a counter is preferable to lifting to transport food item.
- To avoid breakage, soak dishes, rinse with hand sprayer and drip dry—eliminate dish handling.

ADL Area: Housecleaning

Adaptive Equipment

- Heavier work tools are useful. A dust mitt Is easier to handle than gripping a duster.
- Fitted sheets on a bed are recommended.

Adaptive Technique

- Eliminate or store excess household decorations to reduce dusting.

ADL Area: Laundry

Adaptive Equipment

- Premeasured soap and bleach eliminates spills that can occur during measuring.
- Eliminate ironing through selection of no-iron clothing and materials.

ADL Area: Child Care

Adaptive Equipment

- Use a wide safety strap on dressing table or use a bed.
- Use disposable, tape-tab diapers.
- Use Velcro closures for infant clothing.
- Feeding with a spoon is recommended only if incoordination is mild.
- Transporting child: Consider infant carrier or use of bassinet on wheels, stroller, or wagon.

Adaptive Techniques

With mild incoordination:

- Use stabilizing measure such as holding upper arms close to body and sitting while working.
- It is safer to work on the floor while caring for the infant.

Impairment:
Mobility impairment without upper-extremity involvement

Common Diagnoses Resulting in This Impairment:
Paraplegia, osteoarthritis, lower-extremity amputation, bums, leg and knee fractures and replacement

Rationale for Using Compensatory Strategies:
Mobility may be provided by a wheelchair. Wheelchair accessibility includes consideration of work heights, maneuverability, and access to storage, equipment, and supplies.
Other types of mobility devices (walker, crutches) may require increased endurance.

ADL Area: Meal Preparation and Cleanup

Adaptive Equipment

- Transport items using a wheelchair laptray. The laptray can be used as a work surface to protect lap from hot pans.
- Stove controls should be in the front of the stove.
- Use an angled mirror to see the contents of pots.

Adaptive Techniques

- Remove cabinet doors to eliminate need to maneuver around them.

- Place frequently used items on easy-to-reach shelves, above and below countertop level. Increase height of wheelchair to allow use of standard height countertops.

ADL Area: Laundry

Adaptive Equipment

- Use front-loading washer and dryer.

ADL Area: Housekeeping

Adaptive Equipment

- Use self-propelled lightweight vacuums.

ADL Area: Child Care

Adaptive Equipment

For feeding:

- Use plastic baby battles with liners to eliminate the need to sterilize bottles.
- Position the baby in an infant seat. The seat can be held or placed on a table.
- For highchairs, select a chair with a safety belt and a swing-away tray with one-hand release.

For a playpen:

- Use an adjustable-height, portable crib with a hinged door for easy access.

For lifting, carrying, and transporting:

- A converted, lightweight car bed with straps sewn on the side of the bed can be secured to the wheelchair armrests.
- With an older child (4 to 5 months old), touch-fastener seat belt can be attached to the wheelchair.
- Select stroller with the following features: single handle to allow for one-handed steering, brakes, and opening and closing of stroller should be managed easily.

- Attach a safety strap from handle of stroller to waist of parent to prevent stroller from pulling away on an incline.

Adaptive Techniques

Safety consideration for all individuals:

- Use a phrase or certain voice consistently.
- Uses that can be associated with disciplinary action (i.e., "touch my chair" if the child is running ahead).
- Have children play in rooms that have been child-proofed and where access to the parent is not an issue (i.e., child cannot run behind a couch).

Chapter 24

Informed Consumer Guide to Wheelchair Selection

Introduction

A wheelchair can be a wonderful liberator. Someone with a spinal cord injury can get around as quickly in a wheelchair as someone else can walking. For an older person with arthritis, a wheelchair can provide access to the world outside the home. For an active sportsperson, a wheelchair is the means to participate in marathons, basketball, and tennis.

In some respects, a wheelchair is much like an automobile or a pair of shoes. It provides the interface between the body and the world around it. Like shoes, a proper fit is essential if a person is to maximize her/his potential and feel comfortable moving around in the world; like a car, design factors should take into account one's personal needs and interests.

Selecting the appropriate chair, however—particularly for a first-time wheelchair user—can be a bewildering task, due to the variety of options available. The purpose of this guide is to provide the reader with general information about wheelchairs, and to describe the major kinds of wheeled mobility options in the marketplace today. Also included are suggested reading materials that can be used to help determine what kind of wheelchair most accurately meets one's individual needs. Finally, if you are newly injured, you are probably working with an occupational therapist who may have personal experience with specific wheelchairs. This kind of professional knowledge and experience can also be very helpful in assisting you to select the best chair for you.

Types of Wheelchairs

Wheelchairs come in many sizes, shapes, and varieties to meet the diverse needs of a multitude of users with differing levels of physical function and varying interests. People with considerable upper body strength often prefer to use a wheelchair propelled by arm strength, or what is called a manual wheelchair. Some people are unable to propel a wheelchair with their own arm strength and may prefer—or require—a wheelchair powered by batteries. Powered wheelchairs come in several basic styles: The traditional style is similar in appearance to the standard manual wheelchair and has been reinforced to tolerate the added weight of the power and control systems, the plat-form-model powered chair which consists of a seating platform atop a powered base, a round-based powered chair (Hoveround) which emerged on the market in 1993, and three- and four-wheeled scooters.

Manual Wheelchairs

Lightweight Chairs

Everyday Lightweights. The most commonly used everyday wheelchair for active chair users is a lightweight manual wheelchair. *Sports 'n Spokes*, a publication dedicated to sports and recreation for wheelers, conducts an annual survey of lightweight wheelchairs. In its 1993 survey, twenty everyday wheelchairs were listed, with weights varying from a low of 12 pounds to a high of 45 pounds (including wheels), depending upon the type of material used for the frame and the configuration of the chair. Some frames alone now weigh as little as under five pounds!

The options available to today's lightweight wheelchair user are many, allowing one to select a wheelchair that meets the individual's functional needs and personal design preferences. Further information is provided under the heading, "The Selection Process."

Sports Lightweights. Lightweight wheelchairs originally were developed and sold for use in sports, such as basketball, tennis, and road racing. In fact, earlier references to lightweight wheelchairs refer to such chairs as "sports wheelchairs." As wheelchair users were exposed to the lighter-weight chairs, however, they began to realize the "sports" chairs took less energy to propel and were therefore easier to use on an everyday basis, as well.

Sports wheelchairs have continued to become more specialized as wheelchair athletes have become more sophisticated and successful over the years. Most serious athletes have chairs that they use specifically for sports, and separate chairs to use for everyday mobility. Chairs designed specifically for road racing, for example, have only three wheels, with the front wheel extended out from the body to allow for maximum use of aerodynamics. Sports chairs designed for use by tennis players, basketball players, and other athletes, however, have become the everyday wheelchair of choice for many non-athletic wheelchair users who simply prefer the sportier look and comparatively low weight of a sports chair. Sports chairs listed in the *Sports 'n Spokes* Lightweight Wheelchair Survey vary from 14 to 25 pounds including wheels.

Standard Chairs

The most common wheelchair in use prior to the late 1980's was a standard adult wheelchair, a heavy, difficult to maneuver chair, generally available only in an institutional-looking metallic finish. Most standard wheelchairs require a considerable amount of energy to propel, thus making them less practical than a lightweight wheelchair for everyday use for most people.

Specialty Chairs

Because the needs of wheelchair users vary considerably, some individuals require specialized wheelchair designs developed to address their particular needs. People who have had their lower limbs amputated, for example, have a different center of gravity than someone who has a spinal cord injury. A person who has had a stroke may have use of only one arm, and therefore may be unable to propel a wheelchair by turning the wheels on both sides of the chair. A person of large stature may require an oversized chair or one that has been reinforced to handle the additional weight of the individual. Consequently, there are specialized wheelchair configurations available to meet almost any individual need.

Nursing Home/Institutional Wheelchairs

Nursing home residents often require assistance in mobility. If a nursing home resident is generally capable of independent mobility, s/he may wish to use a wheelchair that will allow the fullest measure of independence to be maintained. Thus, it would be important to select a relatively lightweight and easy to use chair. The selection criteria for the chair would be similar to that used in choosing a chair for a more active user.

Many nursing home residents, however, require considerable assistance with activities of daily living, including mobility. Wheelchairs designed for institutional use generally are much less expensive than chairs for active users. Consequently, it often is more cost effective to use an inexpensive chair designed for institutional use if the individual is unable to benefit from the independence afforded by a more expensive wheelchair designed for active, independent wheelchair users.

For a more detailed discussion of the various types of manual wheelchairs, see ABLEDATA Fact Sheet, No. 23 Manual Wheelchairs.

Child/Junior Chairs

Because their bodies are growing and changing, choosing chairs for children and adolescents requires consideration of factors not a part of the adult wheelchair selection process. One of these is the frequency with which a chair must be changed or replaced. Because of the high cost of replacing a chair, and because insurance providers often place limitations on the frequency of chair replacement, purchasing a new chair each year can be financially prohibitive, if not impossible. Growth chairs or chairs with growth kits offer an alternative by allowing adjustments to be made in the existing chair to accommodate a growing child. This may include utilizing replaceable components or designing the chair with features that can be converted from a smaller size to a larger size.

Manufacturers are also responding to the needs of children in having chairs that fit more easily into their environment and social situations. This may be accomplished with a more streamlined appearance and/or a selection of upholstery and/or frame colors. (See also ABLEDATA Fact Sheet No. 22, Wheelchairs for Children.)

Powered Wheelchairs

People who use powered wheelchairs generally have limited strength in their arms, and thus need to use an external power source to enable them to get around. Powered wheelchairs use either gel cell or wet cell batteries that must be re-charged on a regular basis. A powered wheelchair usually is significantly heavier than a manual wheelchair to accommodate both the weight of the battery and the weight of additional adaptive equipment, such as body supports or respiratory equipment.

Today's powered wheelchairs tend to follow one of several design trends. The most traditional design for a powered wheelchair is that of a reinforced standard-looking wheelchair frame with a battery mounted under or behind the seat. Another design being used by some manufacturers today is a more stylized seating unit on a pedestal mounted atop a power platform. A new design, introduced in 1993, utilizes a round platform base (Hoveround) with a seating system affixed to it. Finally, several manufacturers offer power pack attachments which allow manual wheelchairs to be converted to powered chairs. (For more detailed information, see ABLEDATA Fact Sheet, No. 24 Powered Wheelchairs.)

Scooters

An alternative to either a manual or powered wheelchair is a scooter, or three- or four-wheeled cart. Some people like scooters because they prefer to use a form of mobility that does not look like a wheelchair. Others use them because they provide power but often are not as expensive as regular four-wheeled power wheelchairs. Scooters also have a narrower wheelbase and overall profile than many wheelchairs, making them more maneuverable.

A scooter operates much like a golf cart. The user sits in a chair-style seat normally contoured to fit the body. The scooter is propelled through use of a steering mechanism located in front of the user, as if s/he were riding a bicycle. (See ABLEDATA Fact Sheet, No. 5 Powered Scooters.)

The Selection Process

The wheelchair selection process includes several distinct steps:

1. Deciding the level of assistance necessary.

2. Determining how the wheelchair will be used.

3. Selecting the appropriate chair that meets all of the needs outlined in the first two steps.

Anyone choosing a wheelchair for the first time should consider working closely with a wheelchair prescriber, such as an occupational or physical therapist, to help determining how much assistance the wheelchair should provide. While some individuals with quadriplegia, for example, can only use powered wheelchairs, others may find that they are able to use a manual wheelchair or a powered scooter. These alternatives generally are less expensive and may more appropriately fit the individual's lifestyle.

It also is important to determine how the wheelchair will be used. Will it be used indoors, outdoors, and during transport in a van or car? Some people keep a manual wheelchair in their homes, but travel to work or other outside activities in a powered scooter. For many manual wheelchair users, the ability to fold a wheelchair or take it apart easily for travelling in a car is of utmost importance.

Once an individual's needs have been determined, the next step is to choose the "right" chair. New wheelchair users may wish to talk with current chair users about their likes and dislikes. There is nothing like practical experience to provide feedback on specific features that may be desirable, as well as those that should be avoided. Prescribers may also be another source of information, since they often receive feedback from previous clients.

Finally, many written resources on wheelchairs are now available (see below), and ABLEDATA, the premier assistive technology information database, provides up-to-date information on products for people with disabilities, and is a good source for information on specific wheelchairs.

Funding Sources

Funding for wheelchairs or other assistive devices is dependent upon an individual's eligibility for medical, social services, income support or vocational assistance from any of a number of different resources. ABLEDATA Fact Sheet No. 14 Funding Assistive Technology is available to answer questions about funding resources.

Wheelchair Standards

The American National Standards Institute (ANSI) recently approved a complete set of standards for wheelchairs. These standards consist of standard methods of disclosing information (example: How do you measure the width of a seat? Inside to inside of each tube, or width of a cushion, or what?); and standard test methods to test a chair's strength, "tip-ability," turning radius, and so forth.

Copies of the standards themselves are available from RESNA [Rehabilitation Engineering and Assistive Technology Society of North America] for $180 for the complete set. The standards consist of eighteen separate parts, such as standards for brakes, test methods to determine the stability of a wheelchair, standard methods to measure wheelchairs, and so forth. These probably would be of interest only to manufacturers and others who are going to conduct testing themselves, as they are very technical documents. However, there are some good summary documents available that describe the standards for therapists and laypeople.

Invacare, one of the largest wheelchair manufacturers in the United States today, recently began advertising that its wheelchairs had been tested according to these standards. It is expected that other manufacturers also will begin using the standards for testing—and advertising this fact to the public—as consumers and therapists begin to ask for this information. Once standards information becomes more readily available, it can be used by consumers and prescribers to make more informed purchasing decisions.

Beginning at the Beginning . . .

This ABLEDATA "Informed Consumers Guide" is designed as an introduction to the wheelchair selection process. ABLEDATA also offers more detailed information on the specific types of wheelchairs mentioned here in its fact sheets on Powered Wheelchairs, Manual Wheelchairs, Sports Wheelchairs, and Scooters. Individual copies of the Fact Sheets are available from ABLEDATA.

The ABLEDATA database of assistive technology provides information about and descriptions of more than 22,000 products for people with disabilities. Included are all types of wheelchairs currently available in the United States, as well as information about manufacturers and distributors.

Computer users may also search the database themselves and download the search results using the ABLE INFORM computer bulletin board service. ABLE INFORM can be accessed via modem at 301/589-3563 (8-1-n), or through Internet. There is no charge for this service except long-distance telephone charges for calls placed from outside the metropolitan Washington, D.C. area.

Resources and Related Reading

Because of the expanding number of options available, several resources have been developed to assist either an individual select his/her own wheelchair, or to assist a health care provider in selecting the appropriate wheelchair for a client or patient.

How to Select and Use Manual Wheelchairs
A. Bennett Wilson, Rehabilitation Press, 1993. Available from:

Rehabilitation Press
P.O. Box 380
Topping, VA 23169.

Selection of the most appropriate wheelchair and seating system can be simplified if one has information about factors to consider and products on the market. This guide helps new wheelchair users select a wheelchair with the right dimensions and seating system depending upon the degree of disability, goals of the user, and the environment in which the chair will be used. It also provides information about proper use and maintenance of wheelchairs.

Wheelchairs: A Prescription Guide
A. Bennett Wilson and Samuel R. McFarland, Rehabilitation Press, 1986. Available from:

Rehabilitation Press
P.O. Box 380
Topping, VA 23169

This small, straightforward publication addresses in clear language the factors to be considered by people responsible for prescribing wheelchairs. It is filled with illustrations and practical suggestions for making prescription decisions. Although intended primarily for prescribers, the information contained in this guide would be of value to an individual selecting a wheelchair for personal use. The information about manufacturers and product availability is slightly dated because of the swift advances that occurred in the wheelchair industry, but the basic concepts presented remain useful, and up-to-date manufacturer information can be obtained through an ABLEDATA product search.

Choosing a Wheelchair System
Department of Veterans Affairs, 1990. Available from:

Department of Veterans Affairs
Veterans Health Services and Research Administration
Washington, DC 20420.

Ask for the Clinical Supplement #2, Journal of Rehabilitation Research and Development, March 1990.

Price: FREE.

The U.S. Department of Veterans Affairs Rehabilitation Research and Development Service (Rehab R&D) several years ago issued a Clinical Supplement entitled "Choosing a Wheelchair System." This resource was written by people with disabilities who have selected wheelchairs for many years; health care providers who prescribe wheelchairs; and researchers/engineers who participate in the development of new wheelchair designs.

RESNA Video. Available from:

RESNA Third-Party Payor Program
1700 N. Moore Street, Suite 1540
Arlington, VA 22209
703-524-6686

RESNA, an association for the advancement of assistive technology, recently published a series of videotapes directed primarily toward organizations or individuals that provide funding for assistive technology. One of the videos in this series, a thirty minute tape entitled Manual Mobility: Finding the Right Wheels, discusses the options to be considered for someone purchasing a manual wheelchair.

Annual Wheelchair Surveys. Available from:

PVA Publications
2111 East Highland Avenue, Suite 180
Phoenix, AZ 85016-4702
602-224-0500

Price: Call for price and availability

Sports 'n Spokes, a bi-monthly publication for active wheelchair users, publishes an Annual Survey of Lightweight Wheelchairs in their March/April issue each year. The most recent survey (March/April 1994) includes a description of how wheelchairs are tested in order to comply with recently-issued American National Standards Institute (ANSI) standards. Also included are illustrations of a variety of everyday, sports, and junior-sized lightweight wheelchairs from different manufacturers; comparative sizing information; warranty information; delivery time; and retail price. Back issues of the magazine sometimes are available; so are reprints of specific articles.

Homecare Magazine and Team Rehab Reports also publish an annual **"Wheelchair Focus"** that provides similar comparative information. It is published once a year (also in the spring) and can be ordered through Miramar Publishing. Available from:

Miramar Publishing
6133 Bristol Parkway
P.O. Box 3640
Culver City, CA 90231-3640
800-543-4116 or 213-337-1041

Price: Call for price and availability

This Consumer Guide was researched and written by Lynn Bryant and Katherine Belknap, and was produced by ABLEDATA. ABLEDATA is funded by the National Institute on Disability and Rehabilitation Research (NIDRR), with contract number HN-92026001. It is operated by Macro International Inc.

Chapter 25

Technical Considerations in the Selection and Performance of Walkers

The walker is a mobility aid that provides a portable base of support. People of all ages use different kinds of walkers for a variety of reasons. With the correct walker, many people stroll along at the same pace as their companion. Today, walkers are available in a variety of styles and colors and have numerous accessories. It is the purpose of this article to describe the various types and models of walkers and accessories that are available. Our goal is not to recommend or rate the walkers but to help you find the right walker. The ultimate selection of a walker will depend on a cooperative effort between the physiatrist, physical therapist, and medical equipment supplier. Before you purchase a walker you should test it out to decide if it is the right one for you. The physical therapist who supplies your walker should adjust for your height and should check the physical fit of the equipment. Moreover, the physical therapist should demonstrate the proper gait for walking. During the past few years, radical changes have occurred in the design and style of walkers. We expect this trend to continue with more attractive, easier-to-use products to be introduced regularly. If

© 1993 Burn Science Publishers, Inc., *Journal of Burn Care and Rehabilitation*, Vol. 14, No. 2, Part 1, "Technical Considerations in the Selection and Performance of Walkers," by Shahriar A. Nabizadeh, BS, Tad B. Hardee, PT, Michael A. Towler, MD, Van T. Chen, MD, and Richard F. Edlich, MD, PhD., Supported by a generous gift from Mr. Harvey R. Heller, Winter Garden, Florida; reprinted with permission.

you think that your walker is outdated and is not adapting to your lifestyle, talk with your physiatrist regarding alternatives. Today, walkers are as different as their users. Find the best one for you by taking a test walk in your home and community.

—(J Burn Care Rehabilitation *1993;14:182-8)*

Walkers are used to enhance balance and to reduce weight bearing fully or partially on a lower extremity. Of the three types of ambulatory assistive devices (canes, crutches, and walkers), walkers provide the greatest stability. They provide a wide base of stance, improve anterior and lateral stability, and permit the upper extremity to transmit body weight to the floor.[1]

Within the past 2 decades, the function, capability, and design of walkers has changed dramatically. Before this time, walkers were made of tubular aluminum with molded handgrips and rubber tips. Sizes were adjustable for both adults and children. Today notable differences exist between manufactured walkers in their size, style, weight, types of floor contact, breaking action, and platform accessories.

Persons with disabilities are no longer limited to a generic choice of one style but have a wide array of products to choose from. Whether the use of a walker is temporary or permanent, the selection of a walker should not be based only on manufacturing claims, research studies, or testimonies. Purchase should be determined by the results of actual trials, which take into consideration the person's needs, abilities, and living arrangements.

Regardless of the type, selecting the correct size is a critical decision. Although most are height-adjustable, adequate width and depth are important considerations for proper support. The height of a walker is measured similar to that of a cane.[2] The top of the walker should come approximately to the greater trochanter and should allow for 25 to 30 degrees of elbow flexion.

Basically, walkers can be divided into two types. One type has a three-point floor contact, whereas the other has a four-point floor contact. The points of the floor contact can either be a rubber endcap, a rubber endcap with an attached spring-loaded nylon glide, or a wheel. Because breaking action is advisable for walkers with wheels, the ease with which the breaks can be applied is an important consideration. For those with limited use of their hands, push-button or palm-depress hand breaks, which activate with minimal pressure, are worthy of serious consideration. In some walkers seats serve as a breaking mechanism for the wheels.

A folding mechanism for walkers is particularly useful for patients who travel. These walkers can be easily folded to fit into an automobile or other storage space. However, some heavier walkers require considerable effort to fold, and they mandate the assistance of a strong attendant. The patient should be informed about numerous accessories that have been developed for walkers to facilitate their use.

The height of the legs of each walker is usually adjusted to be the same. Moreover, the legs connect to each other in a rigid, secure configuration. However, reciprocal walkers are now designed with two movable joints to permit unilateral progression of one side of the walker. This feature is especially useful with patients incapable of lifting the walker with both hands and moving it forward. This advantage must be weighed against some inherent loss in the stability of the walker. By manufacturing walkers with different heights of the front and back legs, these walkers appear to be especially suitable for climbing and descending stairs.

The purposes of these studies were to identify the biomechanical performance of walker foot-pieces and to describe new innovations in the design of walkers.

Material and Methods

An Instron Universal Testing Machine, Model 1122 (Instron Corp, Canton, Mass.) was used to measure the frictional force of resistances to horizontal movement generated by three different walkers. For each test, the two anterior wheel foot-pieces were identical (Guardian Products, Inc., Model 7731PG, Arleta, Calif.). These wheel foot-pieces are able to negotiate uneven surfaces like doorsills, rough cement, asphalt, or thick carpeting more easily than are rubber cap foot-pieces, which have to be lifted over these barriers.

The first walker had two posterior foot-pieces with endcaps and two anterior foot-pieces with wheels. The endcap of the posterior foot-piece was made of rubber. The second walker had two anterior foot-pieces with wheels, whereas the posterior foot-pieces had rubber endcaps with attached spring-loaded nylon glide. The auto-glide mechanism of the posterior foot-piece was designed so that only the spring-loaded nylon glide contacted the floor during light weight-bearing. As the weight on the walker is increased, the glide retracts, allowing the rubber endcaps to also contact the floor, providing a brake mechanism. The third walker had wheels on all four foot-pieces. These foot-piece wheels remain in a vertical position. Foot-pieces with wheels that pivot on a swivel are also made. Because wheels that pivot are difficult to direct on uneven surfaces, the need exists for the development of a self-damping caster wheel whose direction can easily and reliably be controlled. Each walker was tested without a load, after which the procedure was repeated with a 16 kg load placed on the walker, simulating the approximate weight a patient might place on the walker.

The Instron Tester was calibrated by hanging a 500 gm weight from the load cell mounted on the Instron Tester's crosshead. This crosshead was moved at a controlled speed (10 cm/min), and the frictional force of resistance to horizontal movement was plotted as a function of walker displacement of an attached strip-chart recorder. The walker was connected to the load cell by a cord that passed horizontally from the walker around a frictionless pulley and vertically upward to the Instron load cell. The frictional force was then recorded eight times for each loaded and unloaded walker as the walker was pulled across a smooth, wooden surface at a constant rate (10 cm/min).

For each walker the mean and standard deviations of the frictional forces were calculated. The statistical significance of the data was determined by the Student's t test.

Results

The frictional forces encountered on the loaded walkers were always significantly greater than those on the comparable unloaded walkers ($p < 0.01$). For both the loaded and unloaded walkers, the walkers with four wheels encountered the least frictional forces ($p < 0.01$). The frictional forces encountered by the foot-pieces with the auto-glide mechanism were significantly greater than those of the wheel foot-pieces but were significantly less than those encountered with walkers with rubber cap footpieces ($p < 0.01$).

Discussion

Within the past 2 decades the function, capability and design of walkers have changed dramatically.[3] No longer does selecting a walker remain limited to a generic choice of one type. Today, those who need assistance with mobility have a wide array of products from which to choose. The generic form is made of tubular aluminum with four foot-pieces covered by rubber caps. This generic form can be sub-divided into rigid and collapsible models. The collapsible models are particularly useful for patients who travel. These walkers can be easily made to fit in an automobile or other storage space. Although definite advantages to folding walkers exist, it is important to determine if the patient has sufficient strength to fold the walker. If not, the services of an attendant will be needed.

The endpieces of the walker are important considerations. The endpieces with wheels encounter the least frictional forces with the ground. Consequently, walkers with wheels should be used very judiciously because the stability of the walker is reduced. This disadvantage must be weighed against the special benefits encountered in walkers with wheels. They may allow functional ambulation for patients who are unable to lift and move a conventional walker. In such cases pressure brakes are advocated. Because braking action is advisable for walkers with the ease with which brakes are activated can make a substantial difference. For those with limited use of their hands, push-button or palm-depressed hand brakes, which can be applied with minimal pressure, are models worthy of consideration. For some walkers seats serve as a breaking mechanism; the walker is secured and stabilized as the patient sits (The Merry Walker, Ballard International, Inc., Worthbrook, Ill.).

Walkers with rubber endcaps provide the greatest frictional forces with the ground and ensure secure patient ambulation. These substantial frictional forces necessitate lifting the walker from the floor. The walker should be picked up and placed down on all four legs simultaneously to achieve maximum stability. The nylon-glide attachment reduces the friction and allows the back legs of the walker to slide on the floor. Consequently, the patient does not have to remove the back legs from contact with the floor during ambulation.

The versatility of the generic walker with rubber endcaps has been enhanced by adding attachments and seats to the walker. Platform attachments have been designed when weight-bearing is accomplished through the forearm rather than through the hands and wrists. Arm troughs designed to attach to walker handles support the forearms, affording security, support, and durability (Danmar Products, Ann Arbor, Mich.). A handle has been attached to each back leg of the walker, affording the patient assistance to rise from a seated position (Easy-Up Handle, Crestline Products, Orlando, Fla.). Adopted from the traditional no-wheel "pick up & put" walker, the multipurpose stair walker (Temco Health Care, Passaic, N.J.) has uniquely angled accessory back handles that can be used to help the patient ascend and descend stairs and to walk on level ground while he or she maintains balance. Although the design of stair-climbing walkers is intriguing, the patient should be cautioned to ask for the help of an attendant during stair climbing. Finally, the generic walker with wheels has been designed with a basket that can be rearranged into a seat (Companion Walker; Companion Walker, Calgary, Alberta, Canada). This walker can serve as a seat for a patient who tires easily.

— by Shahriar A. Nabizadeh, BS, Tad B. Hardee, PT,
Michael A. Towler, MD, Van T. Chen, MD, and
Richard F. Edlich, MD, PhD.

References

1. O'Sullivan SB, Schmitz TJ, *Physical rehabilitation: assessment and treatment.* 2nd ed. Philadelphia: FA Davis Company, 1988:293-306.

2. Hartigan C, Morgan PF, Hunter FP Jr., Shotwell RE, Thacker JG, Edlich PF. Ergonomics of support cane handles. *J BURN CARE REHABIL* 1987;8:150-4.

3. American Association of Retired Persons: product report: walkers. American Association of Retired Persons, Washington, DC. 1991;7:1.

Chapter 26

Big Steps Forward for Amputees

David S. Barr of Bodfish, Calif., took an 80,000-mile motorcycle trip that spanned North and South America, Europe, Asia, and Africa. "Only 70 people have ever done anything like it before," Barr said. "There've been more people in outer space than have made this trip."

What makes it more extraordinary is that Barr, 41, is a double amputee. Fighting in Angola in 1981, he lost one leg above the knee and the other below the knee. But that hasn't kept him from riding a two-wheel 1972 Harley Davidson and writing a book about his around-the-world motorcycle trip.

And that is not all. Barr is one of only a handful of double-amputee parachutists who jump with special prosthetics. And he walks 3 or 4 miles a day and mows his own grass.

Advances in prosthetics, and the example set by amputees such as Barr, have shown more and more people that an amputation does not always mean confinement to a wheelchair. At private companies and key centers such as Northwestern University in Chicago and the University of Utah at Salt Lake City, research that sounds like something out of "The Six Million Dollar Man" could give amputees even more control over artificial limbs.

Physical therapist Marie A. Schroeder, chief of the Food and Drug Administration's restorative devices branch, explains that FDA regulates prostheses, but manufacturers do not have to undergo a full review for each new device. Instead, they must register the products and keep a record of any complaints.

FDA Consumer magazine, March 1997; Food and Drug Administration.

"But if there's a significant change in the technology, we could get involved," Schroeder said. For instance, she said, her branch has seen some interest in implantable electrodes for stimulating muscles in spinal cord injury cases. Such devices would require review by FDA. Some innovators are also exploring ways to use computers to design and manufacture custom prostheses, to attach muscles directly to a prosthesis, to develop powered fingers with microelectronics, and even to use brain waves to power prostheses.

For thousands of years, inventors have tried to replicate what nature cannot replace. Prostheses have been used since at least 300 B.C., when crude devices consisting of metal plates hammered over a wooden core, were attached to an amputated limb.

Advances in the science of prosthetics burgeon during and immediately after wars, when large numbers of people need to be fitted with artificial limbs. The technology of modern prosthetics has changed little since shortly after World War II.

"There's a real need for revolution in design," said Giovani M. Ortega, research and development project manager at Sabolich Prosthetics & Research in Oklahoma City, Okla., a division of NovaCare. "The systems that we have, have been around for a long time, and at best there have been only improvements. As far along as we've come, we're still far behind many other industries in terms of implementing new technologies."

Estimates of the amputee population in the United States vary widely, from fewer than 400,000 to more than 1 million. About 9 out of 10 amputations involve the leg, from the foot to above the knee.

Three-quarters of all amputations are the result of disease, often cancer or peripheral vascular disease. The latter is a narrowing of the arteries in the extremities that is often associated with diabetes. Most other amputations are the result of workplace or automobile accidents. And a small fraction, perhaps 3 percent, are due to birth defects that constrict bone growth.

Preventing Amputation

Because so many amputations result from disease, considerable attention has been paid to prevention. For example, the American Diabetes Association recommends people stop smoking, which can speed the progress of peripheral vascular disease. Patients with diabetes should monitor their blood glucose levels carefully, eat a healthy, balanced diet, see their doctors regularly, control their weight, and check their feet each day for small cuts or blisters. Electric blankets and heating pads carry warning labels that say people with diabetes should not use them without talking to their doctors first. This is because people with diabetes may lose sensation in their limbs. Patients can be seriously burned by an electric blanket or heating pad because they cannot feel how hot it really is.

Patients are also advised to develop an exercise plan after consulting with their doctors. Regular exercise maintains strength, flexibility, and blood flow to damaged areas and can help control pain. However, it's important not to stress the legs, feet or joints. Some good exercises are bicycling or easy rowing on a rowing machine. Swimming and aqua aerobics are also good choices.

"We know of many things that can help people avoid amputation, but unfortunately, it's no fun to do daily foot care or wear only proper fitting, well-designed shoes," said Jennifer Mayfield, M.D., chairwoman of the association's Foot Care Council. "Everybody keeps waiting for a magic bullet, and that would be nice, but it's not coming anytime soon."

Richard J. Gusberg, M.D., chief of vascular surgery at Yale University, said one of the first signs of peripheral occlusive disease is claudication, an aching, tired feeling in the leg muscles when they are exercised.

"The vast majority of people with claudication remain stable, or nearly stable, for an indefinite period of time," Gusberg said. In most cases the progress of the disease can be slowed if people control the risk factors, which includes reducing blood pressure, controlling their diabetes through diet or insulin, and reducing cholesterol levels. Regular exercise has also proven effective because it can strengthen circulation, he said.

The drug Trental (pentoxifylline) is approved by FDA for people with peripheral artery disease. Its use can decrease the thickness and stickiness of blood, and can reduce the deformities of red blood cells, so the blood can get through the narrowed arteries, but it is not effective in all patients, Gusberg said. The use of other drugs in treating occlusive disease has largely been abandoned, he said.

If the disease progresses, the patient might develop gangrene, or ulcers in the leg, as blood flow is reduced.

"When people get to that stage, most of them need to be evaluated for a bypass operation," Gusberg said. Replacing the arteries in the lower leg is effective for five years or more in 70 to 80 percent of cases.

Sensory Loss

Another danger with diabetes is a deadening of the nerves in the extremities. John F. Glass, a biologist with FDA's pacing and neurological devices branch, said there are now a variety of devices that measure sensory loss in the affected limbs. In a patient with diabetes, loss of sensation because of nerve damage signals a need for diligence. Even minor injuries, undetected because the feeling is gone and thus left untreated, can become infected easily and lead to gangrene.

"If you're aware of sensory loss, you want to keep a close watch on it," Glass said. "There's a range of measurement devices, from those that detect general loss of sensation, to those that assess the specific degree of sensory loss, or that can quantify sensitivity to pressure or temperature."

Many of the devices are easy-to-use mechanical implements with no significant health risk to patients. One of the simplest is a hand-held device that looks like an old typewriter eraser with thin wires attached to it. The wires are placed on the toes or fingertips to see if there is tactile sensitivity.

Such simple devices are typically not reviewed by FDA before they are made available to the public. They are intended for use by the patient for monitoring only, not self-diagnosis. "Loss of sensation in an extremity could indicate a lot of other conditions or disorders, so we would encourage the patient to see a physician immediately for a complete physical examination," Glass said.

Unavoidable Limb Loss

Precautions such as Glass advocates can often delay the progression of the disease. Sometimes, though, the loss of a limb is unavoidable. In those cases, physical therapy starts a day or two after surgery. Since more than 9 out of 10 amputations involve one or both legs, physical therapy usually involves the use of parallel bars, and later a walker or crutches. Part of the training involves how to fall and get up safely.

There are other adjustments as well. Barr said the loss of both legs, and covering the stumps with plastic, means his body has become much less effective at cooling itself, so he has to be on the lookout for hyperthermia. And he learned other tricks to cope, as well. "I'm constantly on the move, never standing still, always readjusting my balance even when I'm staying in one place, because I don't want one particular area on the stump to get sore," Barr said.

Until recently, patients were not fitted with an artificial limb for four to eight weeks after surgery, but new techniques allow the use of a protective foam over a sterile bandage, and the prosthesis can be fit as soon as the day following surgery.

New Prosthetic Materials

For centuries, wood and leather were the only materials for prostheses, but today's physical therapist has a much wider range available, including advanced plastics and carbon fiber, which are much stronger and lighter and more durable. "The industry is really moving towards composite materials, because they're lighter in weight, easier to work with, and more durable," said Douglas McCormack, vice president of the Amputee Coalition of America.

Silicone-based compounds used to make prosthetic arms, for instance, give the appearance of real skin, unlike the rigid plastic or metal limbs of years ago, and they are more comfortable for the person wearing them. Women can get prosthetic feet with life-like toes for when they wear sandals; men can get legs with the appearance of hair.

But even materials that work out in one application might not work in another. "We tested a silicone foot at one point. On a machine it was subjected to 300 pounds of stress for a million cycles, and it didn't have any problems. But an amputee broke it within a few minutes. It really surprised us. Torque and other stresses can fatigue the material quickly," said Sabolich's Ortega. "You'd be amazed at the toll that a human body puts on even the strongest material."

New computer programs better determine where and what the forces are. But it's not just a question of choosing a material that will withstand those forces. "With some of the new materials being developed, we could make a foot to take any of the pressures that the human body will give it," Ortega said. "The problem is it might not have any springiness. You give up flexibility for strength. You have to balance all the considerations in a prosthetic."

Prostheses are typically sold as components, so that someone who has an above-the-knee amputation would be able to choose leg, knee and foot units, often from different manufacturers, depending on their individual needs.

Most of the units are adjustable. Shock absorbers in knees, for instance, can be made more flexible as a person gains controls over the artificial leg. Ankles can be adjusted to the weight and activity level of the patient.

Arm amputees today can choose between prostheses that are powered by a harness and cable attached to the residual limb, or externally powered devices. Powered arms can be controlled by switches mounted inside or outside the socket, that the patient can activate by flexing certain muscle groups.

Energy Requirements

Some prosthetics research is aimed at providing active devices, which do part of the work of the amputated limb, as opposed to passive devices that are controlled by the residual limb. An amputee with prostheses expends two to three times more energy than a nondisabled person to perform even the simplest activities, such as walking across a room or climbing stairs. "A semi-active system, in which the limb itself performs part of the function, could reduce that energy requirement significantly," said Sabolich's Ortega. "And there would also be a psychological benefit, because the prosthesis would no longer be just a dead limb, but something that is helping."

Ortega said one area Sabolich is researching would provide sensory feedback from the prosthesis to the remaining limb. For instance, in an artificial leg, pressure sensors in the foot would send a mild electrical signal to the thigh muscles when there is pressure on the back, front or sides of the foot.

That kind of feedback would be similar to what they would get with the pressure of the ground against a natural foot, which would make their adjustment to the prostheses go more quickly, Ortega said. Ortega said prosthetic designs are limited only by how large a power pack the amputee can carry.

"The crucial issue when it comes to trying to introduce any new prosthesis is the energy requirements," said Ortega. "Our muscles are so efficient, in terms of the power that they produce versus the fuel that they use, that we have a difficult time matching it. "Scientists are also working to build a better socket—the part of the prosthesis that attaches to the residual limb.

Dudley S. Childress, Ph.D., of Northwestern University's Rehabilitation Engineering Program, is working on applying the industrial practice known as rapid prototyping to socket production.

Sockets are now produced largely by hand. A cast is made of the residual limb, and plaster is poured into the cast to make a positive mold. The mold is then used to create a plastic or laminated polyester socket that fits over the residual limb.

Childress employs a computer-aided design program to measure the residual limb and design a socket. Then, using a modified "plastic deposition technology" called squirt shaping, a computer lays down small amounts of polypropylene to produce the desired shape, to very tight tolerances. In industry, the technology is used to quickly produce prototypes of everything from car parts to military weapons, to test them before starting mass production.

"Essentially, every socket is a prototype, and there are potentially some significant advantages to applying these techniques to prosthesis manufacture," Childress said. "We can make a socket in about 50 minutes, which isn't bad, but as people continue to work with the technology, it may be possible to get that down even faster. "The process would also allow manufacturers to make sockets out of different types of material than have been used in the past, or alter the thickness or characteristics of the material very quickly.

Another innovation being explored at Northwestern is powered prosthetic fingers. That might be difficult if you were going to match real fingers, he acknowledged, but most of the time that's unnecessary. Picking up a spoon and holding a book don't require much power, just control. Small motor technology and power storage capability have both improved vastly in recent years.

"If you want to do something like squeeze orange juice, you need force," Childress said. "But even for people without a prosthesis, that's tiresome, so we have all kinds of devices to do those jobs for us. So the intent of the powered fingers would be to provide prehensile [wrap-around] force."

Childress said his laboratory is also looking at devices that would improve the "feel" of prostheses over current devices. It would be comparable, he said, to the way power steering reduces the muscle power needed to steer a car, but you can still "feel" the road through the wheel.

Cables in artificial fingers and hands would connect to the muscles of the forearm, either through holes in the muscle that are surgically lined with skin, or tendons could be taken outside the residual limb and covered with skin. Either option would give the muscle the sense of how hard it is working and how fast it is moving.

Mundane, but Important, Needs

Joan E. Edelstein, Ph.D., director of Columbia University's physical therapy program, stresses the need for prosthetics research to focus not just on high-technology improvements, but to the more mundane but critical things such as fit, to make them as comfortable as possible, particularly among the elderly, whose needs may not be fully considered.

"Most patients are older people who have lost a limb because of diabetes, and the assumption is that they're going to be relatively undemanding of their prosthesis," Edelstein said. Better prostheses for the elderly might prevent skin breakdown and infections, yet hardly any research dollars are being spent in that area, she said, explaining that, "It's not as glamorous as developing better prostheses for sport, or for children, and they are very difficult problems to overcome. "Research often proceeds along several courses at once, she noted, and you can never know which might yield the next major breakthrough.

— by Robert A. Hamilton

Robert A. Hamilton is a writer in Franklin, Conn.

Chapter 27

Problems Experienced and Perceived by Prosthetic Patients

"No one thanks a surgeon for cutting off an arm or a leg"[1]. Nonetheless, amputation surgery has been practiced widely and described as a standard procedure in early textbooks of surgery[2]. Once amputation has saved a patient's life, his feelings about the procedure and his situation will influence the subsequent course of his life, rehabilitation, personal relationships, income, health and spirit.

Previous investigators have compared the loss of a limb with the loss of a spouse and studied the progression of psychological responses, patients' feelings after an amputation, depression among amputees, psychiatric symptoms, social and psychological adjustment following amputation, psychosocial factors affecting rehabilitation outcome, the effects of age and time, the effects of activities of daily living (ADL) changes, the effects of depression on phantom pain and reasons for psychiatric consultation following amputation[3-11]. One of us (JJN) attended a support group session, Help Amputees Rehabilitate Themselves (HART), and listened to a multitude of patients' practical problems, perceived wrongs and criticisms, and many difficulties relating to work, personal relations, physician relations, etc. We undertook this study by questionnaire to see if the troubles reported in the HART session were widespread or limited. We discovered many problems and issues that are important to a significant proportion of amputees and therefore should be understood by the health professionals caring for these patients.

© 1993 *Journal of Prosthetics and Orthotics*, Vol.5, No. 1, January 1993; reprinted with permission.

Methods

A questionnaire was designed to elicit pertinent information regarding patients' perceptions, problems and feelings related to their prostheses and their lives as amputees. In addition, standardized tests were administered to assess depression and ADL. Ten of these questionnaires were distributed on a pilot basis, and it was observed patients would answer them quickly and completely.

The questionnaires were then distributed by a physicians' assistant (PA) to 94 consecutive patients with amputations who attended the prosthetic clinic of either the Harmarville Rehabilitation Center or the Presbyterian University Hospital/University of Pittsburgh from September 1987 through October 1988. The PA offered to read the questions and explain the intent of questions in case any patients were illiterate, had vision problems or did not grasp the meaning of the questions. Questionnaires were completed at the clinic visit, and the PA collected them.

The information obtained from the questionnaires was entered into computer files, verified and analyzed using Statistical Package for the Social Sciences (SPSS-X). Although 94 questionnaires were returned, not every subject answered every item, and therefore some items have fewer than 94 responses. Informed consent was obtained from each patient according to guidelines of the Institutional Review Board of the School of Medicine, University of Pittsburgh and the Harmarville Rehabilitation Center Inc.

Results

Demographic Characteristics of the Population

Ninety-four patients completed the questionnaire (63 males, 31 females). The mean patient age was 57 (SD = 19.5) (range 19-91). The age distribution was more skewed toward the younger population than expected.

There were 75 white, 14 black and five "other" patients. Thirty-seven subjects had undergone amputation before 1983 and 57 since 1983. Causes of amputation included a significant incidence of trauma.

Amputations included one above-elbow, three below-elbow, one hip disarticulation and one Syme's amputation but most were above-knee or below-knee (left AK, 11; right AK, 14; left BK, 35; right BK, 28).

The social situation of patients was not unusual. The largest percentage were married (41 percent). Twenty-three percent were widowed and 17 percent never married.

The education level was relatively high with a median level of high school graduation or greater. Thirty-two percent had attended "some college," 5 percent graduated from college and 8 percent completed a professional school.

Most patients were unemployed. At the time of the interviews, six were housewives, 14 were employed fully, four were employed part-time; 38 were retired; eight were unemployed, and 24 were disabled from working. Those who were employed had a higher level of education.

Forty-six patients said they did not lose their jobs because of their amputation, but 13 did. There was no difference in education level between these two groups; however, those with above-knee amputations were more likely to have lost their jobs than those with below-knee amputations. The median income was low, between $10,000 and $14,999.

Public transportation was avoided by most patients.

Amputation Experience and Rehabilitation Training

Eighty patients (84 percent) perceived they had no choice regarding prescription of their initial artificial limb; only 14 said they had. Fifty-nine (63 percent) were either somewhat satisfied or very satisfied with the comfort of the prosthesis while 24 reported dissatisfaction. Eighty-six (92 percent) said they perceived their surgeon as sensitive, and five did not. However, 74 (79 percent) said the surgeon did not speak to them prior to surgery, and 20 said he or she did. Fifty-five (59 percent) of the patients reported no discussion with their surgeon following surgery, while 30 (32 percent) did. Of those who had a discussion with the surgeon prior to surgery, 20 said it was helpful, and two said it was not. As for discussions with the surgeon following surgery, 35 (37 percent) said it was helpful, and four said it was not.

Most patients reported they received appropriate rehabilitation training. Vehicle transfers were taught the least (55 percent only), and a significant number of patients reported never having been taught transfers (36 percent), bathing (40 percent), stair climbing (19 percent), walking on an inclined plane (26 percent) or care of the prosthesis (27 percent).

Practical Experience with Prostheses

Most patients (66 of 89 or 74 percent) wore their prostheses eight or more hours a day. Education level did not affect the hours of wear;

however, those who wore their prostheses for longer periods of time had been amputees longer (R = 0.29; P = .003), found their prostheses more comfortable (R = .19, P = .04) and were less depressed (R = -.23, P = .02) than those who wore them for shorter periods. There was a negative correlation between time since amputation and depression (R = -.25, P = .01). Below-knee prosthesis wearers wore their prostheses for more hours during the day than above-knee prosthesis wearers. Most (46 of 94 or 55 percent) received their prostheses after a period of three months postoperatively, and most (57 of 90 or 63 percent) said they were not familiar with the various options available in prostheses at that time.

Many daily activities were affected by wearing a prosthesis. Outstanding among the changes resulting from amputation were the perceptions of a patient's lessened ability to defend humor herself (72 percent) and the limitation on activities by inclement weather (66 percent). Patients were almost universally satisfied with their rehabilitation physician (84 of 86 or 98 percent) and limb company (87 of 90 or 97 percent). Only a few (14 of 94 or 15 percent) attended a support group.

The ability to defend oneself did not vary significantly with age. Younger patients were more likely to feel their choice of apparel was affected as were women. The more highly educated were also more likely to perceive their choice of apparel was affected (T = -3.35, P = .001).

Discussion

Our patients were not unusual regarding etiology, site of amputation, gender, race or employment status. Although most patients were unemployed, a small number lost or changed their jobs because of amputation. Most felt they had little choice regarding their amputation or selection of a prosthesis yet more than two-thirds wore their prosthesis eight or more hours per day. Lack of communication with the surgeon was almost universal, but it did not alter the patients' perceptions that surgeons were "sensitive" to their needs. It appears therefore that patients did not resent the lack of communication with their surgeons.

Quite striking was the number of patients who felt the selection of clothing, choice of transportation, mobility during inclement weather and other activities of daily living, including their ability to defend themselves, were altered for the worse by their amputations. Also impressive is the number of patients who reported they did not receive some aspect of mobility training (transfers, bathing, etc.). We cannot be sure whether this represents a lack of training or just a lack of memory for the training. Health professionals should be aware of these feelings of conspicuousness and vulnerability.

Regarding depression, it is encouraging to see a negative correlation between the time since amputation and depression, suggesting that affect improves over time after this surgery. Moreover, those who wore their prostheses for longer periods of time were less depressed. Several authors have previously studied various psychological, social and personal responses of patients following limb amputations; however, none has discussed pertinent practical problems in detail.

Parkes (1975) compared the results of interviews from 21 British widows and 48 recent amputees. He found amputees had a stronger sense of their limb's presence and a lesser sense of approval for grieving over their loss. MacBride et al. (1980) interviewed 50 amputees and found elevated stress levels and fear of falling, financial failure and ability to perform ADLS. Stress was greater later rather than immediately following amputation[4]. Froggatt and Mawby (1981) found 35 British amputees they interviewed to be ADL independent and rarely complaining of isolation[5].

Kashani et al. (1983) interviewed 65 amputees and found depression prevalent soon after amputation[6]. Shukla et al. (1982) found psychiatric symptoms acutely common in 72 amputees interviewed after amputation in India[7]. Thompson and Haren (1983) interviewed 134 British amputees and found little depression but much social isolation following amputation[8]. Gerhards, Florin and Knapp interviewed 178 German war veterans and found the wives reported performing increased physical work, and the amputees reported vocational satisfaction and participation in sports activities[9].

Frank et at. (1984) studied 66 amputees by questionnaire and found depression decreased with time after amputation[10]. O'Toole et at. (1985) studied 60 amputees' and found the Barthel Index rose (improved), the PULSES Profile fell (worsened) and the ESCROW Scale rose (indicating a decrease in social supports) following amputation[11].

These studies describe many facets of the amputee experience but do not describe the area of personal concerns and practical problems in which we were interested.

Conclusion

We believe our patients' sense of defenselessness and altered appearance in the eyes of the non-amputee world, and their reduced mobility during inclement weather, should be appreciated more by those professionally involved in their care. These patient perceptions may be unique to amputee patients. Practical suggestions can be offered for dressing and mobility problems. In addition, while many rehabilitation training procedures were taught to our patients, a significant minority in each category denied ever having received the training. Perhaps a checklist should be included with the physical therapy schedule of these patients and items initialed by the therapist so they are not forgotten. Health professionals should take inventory to see whether ADL transfers and automobile transfers are taught in their programs.

Most of our patients were recent amputees. Apparently, more experienced amputees have learned to obtain access to prosthetic devices without attending prosthetic clinics. Our review suggests patients are more depressed acutely following their amputation than when assessed months or years later. It may be that amputee patients require a period of mourning for their loss before they can get on with the daily business of prosthetic wear.

— by John J. Nicholas, MD, Lawrence R. Robinson, MD,
Richard Schulz, PhD,Carol Blair, RN,
Richard Aliota, MD,Gerri Hairston, MSW, LSW

References

1. Scott Nettrour MD, initial lecturer in course for residents. "Introduction to Contemporary Prosthetics." 1983. (Division of Rehabilitation Medicine, Department of Orthopedic Surgery, School of Medicine. University of Pittsburgh, 1983-1988). Personal Communication.

2. Bedington T. The first lines of the practice of surgery being an elementary work for students and a concise reference for practitioners. Boston: S. A. Cooper, 1828:382-91.

3. Parkes CM. Psychosocial transitions: comparison between reactions to loss of a limb and loss of a spouse. *Brit J Psychiat* 1975; 127:204-10.

4. MacBride A, Rogers J, Whylie B, Freeman SJJ. Psychosocial factors in the rehabilitation of elderly amputees. *Psychosomatics* 1980; 21:258-65.

5. Froggatt D, Mawby R. Surviving an amputation. *Soc Sci Med* 1981; 15E: 123-8.

6. Kashani JH, Frank RG. Kashani SR, Wonderlich SA, Reid JC. Depression among amputees. *J Clin Psychiatry* 1983; 44:256-8.

7. Shukla GD, Sahu SC, Tripathi RP, Gupta DK. A psychiatric study of amputees. *Brit J Psychiat* 1982; 141:50-3.

8. Thompson DM, Haren D. Living with an amputation: the patient. *Int Rehabil Med* 1983; 5:165-9.

9. Gerhards F, Florin I, Knapp T. The impact of medical, reeducational, psychological variables on rehabilitation outcome in amputees. *Int J Rehab Research* 1984; 7:379-88.

10. Frank RG, Kashani JH, Kashani SR, Wonderlich SA, Umlauf RL, Ashkanazi GS. Psychological response to amputation as a function of age and time since amputation. *Brit J Psyciat* 1984; 144:493-7.

11. O'Toole DM, Goldberg RT, Ryan B. Functional changes in vascular amputee patients: evaluation by Barthel Index, PULSES Profile and ESCROW Scale. *Arch Phys Med & Rehabil* 1985; 66:508.

Chapter 28

Robotics and Rehabilitation

Space, deep-sea, and radioactive explorations called for the development of technology to allow humans to control inaccessible environments. Some of the solutions arrived at are now being transferred to allow severely disabled people to control their environments. Human-scale manipulators, used to increase independence and the quality of life for severely disabled people, have found a place in rehabilitation.

Richard A. Foulds, Ph.D., of the Tufts Rehabilitation Engineering program, introduces the World Rehabilitation Fund's (WRF) 37th Monograph in the International Exchange of Experts and Information Project, Interactive Robotic Aids—*One Option for Independent Living: An International Perspective*, with the following statement:

> In marked contrast to the science fiction androids popularized in the Star Wars films, these real life robots attempt to deal with the down-to-earth problems of employment, education, and daily living. Unlike fictional robots, which are intended to replace human tasks, the rehabilitation robot serves as a direct extension of the disabled user in an attempt to increase the involvement and independence of that person.

The monograph, a state-of-the-art review, contains papers written by rehabilitation robotics research and development experts from the

1990 *Rehab Brief Bringing Research into Effective Focus*, Vol. X, No. 2, ISSN: 0732-2623, National Institute on Disability and Rehabilitation Research, Office of Special Education and Rehabilitative Services, Department of Education, Washington, DC 20202.

United States and abroad. This *Rehab BRIEF* will summarize these papers on uses of robotic aids and philosophical issues relating to their place in rehabilitation.

The Argument for Using Robotic Manipulators

When manual skills are affected by disability, rehabilitation often centers on substituting or compensating for the losses of physical and sensory abilities in the hands. Craig W. Heckathorne, of Northwestern University, observes, "manipulation aids can be divided into two categories: those that are task specific and those that more generally assist in manipulation."

Remote manipulators and robotic devices may be task specific, but they also hold the promise of serving as general manipulation instruments. They can provide action at a distance. They can be used in unstructured environments, or they can carry out preprogrammed tasks within highly structured environments. They can be used to manipulate larger and heavier objects than an individual could handle with orthotic or body-actuated manipulation aids. And they can accommodate characteristics of the environment, supplementing the commands of the user.

Examples of Robotic Uses

The ensuing overview will highlight several projects and give examples of tasks that were completed by individuals using robotic devices. Readers are encouraged to read the original report for more examples, more technical descriptions of the equipment, and more complete discussions of the configuration, price, and accomplishments of specific devices.

From France: Spartacus

The Spartacus project, a 5-year robotics project intended to stimulate the development of industrial robotics in France, conducted a feasibility study to develop and test a telemanipulator, controllable by people with high-level spinal cord lesions.

To optimize performance, a fixed workstation with an arm derived from nuclear manipulators was used to explore the limits of control feasibility and to avoid failure due to mechanical limitations.

The Spartacus project studied manipulation of the mechanical arm by a variety of methods, depending on the physical abilities of the users. Switches or joysticks operated by chin or mouth, breath-operated switches, eye-movement controls, various versions of head movement transducers, and hum, melody, and voice control were all used. Often the arm was controlled with the combination of methods that best served an individual.

These configurations allowed participants to complete the following tasks:

- pour liquids or "play with water";

- obtain objects from shelves;

- open cupboard doors;

- eat;

- light a lamp;

- draw or paint;

- drink-using a special mode that combines tilting and lifting a cup or glass, simultaneously controlled by a single signal (This task was considered a "landmark" since it showed that a certain level of confidence and dexterity in controlling the system had been obtained.);

- turn pages of a journal or a book;

- use a standard dial telephone;

- use an electric range to heat water and prepare a pot of coffee;

- play games;

- shave with an electric shaver; and

- play with "Rubik's Cube."

From the United Kingdom

At the Cambridge University Engineering Department, the potential of robotics to assist the developmental education of disabled children is being investigated. The project provides a facility in which disabled children can manipulate the environment. This includes tasks such as examining the sizes, colors, relationships, and shapes of objects. In one substantial clinical trial, three learning tasks were investigated. Two were basic developmental tasks that are not achievable by children with severe physical disability-yet are considered central to their education. These were a routine to stack blocks in a pile and then break the pile apart and a routine to sort blocks into boxes depending on their shapes and colors.

The third task was the Tower of Hanoi puzzle, consisting of a tower of discs with decreasing diameters, which must be moved to a second location. The rules are that only one intermediate location can be used and at no time can any disc be placed on a smaller disc. The robot enforces the rules but gives the user control over moving the discs.

The color and shape sorting task offers a good example of how the robot works. It picks up each block in turn and presents it to the user to identify either its color or shape. Once the user indicates that he or she has seen the block, the robot tries to sort it. This may be done on a scanning basis, wherein the robot goes to each bin, in turn, and waits for a yes or no response from the user, or by direct selection where the user can indicate the correct sorting bin.

The robot ensures that the block is eventually sorted correctly; if the user gives a wrong command, the robot's response is to appear to try to put the block in the bin, but to refuse and give a negative sound before continuing with the program.

From Canada

The Nell Squire Foundation set out to create a manipulator that could perform tasks done by personal assistants and was approximately human size. The result was a robot called M.O.M. (a Machine for Obedient Manipulation). M.O.M. is designed as a work station manipulator (as opposed to being mounted on the wheelchair) for technical reasons. It is hoped that a "second generation" M.O.M. will incorporate artificial intelligence, giving the user better control and allowing the arm to be mounted on a wheelchair. Presently, M.O.M. can:

- pick up a manual from a bookshelf and place it in front of an individual:
- turn pages;
- pick up, serve, and replace a drink;
- serve up a mouthstick;
- load a diskette in a computer;
- pick up an electric shaver and shave a person;
- brush hair; and
- brush teeth.

The manipulator is lightweight and easily removed from and replaced in its stand. Therefore, it can readily be moved to a new work area—such as a bookshelf or bedside.

The Neil Squire Foundation is testing M.O.M. with disabled people ranging in age from 19 to 80.

From the Netherlands

Dr. A. P. Zeelenberg and his son, who is disabled by muscular dystrophy report, on the use of a wheelchair-mounted robot (the Cobra Manipulator). Remaining slight finger function allows the son to control the robot by using very responsive switches grouped closely together. More expensive pneumatic (sip-puff) or voice command devices are not needed. The manipulator and a specially designed interface mounted on the wheelchair allow the user to eat, turn pages, pick up books, and use remote control devices (for a television set, doors, and other appliances).

The user is able to open interior doors in the house and roll a small table on casters through the rooms. These tasks require good coordination between the right hand driving the wheelchair and the left hand operating the manipulator.

Recreation and work activities are also possible using this simple manipulator configuration. Playing chess, sandpapering wooden components for ship models, drilling holes in electronic printed circuit boards, and soldering components into circuit boards are among the tasks completed by the younger Zeelenberg.

From the United States

An Independent Vocational Work Station

Boeing Computer Services sponsored a project to experiment with a speech-controlled workstation for quadriplegic programmers and analysts. The workstation has a microcomputer system that supports and is driven by two voice-recognition products and a voice-communication product.

This hardware configuration allows single-voice commands to produce the equivalent of multiple keystrokes. The use of graphics, multiple programming languages, and access to different networks also are permitted.

The robotic aid at the station allows the user to:

- display reading material on the reader-board;

- handle filing in a file cabinet;
- handle floppy diskettes;
- adjust a printer according to the operator's commands; and
- perform miscellaneous support activities.

In this application, the location of the robotic aids becomes more than a functional consideration. Safety of the operators becomes critical. Maneuverability of the operator is limited. The operator's attention is frequently on the computer monitor of the readerboard. The robot is expected to carry out assigned tasks without attendance and without posing a hazard to the operator.

The robot's placement determines the design of the sort station. The robot must access the disk drives, printer, reader-board, file cabinet, bookshelves, in/out tray, waste basket, diskette storage, and user's lap and back pack. A robot with two arms was needed to perform all these tasks. A vertical file and shelves were designed for easy access by the robot. Manuals and books are stored in special vertical bookshelves. Modifications of the hardware were also required.

This workstation and special programming of the equipment allow a quadriplegic computer operator to function independently in a business-programming environment at Boeing Computer Services.

Small Robot Arm in the Workplace

The Rehabilitation Engineering Center in Wichita, Kansas, helped develop a workstation that allows disabled people to solder tinning of the electrical leads of small components prior to inserting them into circuit boards. The operation requires picking up the part, dipping it in a liquid flux, then dipping the lead in molten solder, holding for three seconds, inspecting the lead for uniform solder coating, placing the part aside for cooling, and then placing the part in an alcohol bath.

Disabled workers at Center Activities in Wichita, with precisely set up workstations, are performing these tasks on a subcontract with the Boeing Company.

The following observations made by the research staff are of interest:

1. The robotic arm not only performs fine motor tasks but also acts as a "pacer," forcing the worker to be ready for the next cycle of operations. Staff has found pacing to be difficult for many to grasp without some external indicator.

2. Use of a small console with push buttons to control the arm and enter programmed positions suited this project better than entry of programming data.

3. The human element of judgement was necessary in this task. A robot could not have done the work alone.

4. When production rates are required, a programmed repeatable cycle works better than manual manipulation of the robotic arm.

Robot Arm Work Station

The Johns Hopkins University Applied Physics Laboratory is responsible for a robot arm/work table system that enables high-level quadriplegics to execute manipulative tasks with little or no attendant assistance. This research program has now reached a stage where a manufacturing prototype has been fabricated and is in the final stages of evaluation.

The latest model incorporates a low-cost computer with adequate flexibility to permit programming a number of useful manipulation tasks on structured workstations. The robot arm is a 6-degrees-of-freedom, computer-controlled anthropomorphic limb.

Small vertical chin motion provides proportional control over selecting individual Joint motions or prestored motion sequences, while a single pulse—activated by slight rocking fore and aft—causes an event to start or stop.

The work station places components in fixed locations on the work table so that the robot arm can use manual, step-by-step motion or prestored computer-controlled motion to complete tasks.

The Problems of Getting Manipulators to Users

The papers in the monograph offer differing opinions on the level of technology that should be applied to solve rehabilitation problems. There is no general agreement on the type of manipulator that best meets users' needs. One author argues for a powerful device, custom designed to meet the optimal needs of each user; another argues for the use of low-cost technology that will satisfy economic demands, but necessarily will be limiting. One author advocates preprogrammed robot motions to minimize the demands placed on users; another just as strongly advocates maximizing user control.

Reacting to the papers summarizing clinical evaluations, John H. Leslie, Jr., of the Rehabilitation Engineering Center. The Cerebral

Palsy Research Foundation of Kansas. Inc., states that a device (robotic or otherwise) must satisfy two tests to have practical use in a service delivery environment. Use of the device must result in a cost reduction of the overall system-funding base, and the device must improve the quality of life for the disabled person. He also cites the cost to the consumer, reliability of the device, product liability, and potential consumers other than the disabled market (such as elderly people) as important issues.

Leifer, Michalowski, and Van der Loos, of the Rehabilitation R&D Center, Palo Alto Veterans Administration Medical Center, and the Department of Mechanical Engineering, Stanford University, maintain that the use of robots is cost-effective because they can replace human labor which averages about $15 per hour while robot costs average $5 per hour and are decreasing. Prototypes are now being readied for production and marketing.

It appears that robotic manipulators can enhance the lives of some users and may have vocational applications. What will it take to make them available to disabled consumers?

Newman et al. reviewed the literature on technological development and its application to the problems of disabled people (see sources). They summarized government reports, private industry findings, service providers' recommendations, and consumers' requests and demarcated seven general problem areas in bringing technology to disabled consumers: (1) limited market, (2) lack of financial incentive in the development and distribution of technological products for disabled people, (3) inadequate technology transfer, (4) lack of coordination among the relevant disciplines, (5) no mechanism for dissemination of information, (6) no evaluation of or standards for products, and (7) lack of training related to rehabilitation technology.

The fact that this monograph on robotic aids has been produced just 4 years after such problems were summarized indicates that the problems relating to technology transfer, training, coordination, and dissemination are being addressed. The three remaining problem areas, relating to the market, incentives, and evaluation, comprise major obstacles to getting robotic manipulators to disabled consumers who could benefit from them.

Rehabilitation researchers, developers, practitioners, and users who are interested in robotics should look closely at these and start developing solutions if they are convinced of the value of robotic applications.

The Market. Recognizing the limited market and limited buying power of most disabled people, manufacturers often fall to see potential for profit. When they do produce products and recognize a profit, they have a captive market and little competition so there is little incentive to improve a product in response to consumer needs, or to price it competitively. In 1978, La Rocca and Turem pointed out that many of the approximately 400,000 American wheelchair users are dissatisfied with their wheelchairs. Despite the multimillion-dollar revenues, manufacturers have not significantly changed the design of the wheelchair since the 1940's.

Financial Disincentives. Robotic manipulators won't offer manufactures the financial rewards that wheelchairs do. The expense of such product design and development is enormous compared to that based on needs of an average population and a much larger number of potential buyers.

Newman et al. identify additional financial disincentives.

Evaluation for safety, durability, and reliability presents problems in that potential users must be identified and the evaluation may be conducted in a hospital or clinic, thus adding to the costs of development. Product liability insurance is also high. In addition, most manufacturers are not willing to solve the marketing problems encountered with disability products. These include the inability to exploit the usual advertising sources and the requirement that some products be prescribed by a physician. Manufacturers trying to be competitive find that there is no existing marketing system and that it is difficult to collect accurate information on the market. Another problem to be faced is that the manufacturer is often expected to provide modification, maintenance, and repair of products. This includes the training of sales and service personnel, and represents an unrealistic investment in light of the limited market for many of the products. Clearly, costs on the one hand, and market size on the other, minimize the profit potential for private manufacturers.

Evaluation and Standardization. Product evaluation, although expensive, is necessary. Objective determination of durability reliability, safety, and appropriateness can only be made using consumers and professionals in time-consuming tests. In addition, from the papers presented, it appears to be nearly impossible to mass-produce or mass-market manipulators. Devices developed on an individual problem/solution basis cannot be standardized.

Leslie and the other authors are convinced that this technology can provide what all disabled people need the chance to be productive human beings. Perhaps if government, industry, and rehabilitation work together to accomplish the costly research, design, development, production, and dissemination of robotic devices, this can come about.

Sources

World Rehabilitation Fund, Inc., 1986. Interactive Robotic Aids—*One Option for Independent Living: An International Perspective.* Monograph No. 37. New York.

Newman, Shelia Stephens, John E. Schatzlein, and Rayelenn Sparks. 1983. *Technology In Independent Living for Physically Disabled People,* by Nancy M. Crewe and Irving Kenneth Zola, 245-269. San Francisco: Jossey-Bass Inc., Publishers.

Reviewer Comment

Ability to exert control over one's environment is of paramount importance to self-esteem and good mental health. To illustrate: when children master their first bicycles you hear the triumphant scream, "Look what I can do!" Also, in tracing the etiology of emotional illnesses and relapses, one nearly always finds loss of control over circumstances as a causal factor.

A major thrust of rehabilitation is to restore as much control as possible to those in whom it has been diminished by disability. Robotics (and other environmental-control approaches) have just begun to scratch the surface of potential applications. The research expense is often justified in terms of the practical value of promoting vocational productivity. However, there appears to be a more fundamental value—stabilizing and elevating mental health. This can make attainment of "practical" goals in all realms of living more probable.

—by Herbert C. Rigoni, Ph.D., C.I.R.S.

Chapter 29

Study Shows Physical Therapy Robot Aids Stroke Recovery

A Massachusetts Institute of Technology (MIT) robot for physical therapy on the arm and wrists is a promising new tool for rehabilitating stroke victims, as evidenced by results from the first clinical trial of the machine.

In the study, stroke patients who used the machine four to five hours a week improved further and faster, as measured by increased function of the impaired limb, than a second group of patients that did not receive robot-assisted therapy. At the same time, the trial showed that the robot is tolerated well by patients and causes no pain.

Although it's not clear whether it was the robot or the additional exercises that led to the improvements, these results show the feasibility of the robotic technique. This opens the door for further use of the machine, which offers certain advantages over traditional therapy. For example, it can quantify forces and movements that until now have been judged by "touch and feel." Such data would provide a permanent, objective record of a patient's progress that could be used in many ways.

The clinical trial also answered a long-standing question among therapists: manual manipulation of a stroke victim's disabled limb does indeed aid recovery of the use of that limb.

"There had been a great deal of intuitive belief that this works, but until now there was no objective evidence," said Neville Hogan, principal investigator for the work and an MIT professor with dual appointments in mechanical engineering and brain and cognitive sciences.

The work was reported in the March 1998 IEEE Transactions on Rehabilitation Engineering and in a 1997 issue of the *Archives of Neurology*. Professor Hogan's colleagues are Hermano I. Krebs, a research scientist in mechanical engineering, and Drs. Mindy L. Aisen (SB '76), Fletcher H. McDowell and Bruce T. Volpe of the Burke Rehabilitation Center in White Plains, New York. The first clinical trial was held at Burke, and a second, larger trial is currently underway.

To use the robot—named MIT-Manus for the link between its therapeutic focus and MITs motto "mens et manus," or mind and hand—a person sitting at a table puts the lower arm and wrist into a brace that is in turn attached to the "arm" of the robot. With "hand over hand" instruction, a therapist then physically guides the patient through a given exercise. The machine "goes along for the ride" and records the session.

MIT-Manus can then reproduce the exercise and guide the patient through it. And as the patient begins to recover and starts to initiate some movement on his or her own, the robot can measure how much force the patient is applying and adjust the amount of resistance it provides.

All exercises are also visually guided. "Video games provide the visual feedback and constitute a key motivational aspect." Dr. Krebs said. The computer screen on which the games appear sits on the table in front of the patient.

In the first clinical trial, which lasted slightly over a year, two groups of 10 stroke patients received standard therapy. People in the experimental group received an additional daily hour of robot-aided therapy. The others received "sham" robot therapy once a week: they were exposed to the robot but it didn't guide them through exercises. (They moved the robot manually, using their good arm to guide the disabled arm to play the video games.) As a result, the experimental group received many more manipulations.

Although the results of the trial are encouraging, the group size was small. The researchers are therefore conducting a larger trial with 60 patients that should conclude in August of 1998. Among other things, "we want to confirm that the extra therapy [with MIT-Manus] genuinely leads to increased recovery," said Dr. Aisen.

The researchers envision many applications for MIT-Manus. For example, "I think it could assist a therapist by performing repetitive exercises," Dr. Aisen said. "If human therapists were free from the more tedious end of therapy, they could focus on more difficult problems such as training people to get in and out of a car or access a computer—things the robot can't do."

MIT-Manus can also "precisely standardize the therapy delivered, potentially providing a graded exercise program that adjusts to patient response on a continuous basis," the researchers write in the Archives of Neurology.

The work was sponsored by the Burke Medical Research Foundation. *British Medical Journal*, May 10, 1997 Vol. 314, No. 7091, Pg. 1361(2).

Chapter 30

Home Modification and Repair

Home Modification and Repair includes adaptations to homes that can make it easier and safer to carry out activities such as bathing, cooking, and climbing stairs and alterations to the physical structure of the home to improve its overall safety and condition.

Why Is Home Modification and Repair Important?

Home modification and repair can help prevent accidents such as falls. Research suggests that one-third to one-half of home accidents can be prevented by modification and repair.

Home modification and repair can allow people to remain in their homes. Older people tend to live in older homes that often need repairs and modifications. Over 60% of older persons live in homes more than 20 years old. Home modification and repair can accommodate lifestyle changes and increase comfort.

How Can Home Modification and Repairs Promote Independence and Prevent Accidents?

Typical Problems:

- Difficulty getting in and out of the shower

- Slipping in the tub or shower
- Difficulty turning faucet handles/doorknobs
- Access to home
- Inadequate heating or ventilation
- Problems climbing stairs

Possible Solutions:

- Install grab bars, shower seals or transfer benches
- Place non-skid strips or decals in the tub or shower
- Replace with lever handles
- Install ramps
- Install insulation, storm windows and air conditioning
- Install handrails for support

Financial Assistance

Some home modification and repair programs make loans or provide services free of charge or at reduced rates for eligible older people. For more information, contact:

- Farmers Home Administration: Various grants and loans are available for rural, low-income elders.
- Local Community Development Department: Many cities and towns use Community Development Block Grants to help citizens maintain and upgrade their homes.
- Local Welfare or Energy Department: Two programs from the Low-Income Home Energy Assistance Program (LIHEAP) and the Weatherization Assistance Program (WAP) of the U.S. Department of Energy, provide funds to weatherize the homes of lower income persons.
- Physician or Health Care Provider: Funds from Medicare and Medicaid are available for durable medical equipment with a doctor's prescription.
- Local Area Agency on Aging: Funds from the Older Americans Act Title III often can be used to modify and repair homes.
- Local Lenders and Banks: Some lenders offer Home Equity Conversion Mortgages (HECMs) that allow homeowners to turn

the value of theft home into cash, without having to move or make regular loan payments.

Good News for Renters

The Fair Housing Act of 1988 Section 6(a) makes it illegal for landlords to refuse to let tenants make reasonable modifications to their house or apartment if the tenant is willing to pay for the changes. The law also requires new construction of dwellings with four or more units to include features such as wheelchair accessibility, reinforced walls to accommodate later installation of grab bars in bathrooms, and accessible electrical outlets and thermostats.

Where to Get Help

There are several ways to modify and repair your home. You can: 1) do it yourself, or get a friend or relative to help; 2) hire a handyman or contractor; 3) contact a home modification and repair program. Programs can be located through your Local Area Agency On Aging, State Agency On Aging, State Housing Finance Agency, Department of Public Welfare, Department Of Community Development, Senior Center or Independent Living Center.

Using a Contractor

If you need to use a contractor, make certain that the contractor is reliable. Older people are prime target for con artists and fraud. Be especially wary of door-to-door repair salespersons. Consider taking these steps:

- Get recommendations from friends who have had similar projects completed.

- Hire a licensed and bonded contractor. Be specific about the work which you want. Try to get bids from several contractors.

- Ask for references from previous customers and check out the references; try to see some of the contractor's completed projects.

- Insist on a written agreement, with only a small down payment. Have a trusted family member or friend read the agreement. Consider having the agreement reviewed by your lawyer if it is very complicated.

- Make the final payment only after the project is completed.

- Check with your local Better Business Bureau or your city/county Consumer Affairs Office regarding the contractors reliability and performance record.

Additional Information

Home Safety Guide for Older People: Check It Out/Fix It Up by Jon Pynoos and Evelyn Cohen Serif Press, Inc. 1331 H Street NW, Washington, DC 20005 For more information, call: (202) 737-4650 Price: $12.50

Safety for Older Consumers U.S. Consumer Product Safety Commission Washington, D.C. 20207 For more information, call: 1- 800-638-2772 Price: Free

The DoAble Renewable Home: Making Your Home Fit Your Needs (D12470) AARP Fulfillment, Consumer Affairs 601 E Street, NW, Washington, D.C. 20049 For more information, call: (202) 972-4700 Price: Free (single copies).

Eldercare Locator: For information about services to the elderly, call 1-800-677-1116.

Chapter 31

Assistive Listening Devices

What are Assistive Listening Devices?

Like a hearing aid, an assistive listening device makes sounds louder. Typically, a hearing aid makes all sounds in the environment louder. An assistive listening device can increase the loudness of a desired sound (a radio or television, a public speaker, an actor or actress, someone talking in a noisy place) without increasing the loudness of the background noises.

Are Assistive Listening Devices Only for People with Hearing Aids?

No. People with all degrees and types of hearing loss-even people with normal hearing-can benefit from assistive listening devices. Some assistive listening devices are used with a hearing aid. Some can be used without a hearing aid.

What Kinds of Assistive Listening Devices are Available?

There are many assistive listening devices available today, from sophisticated systems used in theaters and auditoriums to small personal systems. Various kinds of assistive listening devices are listed below.

- *Personal Listening Systems:* There are several types of personal listening systems available. All are designed to carry sound from the speaker (or other source) directly to the listener and to minimize or eliminate environmental noises. Some of these systems, such as auditory trainers, are designed for classroom or small group use. Others, such as personal FM systems and personal amplifiers, are especially helpful for one-to-one conversations in places such as automobiles, meeting rooms, and restaurants.

- *TV Listening Systems:* are designed for listening to TV, radio, or stereo without interference from surrounding noise or the need to use very high volume. Models are available for use with or without hearing aids.

- *Direct Audio Input Hearing Aids:* are hearing aids with audio input connections which can be connected to TV, stereo, tape, and radio as well as to microphones, auditory trainers, personal FM systems and other assistive devices.

- *Telephone Amplifying Devices:* Many, but not all, standard telephone receivers come with an amplifying coil. This coil is activated when the telephone receiver is picked up by a person whose hearing aid is in the "T" position. This position allows the aid to be used at a comfortable volume without feedback and with minimal background noise. These phones are called "hearing-aid compatible," and you should be able to get one from your telephone company. Not all hearing aids have a "T" switch so make sure that your aid has one before asking for a hearing aid compatible phone. In addition there are specially designed telephone receivers which amplify sound. Or, special amplifying devices can be purchased that attach to a regular telephone receiver. Most of these devices have volume control dials. Some are recommended only for use where all household members have hearing loss. Some return to standard sound levels automatically and can be used in homes for people with or without hearing loss.

- *Auditorium Type Assistive Listening Systems:* Many major auditoriums and theaters, churches, synagogues, and other public places are equipped with special sound systems for people with hearing loss. Essentially, they consist of a transmitting system which uses one of a variety of method to send sound signals to an individual receiver. (Sometimes there is a rental fee for the receiver.) Some systems must be used with a hearing aid; other systems can be used with or without a hearing aid.

Where Can I Find an Assistive Listening Device?

If you are considering assistive listening devices for personal use, such as personal FM systems and personal amplifiers, you should seek the help of an audiologist who has expertise in working with assistive listening devices to determine which device is best for you. An audiologist is a professional specially trained to identify and help people with hearing problems. The audiologist you select should hold a Certificate of Clinical Competence (CCC) in Audiology from the American Speech-Language-Hearing Association (ASHA). In many states a license is also required. For further information about assistive devices, including:

- Lists of certified audiologists in your area,

- Lists of assistive listening device "showrooms" in the United States

- Information about TTYs, Telecaption Decoders, and signaling/ alerting devices,

- Other information about assistive listening devices, contact ASHA and ask for our ALD packet (single copy free).

American Speech-Language-Hearing Association
10801 Rockville Pike
Rockville, MD 20852
800-638-8255 (Voice or TTY)
301-897-5700 (voice or TTY)
301-571-0457 Fax
E-Mail: irc@asha.org
http://www.asha.org

Part Four

The Role of Family in the Rehabilitation Process

Chapter 32

The Role of Family in Rehabilitation

A wife may help her spinal-cord-injured husband to prevent the development of pressure sores. A husband may join his arthritic wife in her daily exercise and ambulation routine.

Often rehabilitation counselors must consider ways to involve the family in a client's rehabilitation, and must decide whether the family will aid or hinder the client's rehabilitation process. Traditionally, research on disability and rehabilitation has centered around the client's medical treatment, which has had little or no family involvement and the effect on the client's disability on the family. In short, attention has focused on the disability's effect on the family, rather than the family's effect on rehabilitation.

This traditional pattern is changing, partly because of economics. Family care is much less expensive than long-term institutional care. And family reinforcement is essential to maintain rehabilitation gains after a patient is discharged from an institution.

It is also possible for a counselor to provide services to family members as part of a client's rehabilitation. The Rehabilitation Act of 1973, as amended, authorizes provision of services to members of a handicapped person's family when such services are necessary to the adjustment or rehabilitation of the handicapped individual. Thus the counselor can provide such services as group counseling to help the

1978 *Rehab Brief Bringing Research into Effective Focus,* Vol. I, No. 14, Sept. 15, 1978. Rehabilitation Services Administration, Office of Human Development Service, Department of Health, Education and Welfare, Washington, DC 20202. Despite the old date on this document, it contains information that families will still find helpful.

family adjust to the disability and aid in rehabilitation of a family member.

However, relatively little research has been done to show the family's effectiveness in assisting a client's rehabilitation. The research that is available indicates that a client's family can aid rehabilitation by assisting treatment and by reinforcing the client's rehabilitative behavior.

Spouse Stress Reaction

If the family is to provide support and reinforce rehabilitative gains, it must first be there. It is imperative that the family not disintegrate from the stress of dealing with the disability. Therefore, considerable research has focused on the spouse stress reaction to disability.

Several studies point out different sources of stress experienced by spouses of disabled persons. Frequently, stress is a result of the progressive or unpredictable nature of a client's disability. However, sometimes stress is the result of poor communication between the spouse and the client's physician, who may not explain clearly to the spouse the nature of the disability and any home-care instructions. The stress surely will be family's financial support and now leaves the spouse intensified if the disabled person had been providing them with financial and home responsibilities, plus the burden of caring for the disabled spouse.

Research concludes that most spouses are able to adjust to this increased stress. A number of studies suggest that the quality of marital interactions prior to disability is, in most cases, a better predictor of spouse adjustment to a disability than is the nature of the disability itself.

The Family in a Supportive Role

A follow-up study of inpatients from the Spain Rehabilitation Center in Birmingham, Alabama, documented the patients' perception of the importance of the family in the daily adjustment of severely disabled persons. The study assessed the status of former patients in physical, social, psychological, and vocational areas.

Results of the study showed that the former patients were "moderately successful" using a ten-variable operational definition of success, and that the degree of success was related to the patient's age, medical diagnosis, and environmental factors outside the hospital.

The study found that the significant characteristics of the successful group seemed to be associated with the patient's perception of the family's response to his or her condition in addition to such other factors as medical diagnosis, vocational status, services the patient received in the community, and the patient's own perception of his or her limitations.

Another study examined the relationship between spouse companionship support and the degree of vocational rehabilitation success of the handicapped spouse. The study used a sample of all persons who had received service during a 2-year period through the vocational rehabilitation program of the Cedar Rapids District, Iowa Division of Vocational Rehabilitation.

Results of the study supported the hypotheses that the greater the degree of "dubious" support from the spouse, the less the employment success of the handicapped person. Ironically, according to this study, "dubious" support is given by the spouse who is much concerned about the handicapped spouse, who frequently talks about goals and plans, or who frequently encourages the handicapped spouse in his or her work. The findings suggest that what at first may appear to be the spouse's very active encouragement of vocational activity may actually be care and concern that expresses the spouse's anxiety about the disability. The study did not deal with other factors that might have caused both dubious support and lack of employment success, such as a progressive or terminal illness.

Family Communication Skills

A study by the West Virginia Rehabilitation Research and Training Center examined specific factors related to communication and conflict in families of vocational rehabilitation clients. The study used separate simultaneous interviews with 150 clients and a significant other (family member).

The most pervasive finding of the study was that clients reported more discussion of their problems and more agreement with significant others than the reported with clients. Researchers for this project feel that the prospect of long-term disabling conditions and the accompanying disruptive influence on the family may create a climate for competing or conflicting expectations. The client's feelings that he or she has successfully communicated problems and beliefs are not shared by the significant other. This apparent disagreement may indicate that the family does not usually possess the communication skills required for full family support in the rehabilitation process.

247

Rehabilitation of the Family

If the family is to play a role in the rehabilitation of a client, then the family must be prepared for that role.

A demonstration project in family rehabilitation worked with disabled, rural, poor farm workers and migrants of south-central Arizona. Supported by the Ford Foundation, Arizona's Job College's Family Rehabilitation Project in Casa Grande provided a residential vocational and educational program for up to 120 families at a time. The entire family lived in project facilities an average of one year, during which the disabled client and spouse received rehabilitation services in an individualized plan. Children participated in school or day care activities.

The results of this demonstration show, for many clients, a wide range of job placement, improved job retention, durability of rehabilitation gains, sizeable increases in family income levels, and substantial improvement in family, social, and community participation. The families' children had improved school grades, health, and nutrition.

Implications for Rehabilitation Counselors

- This BRIEF has not attempted to address the complex nature of family relationships and the bearing of such complexities on the family's role in rehabilitation. The counselor will need to consider these complexities when deciding what role of the family to encourage in the rehabilitation of a client.

- The counselor may need to consider providing services to improve marital interaction of couples whose marriages have been impaired by the occurrence of a disability.

- The counselor may be able to clarify physician instructions and thereby relieve stress caused by poor communication between the family and the client's physician or other health care personnel.

- If time is available, counselors can conduct a separate interview with the client's significant other to establish common ground for joint and family counseling. Such counseling can serve to decrease anger or disappointment and to facilitate constructive discussion of problems and misconceptions.

- The counselor may set up supportive services, such as support groups for spouses that may be of particular help to two groups of spouses. Spouses of clients with a sudden onset disability, such as a heart attack, continue to experience particular stress for as long as a year. Spouses of clients with progressive, deteriorative disabilities may experience increasing stress as the client's condition worsens.

- Through counseling with key family members or securing counseling services for them, the counselor may be able to influence the family's reaction to the client's condition in a way which leads to acceptance and support, rather than rejection.

- The counselor can caution the family to avoid communicating excessive concern about the disability to the client and to encourage the client to be as independent as possible.

- The counselor may need to help secure direct services for the spouse and other family members or both in order to keep the family intact.

- With the cooperation and guidance of the client's physician, the counselor can encourage the client's family to provide many types of home treatment assistance that will augment the client's rehabilitation progress. The counselor can also teach the family ways to reinforce rehabilitation gains of the client.

Much of this BRIEF was based on a literature review paper prepared by Kathleen Shea Abrams, a doctoral candidate in the Department of Clinical Psychology, University of Florida.

Chapter 33

Caring for the Caregiver

In spite of the growing attention focused on assisted living, nursing homes, and other care for people with chronic illness and problems related to aging, about 80 percent of late-life care is provided by unpaid family members. About 7 million elderly are receiving regular care.

Many who assist the ill or elderly don't think of themselves as caregivers, particularly if they are employed or don't live with the person they are helping. What they also do not recognize is the stress the additional concerns and responsibilities may be adding to their lives.

Are You a Candidate for Caregiver Stress?

- Do you frequently call or visit an older relative just to make sure the person is all right?

- Do you coordinate with your siblings to help your parents with everyday tasks?

- Do you awaken in the night to help your spouse take medication?

- Do you arrange your schedule to fit in with your parent's doctor appointments?

The quality of life for both the caregiver and the person receiving care can be improved by taking advantage of available community resources.

© American Occupational Therapy Association, Inc., 4720 Montgomery Lane, Bethesda, MD, 20814-3425, undated; reprinted with permission.

Finding Assistance

People take on the role of caregiver with varying definitions of responsibility and perceptions of the needs of the person receiving care. It is extremely helpful to have the assistance of a health professional in understanding the course and effects of a particular condition or disease.

Ask an Occupational Therapist

How much direct help does the person really need?

It is not always easy for the individual receiving care or the caregiver to decide which daily tasks a person is able to perform or should be encouraged to do.

The occupational therapist can provide important information based upon health status, abilities, interest, and the person's environment.

Is there equipment to help the person manage more tasks on his or her own?

Simple devices can help people to bathe, dress, eat, prepare meals, and manage other tasks when they must deal with weakness, poor grasp, using a wheelchair or walker, and other problems. The therapist can identify equipment for the individual's needs, recommend sources of supply, and help the person learn to use the items.

Can the home be made safer and more convenient for the individual and the caregiver?

The occupational therapist can make recommendations for adapting or modifying furniture and other items in the home to improve the daily routine and make the environment safer for the individual and the caregiver.

Caregivers can also learn safe techniques for moving or assisting the person for whom they are caring.

How can daily life in the home better meet the needs of family members?

Although the effects of illness on a person's behavior will vary, an occupational therapist can help develop a routine built on the person's abilities and interests and the caregiver's strengths and needs. For example, if the person needing care insists on dressing independently, he or she may spend a great deal of time at this task. On the other hand, he or she may find eating to be difficult and welcome or require assistance.

How can the caregiver find assistance for an adult who cannot be left alone in the home?

Contact the local Area Agency on Aging, ask your physician, ask your clergy, check with your local library, call a local nursing home. Various respite care programs have volunteers who will spend an hour or two with your family member so you can run errands, take care of your health, or just get a break. Some nursing homes also offer temporary care for a price, so an individual or family can travel or relax at home.

Adult daycare programs, many with transportation, provide meals and activities for those in fairly good health needing supervision but not nursing care.

Dealing with the Emotional Stress of Caregiving

Being ill and unable to control your life can be a frightening experience. Dependence and illness can have profound effects upon relationships.

Talk with the individual's doctor and yours to make sure you understand the effects of particular health problems.

Spouses and family members find important help for their concerns in support groups as do people with similar health problems such as stroke, diabetes, multiple sclerosis, etc. Many such groups are available in hospitals and health care facilities. Caregivers are also finding information and support through websites and list servers on the Internet.

Mental health problems such as depression can complicate caregiving for the person with illness and the caregiver. Report feelings of hopelessness, helplessness, avoidance, and changes from familiar patterns of behavior to the primary physician. The caregiver may also find professional counseling helpful in coping with stresses.

The purpose of this fact sheet is not to offer medical advice. To discuss your particular problem or condition, contact your primary physician. Information may be reproduced for purposes of education.

Resources

Eldercare Locator—nationwide assistance to help older persons and caregivers locate community resources. 1-800-677-1166, Monday-Friday, 9 am-11 pm EST.

The Area Agency on Aging located in every community, provides information on local resources for older adults. Check the telephone book or call the Eldercare Locator.

American Association of Retired Persons Caregiver Resource Kit, free, #D15267. Order from AARP Fulfillment, 601 E Street NW, Washington, DC 20049.

Chapter 34

Help for Family and Friends of the Individual with Brain Injury

Even a mild brain injury may have significant health consequences including fatigue, decreased information processing, and difficulties with attention, short-term and long-term memory, headache, sleep disturbance, dizziness, anxiety, depression, irritability, changes in sex drive, and personality change. Most people with a mild brain injury have a good prognosis, although the process of recovery may take many months.

Different types of problems may follow moderate to severe brain injury.

Confusion

Early in recovery the individual may be confused or disoriented. Redirect the confused person away from what is agitating him or her rather than attempt to persuade him or her out of being agitated. It is often helpful to restructure the person's surroundings to reduce noise level and visual stimulation.

Communication Difficulties

Following brain injury, some people find it difficult to control the muscles involved in breathing and speaking. Some have slow and hesitant speech or may be able to say words easily without making sense. Seek guidance from the rehabilitation team in communicating with the person with a brain injury.

Sensory Disturbances

A person with brain injury may lose sensation in parts of the body or may be more sensitive to certain sensations.

Visual problems may include double vision, inability to see things on one side of the body, or lack of visual acuity.

Loss of smell and alternation in taste may cause those with brain injury to complain about the taste of food and refuse to eat.

Memory Problems

Short-term memory may not be affected by brain injury while the ability to transfer information into long-term memory is often impaired. The inability to remember new information for more than a few minutes may persist.

The occupational therapist can instruct the client in the use of memory aids, and reorder the person's living arrangements to reduce demand upon the impaired memory.

Psychiatric Disorders

Anxiety and depression may follow brain injury. Damage to parts of the brain and changes in brain chemistry following trauma, may make psychiatric disorders such as psychosis, obsessionality, mania, and paranoia more likely to occur. Seek assistance from a psychiatrist with experience in treating people with brain injury.

Alcoholism and Drug Abuse

For the person with brain injury, alcohol use increases the potential for seizures and impairs reasoning, judgment, and safety awareness. Because the injured person may be unable to control the impulse to drink, removing alcohol from easy access can help.

Denial of Symptoms

The person with brain injury may lack awareness of any change in personality or abilities. Helping can be difficult when the person cannot see limitations and becomes angry.

Treat all activities as a means of learning if the injured person can perform safely and effectively. Give immediate feedback. Discuss limitations in the context of brain injury and recovery.

Personalty Change

The person with a brain injury often becomes self-centered and loses the ability to provide the caring and nurturing required for a loving relationship. Others become emotionally reactive, anxious, and demanding.

Family members need to set rules for themselves and the injured person and stick to them. A support group can help the injured person to get impartial feedback on behavior and its impact on others.

Behavior Disorder

In the early stages of recovery, a person may be verbally and physically aggressive, irritable, and angry at imaginary or real slights. The family should be prepared to get help immediately if the situation appears dangerous. Avoid taking anger personally. Be specific and concrete about expectations. Get assistance and counseling for the injured person and the family.

Planning and Self-Control

Following a brain injury, a person may demonstrate impaired judgment such as awareness of an appointment but inability to manage transportation. Some may require 24-hour supervision. Others can make use of ongoing case management to live more independently.

Rehabilitation

Rehabilitation programs evaluate and treat cognitive, language, and behavioral problems that interfere with the individual's return to the community. Teaching clients to translate skills learned in the clinic into their real-life setting holds the best potential for long-term success.

Information taken from "Coping with Brain Injury—A Guide for Family and Friends," by Gordon Muir Giles, published by the American Occupational Therapy Association.

To purchase, call 301-652-2682 or write AOTA Products, P.O. Box 31220, Bethesda, MD 20824-1220.

The purpose of this fact sheet is not to offer medical advice. To discuss your particular problem or condition, contact your primary physician. Information may be reproduced for purposes of education.

Resources

Brain Injury Association Inc.
105 North Alfred Street
Alexandria, VA 22314
703-236-6000
703-236-6001 Fax
http://www.biausa.org

Part Five

Financial Considerations

Chapter 35

Managed Care's Effect on Physical Medicine and Rehabilitation

Physical medicine and rehabilitation (PM&R) faces a serious challenge from managed care, and physiatrists—PM&R physicians—must adapt their practices to new market conditions. Physiatrists' access to patients, clinical decision-making autonomy, reimbursement levels, and administrative burdens will all be affected by the changes in health care delivery sweeping the country. How physiatrists can deal with these changes proactively and turn them to their advantage is the subject of a 125-page monograph titled *Adapting to a Managed Care World: The Challenge for Physical Medicine and Rehabilitation*, developed as part of the PM&R Workforce Study commissioned by a coalition of four PM&R organizations including the American Academy of Physical Medicine and Rehabilitation (AAPM&R).

"The managed care monograph provides welcome insights for physiatrists, showing them what they must accomplish to stay abreast of rapidly moving developments in the modern health care era," said AAPM&R President Martin Grabois, MD. The monograph is the second of two products of the PM&R Workforce Study, the first being the PM&R Workforce Model, a valuable interactive mathematical model for assessing supply and demand implications for PM&R over the next 20 years.

In 1994, the AAPM&R, American Board of PM&R (ABPM&R), Association of Academic Physiatrists (AAP), and American Physiatric Education Council (APEC) contracted with Lewin-VHI of Fairfax,

Virginia, to estimate the need for physiatrists in the United States through the year 2005, as well as to assess whether physiatry will be a shortage or surplus specialty. This recently completed PM&R Workforce Study concluded that PM&R, while still a shortage specialty, must undertake a massive national education effort to enhance its visibility to payers, providers, and the public, or be subject to the same consequences as other specialties in today's cost-cutting climate.

The information in the monograph draws from interviews with approximately 50 physiatrists representing a variety of market and practice structures, interviews with payer representatives, and literature from professional associations and other sources. While the monograph does not summarize the results of a statistically valid survey, it does present the general effects of managed care on the practice of PM&R.

Adapting to a Managed Care World covers the following topics:

- An overview of managed care activity with specific focus on trends in managed care enrollment for patient groups that physiatrists most frequently treat, e.g., Medicare and workers' compensation

- An overview of managed care's impact on physiatry, including changes in the types of services provided, patients treated, and types of physiatric practices

- A discussion of practice contracting strategies that successful physiatrists have employed in highly penetrated managed care markets and

- Case studies and vignettes of managed care markets and physiatric practices across the country with an emphasis on the experiences of physiatrists in highly penetrated managed care markets and the lessons they have learned.

Appendices in the monograph include definitions of managed care and managed care models, a glossary of managed care terms, detailed HMO penetration and physiatrist supply tables, and cost-effectiveness and managed care bibliographies.

While the steadily increasing enrollment of the population into managed care presents tremendous uncertainty and vulnerability for physiatrists, the monograph concludes that managed care also presents a wide range of new opportunities. "Physiatrists who successfully convince case managers and primary care 'gatekeepers' of their cost-effectiveness will likely secure access to managed care referral streams. The outcome of these forces will shape the demand for PM&R specialists for decades to come."

Copies of *Adapting to a Managed Care World: The Challenge for Physical Medicine and Rehabilitation* are available from the AAPM&R National Office. The book costs $12 for AAPM&R and AAP members and $150 for non-members, and prices include shipping and handling. Please make your check or money order payable to AAPM&R, and mail to AAPM&R, One IBM Plaza, Suite 2500, Chicago, IL 60611-3604.

The AAPM&R is a national medical specialty society of more than 5,600 physiatrists (pronounced fizz ee a' trists or fizz eye' uh trists) whose patients include people with physical disabilities and chronic, disabling illnesses. These physical medicine and rehabilitation physicians diagnose and treat all impairing conditions secondary to disorders involving the neuromusculoskeletal system. Treatment used by physiatrists includes medical therapies, the use of injections, physical agents, and other interventions with the goals of minimizing pain, weakness, and numbness and restoring function.

For more information or referral to PM&R physician spokesperson, credentialed media and freelancers may contact John Wilson, director, marketing and communications, by phone at (312) 464-9700, fax at (312) 464-0227, website: http://www.aapmr.org.

Chapter 36

Social Security Administration—How Can We Help with Vocational Rehabilitation?

How Social Security Can Help with Vocational Rehabilitation

The Social Security Administration (SSA) can help people with disabilities get the vocational rehabilitation services they need to return to work or to go to work for the first time. We can put them in touch with agencies that provide services such as job counseling, training and job placement. SSA doesn't provide these services, but we can help pay for them when certain conditions are met.

We can continue to assist a person with a disability even after he or she goes to work. There are special provisions of the law, called work incentives, which help the individual to continue working. These work incentives allow us to continue cash payments and health insurance coverage even though the individual has returned to work.

This text provides more information about how SSA can help people with disabilities successfully return to work or go to work for the first time.

Referring People with Disabilities to State Vocational Rehabilitation Agencies

When a person files an application for disability benefits, specially trained employees at the state Disability Determination Services

U.S. Social Security Administration, SSA Publication No. 05-10050, June 1997, ICN 460280.

(DDS) office review the application to see whether the person's medical condition qualifies him or her for disability benefits. At the same time, they also evaluate the person's rehabilitation potential. If it appears that the person may benefit from vocational rehabilitation services, they refer the applicant to the state vocational rehabilitation agency.

SSA sends information about the applicant's medical condition and work history to the rehabilitation provider. Rehabilitation counselors evaluate this information. They may contact the person to obtain further information and may request that the individual come in for an interview.

At that time, the counselor will try to find out more about the person's interests and employment goals. Clients are given an opportunity to discuss how the counselor can work with them to achieve their job goals. If the counselor believes the vocational rehabilitation agency can provide the rehabilitation services that are needed, the counselor and client will jointly develop a written plan describing the job goal and the services the vocational rehabilitation agency will provide to reach that goal. This written plan is tailored to the needs of the client.

Use of Alternate Vocational Rehabilitation Service Providers

SSA first refers persons to the state vocational rehabilitation agency for consideration. If the state agency is unable to serve the individual, we may refer that individual to an alternate participant in our vocational rehabilitation program. An alternate participant is any nonstate public or private agency that is qualified to serve Social Security disability beneficiaries. Such providers must be licensed, certified or accredited to provide vocational rehabilitation services within their state and meet other requirements that assure us they can provide clients with the necessary help. SSA pays these alternate providers for the costs of their services under the same conditions that apply for state vocational rehabilitation agencies.

Paying Providers for Vocational Rehabilitation Services

The Social Security Act allows SSA to pay for vocational rehabilitation services they furnish to people receiving Social Security disability benefits or Supplemental Security Income (SSI) payments based on disability or blindness if certain conditions are met. The vocational rehabilitation services must result in the person's return to work for at least nine continuous months at a substantial earnings level. The earnings levels change from year to year. Check with your local Social Security office for current information.

Types of Vocational Rehabilitation Services

Vocational rehabilitation providers furnish a wide variety of services to help people with disabilities return to work. These services are designed to provide the client with the training or other services that are needed to return to work, to enter a new line of work or to enter the workforce for the first time. Examples of the types of services that may be offered by vocational rehabilitation providers include:

- various types of tests and assessments to evaluate the client's physical or mental condition, skills and abilities;
- counseling and guidance, including counseling to family members;
- wheelchairs, specially modified vans, prosthetics and other devices to help restore the individual's availability to work;
- training;
- transportation;
- job placement;
- post-placement services; and
- other goods and services necessary to achieve the planned job goals of the person's rehabilitation program.

Refusal to Accept Rehabilitation Services

Most people with disabilities want to work and will cooperate with the rehabilitation provider during the course of their rehabilitation program. However, the law provides for the suspension of Social Security benefits if a person fails to cooperate with the rehabilitation agency without a good reason for doing so. If a rehabilitation provider offers services to a person with a disability, the person must accept the services to continue receiving Social Security benefits unless we determine that there is a good reason for not accepting services.

Benefits While Participating in a Vocational Rehabilitation Program

A person who medically recovers while participating in an approved rehabilitation or training program may continue to receive benefits until the vocational rehabilitation program ends if SSA finds that the program is likely to help the individual become self-supporting. This continuation of benefits is available to persons who participate in either an approved state or private vocational rehabilitation program.

Social Security Work Incentives

Once a person with a disability has returned to work, special rules called "work incentives" will help serve as a bridge from reliance on benefits to financial independence achieved by returning to work. With these incentives, the individual can continue to receive cash payments and health insurance coverage (for a period of time) until he or she is able to work regularly.

There are different work incentives for persons who receive Social Security disability and SSI benefits. There are also special work incentives for persons who are blind and for students with disabilities. The purpose of all of these work incentives is to provide support and assistance to people with disabilities while they attempt to work.

Some of the ways that these incentives help people with disabilities to work is by allowing them to:

- test the ability to work for a specified period of time without losing any benefits;

- deduct from earnings the cost of certain impairment-related work items or services needed to work in determining whether earnings are too high to continue receiving benefits;

- continue Medicare coverage if disability benefits stop because earnings are too high;

- continue to receive SSI payments until the earnings we count exceed the SSI limits; and

- continue Medicaid coverage if the person depends on Medicaid to work even if earnings exceed the SSI limits until the person's earnings are sufficient to replace lost benefits.

For More Information

Persons with a disability who want to work do not have to be referred to a rehabilitation agency or wait for an agency to contact them. They may contact the rehabilitation agency in their state directly at any time. Your Social Security office will be glad to provide the location and phone number of the nearest office of the state vocational rehabilitation agency. Individuals then can let the agency know of their interest in receiving rehabilitation services to help them return to work. The address and phone number of the state vocational rehabilitation agency also can be found in the phone book.

For more information about how work may affect disability benefits, call or visit any Social Security office. You may wish to ask for our publication *Working While Disabled—How We Can Help* (SSA Publication No. 05-10095) or *If You Are Blind—How We Can Help* (SSA Publication No. 05-10052). You can find the address and phone number of your local Social Security office in your phone book. You also can call our toll-free number, 1-800-772-1213, between 7 a.m. and 7 p.m. any business day.

People who are deaf or hard of hearing may call our toll-free "TTY" number, 1-800-325-0778, between 7 a.m. and 7 p.m. business days.

Chapter 37

Medicaid Services

Rehabilitation Services

Rehabilitation services are an optional Medicaid benefit that must be recommended by a physician or other licensed practitioner of the healing arts, within the scope of practice under State law, for the maximum reduction of a physical or mental disability and to restore the individual to the best possible functional level. The services may be provided in any setting and generally include mental health services such as individual and group therapies and psychosocial services. In addition, States also provide services aimed at improving physical functional abilities, including physical, occupational and speech therapies.

Contact:
Linda Peltz (410) 786-3399 or lpeltz@hcfa.gov.

Physical Therapy, Occupational Therapy, and Services for Individuals with Speech, Hearing and Language Disorders

All of these services are optional Medicaid services States may choose to provide. Physical therapy services are prescribed by a physician or other licensed practitioner of the healing arts within the scope of his or her practice under State law and provided to a recipient by

1998 Health Care Financing Administration.

or under the direction of a qualified physical therapist. Included are any necessary supplies and equipment.

Occupational therapy services are prescribed by a physician or other licensed practitioner of the healing arts within the scope of his or her practice under State law and provided to a recipient by or under the direction of a qualified occupational therapist. Included are any necessary supplies and equipment.

Services for individuals with speech, hearing, and language disorders means diagnostic, screening, preventive, or corrective services provided by or under the direction of a speech pathologist or audiologist, for which a patient is referred by a physician or other licensed practitioner of the healing arts within the scope of his or her practice under State law. Included are any necessary supplies and equipment.

Qualifications for providers of physical therapy, occupational therapy and services for individuals with speech, hearing, and language disorders, are specified in Federal regulations.

Contact:
(410) 786-3399 or lpeltz@hcfa.gov.

Home Health Services

Home health services are a mandatory benefit for individuals who are entitled to nursing facility services under the State's Medicaid plan. Services must be provided at a recipient's place of residence, and must be ordered by a physician as part of a plan of care that the physician reviews every sixty days. Home health services must include nursing services, as defined in the State's Nurse Practice Act, that are provided on a part-time or intermittent basis by a home health agency, home health aide services provided by a home health agency, and medical supplies, equipment, and appliances suitable for use in the home. Physical therapy, occupational therapy, speech pathology, and audiology services are optional services that States may choose to provide.

To participate in the Medicaid program, a home health agency must meet the conditions of participation for Medicare.

Contact:
(410) 786-5921 or wcoons@hcfa.gov

Part Six

Common Disorders and Specific Issues in Rehabilitation

Chapter 38

After the Traumatic Injury

Let's face it, sports can be a blast. But an injury? Well, that's another story. Not only can an injury be painful, but having to put your active life on hold while recuperating is no fun at all. Yet, doctors, physical therapists, and trainers all agree it is very important to allow enough time for an injury to heal properly before returning to physical activities.

Athletes anxious to get back into the game risk further and/or worse damage to the injured area when they become too impatient for the healing process to complete its course. According to Dr. Craig Young, primary care team doctor for the Milwaukee Brewers and the Milwaukee Ballet Company, if an injured person returns to the activity too soon, that person risks permanent damage. In an athlete's case, that can ruin a career. Not only do injured athletes miss the season, but everyday movements they take for granted can become very painful. For example, a knee injury can make ordinary movements such as walking, getting up, or sitting down sheer torture; tendinitis or tennis elbow can make turning a doorknob or holding a toothbrush a painful procedure; and a rotator cuff injury in the shoulder can make getting dressed a real chore, especially when putting on anything with sleeves.

The one good thing about pain is that it is your body's way of telling you something—like "Lay off!" Here is an example of what happened to Roger Jackson when he didn't listen to his body's message.

Not Knowing When Enough Is Enough

Roger was on a spring skiing trip with his senior class in Winter Park, Colorado, when the edge of his ski caught an icy patch and he toppled over. He was going pretty fast and took a hard spill. All 200 pounds of him landed shoulder first on the ice—well, it seemed that way. Roger knew he fell hard, but he was amazed that his legs felt fine, all things considered. So he got up and decided to finish the run.

He felt a little shaken and there was pain in his right shoulder. He was relieved his legs were OK, and so he continued skiing. However, each time he planted his poles, he saw stars. Well, it was only the second day of his ski trip, and he didn't want to miss a thing, so he kept skiing. His fall had weakened him, and he noticed his skiing wasn't up to par, but he kept on going. Because he wasn't skiing well, he took some more falls. Some falls were minor, but he wiped out on a few—several times hitting his injured shoulder.

Back Home

When he got home, he was a mess. He could no longer play tennis, baseball, or basketball. He couldn't even drive. Turning the steering wheel, combing his hair, putting on a sweater were all painful chores.

His doctor told him he had a rotator cuff injury and recommended physical therapy to strengthen the muscles around the joint. Although Roger had lifted weights before his accident, he was surprised to learn he would be using "wimpy small weights" while working with the physical therapist. "There is a fine line between building strength and overdoing," the therapist said. "People have to be very careful when rehabbing to use weights light enough so that they don't reinjure themselves. When you are in a weakened state is when you are most vulnerable to injury. And the reinjury can prove to be worse than the first one."

Beginning Rehab

Roger began rehabilitating his shoulder by lying face down with his right arm dangling over the therapist's table. He lifted his arm slowly and held it parallel to the floor for 10 counts, then repeated the motion five times. He did this with his arm held out in front, out to the side, and extended back. When his shoulder got stronger, he was given a half-pound weight to hold as he did his lifts. He gradually built up to a 2-pound weight. This came as quite a surprise to someone who could previously bench-press 200 pounds.

Next he used rubber tubing and pulleys to add to his strengthening and increase his range of motion. Roger was told to repeat the routine at home five times each day. Because he stuck to a gradual rehab program, Roger made a successful recovery.

Soreness Is OK, But Not Pain

Physical therapist Peter McMenamin says, "How much weight to use and the amount of resistance is really critical when recovering from an injury. Rehab is the time to start challenging the tissue." You start working and building up the muscles gradually to avoid further injury.

The other key thing to remember about rehabilitation is making sure you don't over-stress the tissue. "Sharp pain must be avoided. Load the tissue step by step in order to promote strengthening, but don't overwhelm it. Sharp pain means you are overwhelming the tissue." Frequent movement, proper stretching, and light loads are emphasized in recovery. McMenamin warns that recovering injuries should be supervised by a physical therapist—or in a team sport, by a certified athletic trainer, not a health club trainer. "Health club trainers are taught to work with healthy populations."

You Can Still Work Out

Don't worry; you don't have to turn into a couch potato while recovering from an injury. On the contrary, Dr. Young advises injured folks to work the uninjured areas so they won't get weak. "Maintain cardiovascular fitness, strength, and flexibility in the uninjured body areas, so that you won't get injured when you start back," he says. If you don't, you'll be weak. It is when you are weak that the chances of injury become greater.

Proper recovery is especially important during your teen years. McMenamin stresses the need for proper diagnosis and gradual rehabilitation during these years of growth. Because the growth plate (a zone of new cartilage near the end of each bone, where new bone cells are laid down to make the bone longer) is soft, it can fracture easily. "A fracture through the growth plate will not necessarily be seen on X-rays. If it is not detected, it can result in malformation during remaining growth years, especially under age 16." The patience you exercise after an injury and during rehabilitation can make the difference between a complete and successful recovery and a lifetime of limitations.

What to Do When the Cast Comes Off

When a bone is fractured, the first priority is to stabilize and protect the injured area. This is best done by wearing a cast. The treatment, however, doesn't stop there. Once the cast is removed, rehab begins.

Anyone who has been in a cast for an extended period of time knows how weird it feels when the cast comes off. The area where the cast was worn feels weak and stiff, and the skin doesn't look too good at first.

Here are some helpful suggestions from Dr. Craig Young, medical director of sports medicine at the Medical College of Wisconsin:

- When a cast is removed, there is a loss of flexibility, because the joint was held in one position for a long period of time. That is why a person experiences a stiff feeling in that area. It is important to work on range-of-motion exercises, flexibility, and strengthening. For example, when rehabilitating a broken wrist after the cast is removed, a good way to alleviate stiffness and increase the range of motion would be to extend the arm out in front, thumb up, bend the wrist turning the hand inward, then bring the hand to center; slowly repeat several times, each time working on increasing the movement. Next, with the arm extended in front, thumb up, move the hand outward, come back to center, and repeat. Then with the arm extended in front and the thumb up again, bend the wrist moving the hand downward, bring the hand in a center position, then bend the hand upward, also gently trying to increase the range of motion. Gentle stretching is important.

- It also is a good idea to do isometric exercises (pushing against an immobile object) to bring back strength to the area. Isometrics is a good way to fire up the muscle and regain strength.

— by Phyllis Gerstein

278

For More Information

American Physical Therapy Association
1111 North Fairfax Street
Alexandria, VA 22314
703-684-APTA
703-684-7343 Fax
http://www.apta.org
Pamphlet: *"Taking Care of Your Knees,"* single copy free with a self-addressed, stamped business-size envelope.

American Running & Fitness Association
4405 East West Highway, Suite 405
Bethesda, MD 20814
301-913-9517
800-776-ARFA
301-913-9520 Fax
http://www.arfa.org
Pamphlets: *"Stress Fractures," "Running Injuries,"* single copy of each free with self-addressed, stamped business-size envelope.

American Academy of Orthopaedic Surgeons
6300 N. River Road
Rosemont, IL 60018-4262
847-823-7186
800-346-AAOS
847-823-8125 Fax
E-mail: webhelp@aaos.org
http://www.aaos.org
Pamphlets: *"Sprains and Strains," "Shoulder Pain," "Fractures,"* single copy of each free with self-addressed, stamped business-size envelope. Include pamphlet name on envelope request.

Chapter 39

Rehabilitation Process of Persons with Spinal Cord Injury

Spinal cord injury (SCI) can occur at any time to any individual. Acute SCI is an unexpected event that can result from a fall or a car accident, no matter how minor. It can occur from diving into too shallow water, or it can occur because of a wrong move during a sports event, and it often persists for the lifetime of the person who acquires it. Young, Burns, Bowen, and McCutchen (1982) point out that most spinal cord injuries occur predominantly in younger people, with the most common age being 19, and that fifty percent of all injuries occur to individuals under the age of 25. Though young age is not a determining factor in acquiring an SCI. It can also occur during birth, or from a fall at age one hundred and one. Although over eighty percent of SCI persons in the United States are young men in the prime productive years of their lives, they come from all races, places, ages, occupations, educations and income brackets (Corbet, 1985). An SCI plays no favorites and it may even be a result from disease (Chronic SCI).

According to the *New England Journal of Medicine* (1991) the incidence of acute spinal cord injury in the United States today is about 10,000 per year. With the latest advances in medical treatment and technology, less than 10 percent of these persons die following their injury, as compared to years ago.

Once an injury to the cord has occurred, whether the result of an accident or chronic illness, and a person develops paralysis, there are certain steps that need to be taken in relation to the rehabilitation of the person. This rehabilitation will enable the SCI person to return to the environment of social and vocational functioning as best as can be managed. It should be mentioned here that not all spinal cord injuries result in extensive rehabilitation, though for the purpose of the present paper I will be focusing on those who do need extensive rehabilitation to enable them to return to the community following their injury and be productive members of society.

Before returning to the world outside the rehabilitation center, however, the SCI patient must learn a number of things to aid them in this enormous step towards independence.

One of the first experiences one has after an SCI are emotional in nature. No two people experience the exact same feelings following a spinal injury. What the SCI person feels is totally unique to them. Some feel stunned after their injury, as if what was happening to them was not real. Other people are actually happy after their accident for the main reasons that they are still alive and still have their mental faculties intact.

During the initial phase of rehabilitation the strongest emphasis is on the SCI patient regaining as much strength and movement as is possible in either their arms and/or legs, depending on the locality and severity of their injury. A full understanding of SCI and what it entails is another factor to be learned during the beginning stages of rehabilitation.

In order to understand the effects of SCI, it is important to first understand the structure of the spine and spinal cord. The hard bony frame located from the base of the neck to the tail bone is called the spine, which is divided into segments called vertebrae. The vertebrae make up the spinal column by joining each other from end to end. It is within the spinal column that the spinal cord is enclosed. The spinal cord connects to the base of the brain and runs down the spinal column to the first lumbar vertebrae. The very end of the spinal cord contains a group of nerves called the Cauda Equina. The two major functions of the spinal cord are to carry nerve messages to and from the brain and body, and to carry nerve messages within the cord itself. These nerve messages are responsible for motor movement and sensation. (Harmarville Rehabilitation Center, Inc. (1983).

An injury to the upper spine, in the cervical vertebrae's of 1 through 8 results in quadriplegia, while an injury from the first thoracic vertebrae or lower results in paraplegia.

Once a person acquires a spinal cord injury, extensive rehabilitation is needed in order to return that person to their optimal functioning. Cull and Hardy (1977) say that the two most important areas of function for the SCI person are in mobility and transportation and in communication. Mobility and transportation refer to the patient's ability to move about freely in their immediate surroundings. To do this the patient would have to be able to be independent in mobility. For the SCI patient this can only be done with the assistance of devices such as a walker, leg braces, or in most cases a wheelchair, depending on the severity of their injury. Communication skills for the SCI patient, i.e., writing, typing, reading, and using the telephone can be accomplished by using adaptive devices. For example, a splint which fits over the fingers on the hand will enable the SCI person to hold a pencil in which to write with.

Other types of rehabilitation include physical, and occupational therapy. Physical therapy includes an exercise program geared toward muscle strengthening, while occupational therapy involves the redevelopment of fine motor skills.

During the rehabilitation process bladder and bowel management programs are also initiated. Because the bladder and bowel functions are located in the Sacral region of the spinal cord, below the level of injury in both quadriplegia and paraplegia, control of these functions are lost after injury (Hanak and Scott, 1983). Therefore, to avoid complications, a strict regimen is applied to control of these areas in order to ensure proper emptying at appropriate times.

As with any type of physical injury, medications are needed to keep such systems regulated and for preventive measures of other conditions brought about from the initial injury.

For the spinal cord injured person, when dealing with the bladder management program, for example, autonomic dysreflexia (the elevation of the blood pressure due to complications below the level of injury), can occur if the bladder does not fully empty. Some preventative medications that aid in the emptying process are dibenzyline and ismelin. These medications are prescribed by the physiatrist and are for relaxing the sphincter muscle of the bladder to enable proper emptying. Therefore, avoiding the pressure of a full over distended bladder, which causes undue complications below the level of injury, while at the same time avoiding autonomic dysreflexia.

If autonomic dysreflexia occurs and the source is not found, the blood pressure will continue to rise, causing a cerebrovascular accident (CVA) or even death. In this case, certain emergency medications can be used to lower the blood pressure before a CVA can occur. Such emergency medications are Hyperstat, Apresoline, Levophed, and Aramine (Harmarville, 1983).

A person with SCI may need to use a variety of other medications to counteract conditions caused by the injury. In addition to bladder management medications, the need to reduce spasticity (involuntary muscle movements) also requires medications. The medications used primarily for spasticity are muscle relaxants called Baclofen (Lioresal) and Valium. These muscle relaxants serve their purpose for reducing spasms, though they do cause the side effects of drowsiness, and possible heart deterioration with the use of Baclofen. An antibiotic such as Macrodantin may also be used on a daily basis to help prevent urinary tract infections from occurring.

There is much emphasis, during rehabilitation, on reeducating the SCI patient as to the basic survival skills originally learned as an infant, e.g. grooming, and toileting. The physical limitations placed on a person with SCI are the reasons this reeducation needs to be initiated. In addition to the redevelopment of basic survival skills, there is a need to reevaluate the work setting of a person with SCI (Cull & Hardy, 1977).

Vocational rehabilitation enables an SCI patient to return to the work world once a return to the community as been established. A vocational counselor works directly with the patient in determining what the future holds for the person, whether in the work place or returning to school.

An initial interview between the patient and the vocational counselor enables the counselor to "determine the patient's attitude toward his disability and future" (Ruge, 1969). Ruge (1969) goes on to state that if the patient reflects feelings of denial about the permanence of his disability, it is best to reschedule his vocational evaluation until he is able to accept the reality of his condition.

If an SCI patient was attending school or previously employed before the disability, the vocational counselor will contact the school or employer to recommend alternative methods for continuing, if necessary. Some of these alternative methods may be modifications, scheduling, and transportation or parking availability.

If the patient was unemployed, or unsure of a career decision, the counselor will administer tests to define the skills and interests of the patient. From there the patient and counselor can work out a plan for future employment or schooling. Gainful employment can be an important goal to set while in rehabilitation. Unfortunately, in a study on SCI persons' vocational resettlements, Crisp (1990) has indicated a very low rate of employment, usually below 40 percent of SCI persons find employment.

Before a person with a spinal cord injury can even attempt to find employment following discharge from the rehabilitation facility, they must acquire a new set of social skills that will enable them to interact with the world outside the rehabilitation center. The ability to groom oneself or to transfer from bed to wheelchair or to apply feeding devices, does not ensure that the person will function completely once outside the rehabilitation center (Trieschmann, 1980).

Once a person acquires an SCI and then ultimately moves on to a rehabilitation facility, they find consolation, safety, and a togetherness bond between themselves and others within the rehabilitation center. While in the rehabilitation center SCI persons feel they are no different than the others around them. They all have a disability. The environment which surrounds them suits all their needs. Behind the walls of the center, and within their cliques of "others like them," SCI persons feel just as "normal" as they did while in a clique of able-bodied person's before their disability. Only when SCI persons are faced with their first "Outing" into the public, usually through recreational therapy, does the anxiety of leaving the protective walls of the center hit them. They may not want to go. Some may refuse to go, and others who are hesitant may eventually give in and opt for a change of scenery.

This social outing for the SCI person provides for a high dose reality check. They find that not everything out in the public is as accessible as behind the walls of the rehabilitation center. For the first time they may notice people staring at them. If they use adaptive devices to eat with, they may feel self-conscious and disinclined to use them in front of other "normal" people, for fear of being stared at.

The social encounters a person with SCI faces are the only type of rehabilitation—and maybe just the most important type of rehabilitation—that cannot be attained behind the protective walls of the rehabilitation center. The only way a person with an SCI can attain a societal role is through the actual experience of being one with society, of contributing to society, and dealing with what society contributes to them.

Once a person with a spinal cord injury is discharged from the rehabilitation center and is a functioning part of society, other factors and social implications may come into play. For instance, social isolation (Trieschmann, 1980) may occur because of the need for the SCI person to have assistance in transportation to everywhere they may want to go. They may feel as if they are being a burden on the people they depend on, and therefore decline to ask for assistance in travel. Therefore, isolating themselves within their home, and away from the community.

In conclusion, spinal cord injury affects every aspect of an individuals life. It is only through the retraining and reeducation provided through rehabilitation and actual experience that a person with a spinal cord injury can obtain a maximal role in society.

— by Jerry Carter

References

Corbet, B. (1985). *National Resource Directory Massachusetts*: National Spinal Cord Association.

Crisp, R. (1990). Return to Work After Spinal Cord Injury. *The Journal of Rehabilitation*, 56, 28.

Cull, J. G., & Hardy R. E. (1977). Physical Medicine and Rehabilitation Approaches in Spinal Cord Injury Springfield Illinois: Thomas.

Hanak, M., & Scott, A. (1983). Spinal Cord Injury New York: Springer Publishing Company.

Harmarville Pamphlet (1983). Autonomic Dysreflexia Pittsburgh. Harmarville Rehabilitation Center, Inc. (1983). Learning and Living Pittsburgh: Harmarville.

Ruge, D. (1969). Spinal Cord Injuries Springfield Illinois: Thomas. Trieschmann, R. B. (1980). Spinal Cord injuries New York: Pergamon Press. Walker, M. D. (1991). Acute Spinal-Cord Injury. *The New England Journal of Medicine*, 26, 1885-87.

Young, J., Burns, P., Bowen, A. M., and McCutchen, R. (1982). Spinal Cord Injury Statistics Phoenix, Arizona: Good Samaritan Medical Center.

Chapter 40

Spinal Cord Injury Treatment and Rehabilitation

One mystery doctors would like to see solved quickly is why—far from healing itself—the spinal cord self-destructs following injury. Usually the spinal cord is not severed in an accident, but only crushed or bruised. However, in the next few hours (the acute stage) the injury gets worse. First the spinal cord swells. Then blood pressure drops off sharply in the damaged area, starving cells of their precious blood supply. Hemorrhaging begins in the center of the cord and spreads outwards. Nerve cells die, and their dying produces a gap in the cord with scar tissue forming on either side of the gap. Now the connections in the cord are well and truly broken and the result is paralysis and loss of sensation below the break.

Many investigators, including scientists at the Spinal Cord Injury Clinical Research Centers supported by the National Institute of Neurological Disorders and Stroke (NINDS) at Yale, New York and Ohio State Universities, and at the Universities of South Carolina and Texas are trying to solve this problem. One of the intriguing leads they are following involves drugs.

- **Steroids.** One family of drugs that may help prevent the cord's self-destruction is the steroids. These drugs have been used effectively to reduce the redness and swelling associated with a variety of illnesses or injuries. But their benefit in the case of spinal cord injury is not clear: Researchers at several NINDS-supported Spinal Cord Injury Clinical Research Centers have

1997; National Institute of Neurological Disorders and Stroke.

noted that small doses of steroids have little or no effect. On the other hand, larger doses may reduce the cord swelling but may retard healing. A collaborative study of the effectiveness of the steroid methylprednisolone is now under way at the five NINDS Spinal Cord Injury Clinical Research Centers and at the Universities of Miami and Puerto Rico.

- **DMSO.** NINDS-supported research scientists are also examining the properties of the controversial chemical, dimethyl sulfoxide (DMSO), a common industrial solvent thought to have healing and pain-relieving effects. DMSO is being tested on animals in experiments at five universities in the United States. As with all experimental drugs, the investigators are concerned with the safety and side effects of the drug as well as with determining its effectiveness.

- **Endorphin blockers.** A major discovery in the past decade concerns a class of brain chemicals called endorphins—referred to as "the brain's own opiates" because they relieve pain. Now it appears that the endorphins are also involved in the production of shock. In shock, there is a sharp drop in blood pressure that can be life-threatening. During the acute stage of spinal cord injury, the cord also undergoes "spinal shock"—when blood pressure drops off sharply. Some investigators now think that endorphins are released by the brain at the time of injury—probably to relieve the victim's pain—but unwittingly cause more damage by contributing to shock. Suppose you inject a drug that blocks the actions of endorphins, the investigators reasoned. Would that treatment prevent spinal shock in laboratory animals with induced spinal cord injuries? Simulating the course of events in a real-life accident, the scientists injected an endorphin-blocking drug about 45 minutes after the spinal cords had been severed in laboratory animals. Not only did most of the animals avoid shock, but they also recovered from the injury. Many were able to walk again—some with no trace of injury. It is too soon to tell whether these results are applicable to human spinal cord patients, but the research is considered highly promising and is being followed closely.

Besides drugs, some specialists have tried cooling the injured cord to prevent secondary damage. If initiated soon after injury, the cooling should slow down metabolism and so might forestall tissue destruction.

Surgery during the acute stage may also be necessary to relieve pressure on the cord or reduce swelling. Damage to the bones of the spinal column—the vertebrae—might also need to be repaired, and the spinal column fixed in place around the cord.

Cool Head and Efficient Hands

Spinal cord injury represents a major medical emergency than demands knowledgeable handling at the scene of the accident and rapid specialized transport to medical facilities designed to treat trauma patients. The United States is considered the world leader in research on spinal cord injury, and the clinical research conducted at the five National Institute of Neurological Disorders and Stroke (NINDS) supported Spinal Cord Injury Clinical Research Centers reflects this expertise.

It is not unusual for a spinal injury victim to be taken first to a nearby hospital emergency room for immediate care of bleeding or other life-threatening conditions, and later be moved to an appropriate medical facility. Treatment might be at one of over 300 regional trauma centers, for example, special spinal cord injury units, or major medical centers equipped to treat spinal cord injury. In some cases, patients may qualify for participation in clinical research projects conducted at the NINDS-supported Spinal Cord Injury Clinical Research Centers. In any case, a multidisciplinary team at the center will be alerted to the arrival of a patient and prepared to make a rapid but meticulous diagnosis. First steps will include an evaluation of lung function — especially important in the case of injuries in neck and chest regions. An anesthesiologist stands by ready to provide emergency respiratory aid.

An examination of the injury will determine what measures will be employed to relieve pressure on the cord, and how to stabilize the spinal column so that it does not move and is properly aligned around the cord. Traction and weights may be used, as well as special bed frames, to prevent movement.

A neurological examination will determine the extent of nervous system damage. All efforts will be made to preserve whatever movements the patient can make or sensations he or she can feel. Neurologists will test reflexes and question the patient, but also rely on a battery of electrical and other tests to determine the extent of damage to spinal cord nerves. At the Medical College of South Carolina, NINDS-supported specialists are refining electrophysiological tests to aid diagnosis and also to determine rapidly whether the cord has been partially or completely severed.

It is during this stage that drugs, cooling, surgery, or other techniques may be used to help prevent secondary damage to the cord. If, after 48 hours, the patient is unable to move or feel sensations below the level of injury, the resulting paraplegia or quadriplegia is considered "complete."

Man-Made Aids

Once the patient is out of danger, long-term treatment and rehabilitation can begin. Of growing importance in treatment are electronic aids that allow patients to regulate vital organs like the lungs or bladder, whose nerve supply may be impaired. Man-made devices that work by direct stimulation of nerves and muscles are one approach to the problem. The NINDS currently supports the development of a wide range of such devices, technically known as neural prostheses.

A Yale University research scientist has reported success with a new electronic device—the Diaphragm Pacer—designed to help paraplegics who have lost automatic control of their breathing muscles. Normally these patients have to be maintained on mechanical respirators. The system consists of an external radiotransmitter and antenna, a receiver implanted under the skin, and an electrode placed on the phrenic nerve. The phrenic nerve controls the diaphragm, the main breathing muscle. The transmitter's signals are picked up by the antenna, beamed to the receiver, and converted to electrical impulses which are sent to the phrenic nerve. The signals are beamed in an on-off pattern designed to match the normal breathing cycle. Electrophrenic electrodes have been implanted in over 200 patients so far. In clinical tests over a period of 8 years, the system has been found to be safe and effective.

Other neural prostheses designed to make life safer and more manageable for spinal cord injury patients are being developed:

- **Bladder control**. Urinary tract problems are a frequent complication of spinal cord injury, and serious infections are a major cause of death. At the University of California at San Francisco, a device designed to enable a patient to empty the bladder voluntarily is being tested on animals. This prosthesis involves electrical stimulation of the sacral nerve roots at the base of the spine. If the bladder device proves safe and effective, bladder infections could be reduced and perhaps eliminated.

290

- **Hand control**. At Case Western Reserve University in Cleveland, Ohio, investigators report that electrodes implanted in paralyzed finger and thumb muscles have enabled patients to grasp and hold pens, pencils, spoons, forks and other small objects. Plans call for further experiments aimed at the control of wrist and elbow muscles.

Paraplegic patients face other complications besides breathing difficulties and loss of bladder and bowel control. There may be painful muscle spasms, and bone and joint problems. Common illnesses present serious hazards. Flu or pneumonia, for example, can be fatal.

Pressure sores are a common problem. Sensations that ordinarily signal danger from heat, cold, or pressure may be lost below the level of injury. That loss, combined with reduced mobility, poor blood circulation, and inadequate nutrition, can give rise to troublesome skin ulcers. Careful daily inspection of the skin is necessary to prevent the sore and detect other problems.

The overall adjustment to a new life style is the overwhelming problem for the paraplegic, however. As one paralyzed veteran put it:

"The impact on the patient is traumatic, to say the least. There is the realization that a once whole and healthy body is no longer fully functional and is plagued with a myriad of secondary disabilities. The psychological/emotional problem of learning to accept this condition and learning how to cope with it is devastating in itself."

It is a tribute to human resourcefulness and strength that the great majority of paraplegics do adjust. They return to work, drive their own cars, and have fulfilling family and social lives.

Aiding and abetting them on their route to recovery are facilities designed to provide follow-up treatment once patients have passed the acute stage. Such treatment is available at regional spinal cord injury centers, rehabilitation institutes, veteran hospitals, departments of physical medicine or rehabilitation medicine in medical centers, and in clinics operated by nonprofit organizations such as the National Easter Seal Society.

The aim of a spinal cord injury rehabilitation program is to teach patients how to become independent. A variety of services and therapies are offered. Patients are often provided with self-care handbooks. An excellent example is one used at the New York University Institute for Rehabilitation Medicine, "Spinal Cord Injury—A Guide For

Care." No aspect of everyday living in a wheelchair is omitted. Here, for instance, are a few of the handbook's instructions on protecting skin and preventing pressure sores:

- Bathe daily and dry thoroughly, especially between toes and in the groin area. Make sure soiled skin is cleansed and dry thoroughly after bowel and bladder accidents.

- When sitting, buttock pressure should be relieved every 15 to 30 minutes by doing one-minute pushups or by shifting your weight from side to side. If you are unable to do this, ask for assistance.

- If you recline on a couch for long periods, use your air mattress or sheepskin under you.

The booklet tells patients what they need to know about nutrition, medication, foot care, and prevention of kidney and bladder complications. The assumption is that the patient will be independent. Tips range from how to negotiate a wheelchair to what to do about colds, asthma, allergies, or smoking.

Physical therapy is a major part of the treatment program in rehabilitation centers. If the patient is not yet permitted out of bed, a therapist will start bedside treatment. The degree of healing of fractured bones, the presence of pressure sores or infection, and the patient's general strength may limit the amount of exercise possible. But physical therapists will encourage patients to do as much as they can. A full physical therapy program often includes:

- **Progressive regressive resistive exercises**. These are exercises done with weights, pulleys and special exercise machines. They are part of a vigorous advanced program to strengthen muscles.

- **Tilt table**. A table that can be positioned at various angles to the horizontal helps the cardiovascular system readjust to upright position after a patient has been in bed for extended periods.

- **Mat class**. Working on a mat, the patient relearns and practices the skills needed for independent living: changing position in bed, getting dressed, moving from one place to another.

- **Wheelchair class**. The patient learns to handle a wheelchair, especially on curbs, ramps, stairs, and in a car. A patient's ability to negotiate these obstacles depends, of course, on the extend of impairment.

- **Driver evaluation & training**. Most patients ask "Will I ever be able to drive my own car?" The center says yes—in the vast majority of cases.

At most rehabilitation centers, treatment is coordinated by a team that includes neurosurgeons, urologists, internists, physical therapists, and vocational rehabilitation specialists. Some patients may be ready to leave after a month's stay in a center. For others, rehabilitation takes longer, because a great deal more is involved than just physical problems.

There are days during rehabilitation when most spinal cord injury patients feel hopeless and helpless, unable to see much point in living. At the New York University Center, when a patient has these feelings, a volunteer, perhaps a successful advertising agency executive, is likely to wheel in for a visit. The executive tells the despondent patient that he, too, was once consumed with anger. In a rage, he demanded: "Why me? Why did this have to happen to me?" He talks about how he overcame his despair. He says, "I made it; you can, too." The executive himself was once a patient at the center.

A major factor in successful rehabilitation is motivation. It requires motivation, first, to accept irreversible facts. It takes still more motivation to make the most of what has not been injured—talent, creative energies, intellectual resources. In addition, rehabilitation experts say that three factors always seem to be present: The patient has some definite activity—a job, a career, plans for an education— waiting to be undertaken as soon as he or she leaves the center.

NINDS

The National Institute of Neurological Disorders and Stroke (NINDS) supports and conducts research on brain and nervous system disorders. NINDS is one of the 17 research institutes of the Federal Government's National Institutes of Health, an agency of the Public Health Service within the U.S. Department of Health and Human Services.

Neurological disorders, which number more than 600, strike an estimated 50 million Americans each year. By supporting and conducting neurological research, the NINDS seeks better understanding, diagnosis, treatment and prevention of these disorders. To achieve this goal, the institute relies on both clinical and basic research. Some key areas of NINDS research include AIDS, amyotrophic lateral sclerosis (ALS), Alzheimer's disease, developmental disorders, epilepsy, neurogenetic disorders, head and spinal cord injury, multiple sclerosis, pain, Parkinson's disease, sleep disorders, and stroke.

If you have a personal concern about neurological disorders, please consult with your healthcare provider. For more information on neurological disorders and stroke call the National Institute of Neurological Disorders and Stroke at 1-800-352-9424.

Chapter 41

Questions and Answers about Hip Replacement

What Is a Hip Replacement?

Hip replacement, or arthroplasty, is a surgical procedure in which the diseased parts of the hip joint are removed and replaced with new, artificial parts. These artificial parts are called the prosthesis. The goals of hip replacement surgery are to improve mobility by relieving pain and improve function of the hip joint.

Who Should Have Hip Replacement Surgery?

The most common reason that people have hip replacement surgery is the wearing down of the hip joint that results from osteoarthritis. Other conditions, such as rheumatoid arthritis (a chronic inflammatory disease that causes joint pain, stiffness, and swelling), avascular necrosis (loss of bone caused by insufficient blood supply), injury, and bone tumors also may lead to breakdown of the hip joint and the need for hip replacement surgery.

Before suggesting hip replacement surgery, the doctor is likely to try walking aids such as a cane, or non-surgical therapies such as medication and physical therapy. These therapies are not always effective in relieving pain and improving the function of the hip joint. Hip replacement may be an option if persistent pain and disability

1997 National Institute of Arthritis and Musculoskeletal and Skin Diseases; National Institutes of Health; Public Health Service; Department of Health and Human Services.

295

interfere with daily activities. Before a doctor recommends hip replacement, joint damage should be detectable on x-rays.

In the past, hip replacement surgery was an option primarily for people over 60 years of age. Typically, older people are less active and put less strain on the artificial hip than do younger, more active people. In recent years, however, doctors have found that hip replacement surgery can be very successful in younger people as well. New technology has improved the artificial parts, allowing them to withstand more stress and strain. A more important factor than age in determining the success of hip replacement is the overall health and activity level of the patient.

For some people who would otherwise qualify, hip replacement may be problematic. For example, people who suffer from severe muscle weakness or Parkinson's disease are more likely than healthy people to damage or dislocate an artificial hip. Because people who are at high risk for infections or in poor health are less likely to recover successfully, doctors may not recommend hip replacement surgery for these patients.

What Are Alternatives to Total Hip Replacement?

Before considering a total hip replacement, the doctor may try other methods of treatment, such as an exercise program and medication. An exercise program can strengthen the muscles in the hip joint and sometimes improve positioning of the hip and relieve pain.

The doctor also may treat inflammation in the hip with nonsteroidal anti-inflammatory drugs, or NSAIDS. Some common NSAIDs are aspirin and ibuprofen. Many of these medications are available without a prescription, although a doctor also can prescribe NSAIDs in stronger doses.

In a small number of cases, the doctor may prescribe corticosteroids, such as prednisone or cortisone, if NSAIDs do not relieve pain. Corticosteroids reduce joint inflammation and are frequently used to treat rheumatic diseases such as rheumatoid arthritis. Corticosteroids are not always a treatment option because they can cause further damage to the bones in the joint. Some people experience side effects from corticosteroids such as increased appetite, weight gain, and lower resistance to infections. A doctor must prescribe and monitor corticosteroid treatment.. Because corticosteroids alter the body's natural hormone production, patients should not stop taking them suddenly and should follow the doctor's instructions for discontinuing treatment.

If physical therapy and medication do not relieve pain and improve joint function, the doctor may suggest corrective surgery that is less complex than a hip replacement, such as an osteotomy. Osteotomy is surgical repositioning of the joint. The surgeon cuts away damaged bone and tissue and restores the joint to its proper position. The goal of this surgery is to restore the joint to its correct position, which helps to distribute weight evenly in the joint. For some people, an osteotomy relieves pain. Recovery from an osteotomy takes 6 to 12 months. After an osteotomy, the function of the hip joint may continue to worsen and the patient may need additional treatment. The length of time before another surgery is needed varies greatly and depends on the condition of the joint before the procedure.

What Does Hip Replacement Surgery Involve?

The hip joint is located where the upper end of the femur meets the acetabulum. The femur, or thigh bone, looks like a long stem with a ball on the end. The acetabulum is a socket or cup-like structure in the pelvis, or hip bone. This "ball and socket" arrangement allows a wide range of motion, including sitting, standing, walking, and other daily activities.

During hip replacement, the surgeon removes the diseased bone tissue and cartilage from the hip joint. The healthy parts of the hip are left intact. Then the surgeon replaces the head of the femur (the ball) and the acetabulum (the socket) with new, artificial parts. The new hip is made of materials that allow a natural, gliding motion of the joint. Hip replacement surgery usually lasts 2 to 3 hours.

Sometimes the surgeon will use a special glue, or cement, to bond the new parts of the hip joint to the existing, healthy bone. This is referred to as a "cemented" procedure. In an uncemented procedure, the artificial parts are made of porous material that allows the patient's own bone to grow into the pores and hold the new parts in place. Doctors sometimes use a "hybrid" replacement, which consists of a cemented femur part and an uncemented acetabular part.

Is a Cemented or Uncemented Prosthesis Better?

Cemented prostheses were developed 40 years ago. Uncemented prostheses were developed about 20 years ago to try to avoid the possibility of loosening parts and the breaking off of cement particles, which sometimes happen in the cemented replacement. Because each person's condition is unique, the doctor and patient must weigh the advantages and disadvantages to decide which type of prosthesis is better.

For some people, an uncemented prosthesis may last longer than cemented replacements because there is no cement that can break away. And, if the patient needs an additional hip replacement (which is likely in younger people), also known as a revision, the surgery sometimes is easier if the person has an uncemented prosthesis.

The primary disadvantage of an uncemented prosthesis is the extended recovery period. Because it takes a long time for the natural bone to grow and attach to the prosthesis, people with uncemented replacements must limit activities for up to 3 months to protect the hip joint. The process of natural bone growth also can cause thigh pain for several months after the surgery.

Research has proven the effectiveness of cemented prostheses to reduce pain and increase joint mobility. These results usually are noticeable immediately after surgery. Cemented replacements are more frequently used than cementless ones for older, less active people and people with weak bones, such as those who have osteoporosis.

What Can Be Expected Immediately After Surgery?

Patients are allowed only limited movement immediately after hip replacement surgery. When the patient is in bed, the hip usually is braced with pillows or a special device that holds the hip in the correct position. The patient may receive fluids through an intravenous tube to replace fluids lost during surgery. There also may be a tube located near the incision to drain fluid and a tube (catheter) may be used to drain urine until the patient is able to use the bathroom. The doctor will prescribe medicine for pain or discomfort.

How Long Are Recovery and Rehabilitation?

On the day after surgery or sometimes on the day of surgery, therapists will teach the patient exercises that will improve recovery. A respiratory therapist may ask the patient to breathe deeply, cough, or blow into a simple device that measures lung capacity. These exercises reduce the collection of fluid in the lungs after surgery.

A physical therapist may teach the patient exercises, such as contracting and relaxing certain muscles, that can strengthen the hip. Because the new, artificial hip has a more limited range of movement than an undiseased hip, the physical therapist also will teach the patient proper techniques for simple activities of daily living, such as bending and sitting, to prevent injury to the new hip. As early as 1 to 2 days after surgery, a patient may be able to sit on the edge of the bed, stand, and even walk with assistance.

Usually, people do not spend more than 10 days in the hospital after hip replacement surgery. Full recovery from the surgery takes about 3 to 6 months, depending on the type of surgery, the overall health of the patient, and the success of rehabilitation.

How to Prepare for Surgery and Recovery

People can do many things before and after they have surgery to make everyday tasks easier and help speed their recovery.

Before Surgery

- Learn what to expect before, during, and after surgery. Request information written for patients from the doctor or contact one of the organizations listed near the end of this fact sheet.

- Arrange for someone to help you around the house for a week or two after coming home from the hospital.

- Arrange for transportation to and from the hospital.

- Set up a "recovery station" at home. Place the television remote control, radio, telephone, medicine, tissues, wastebasket, and pitcher and glass next to the spot where you will spend the most time while you recover.

- Place items you use every day at arm level to avoid reaching up or bending down.

- Stock up on kitchen staples and prepare food in advance, such as frozen casseroles or soups that can be reheated and served easily.

After Surgery

- Follow the doctor's instructions.

- Work with a physical therapist or other health care professional to rehabilitate your hip.

- Wear an apron for carrying things around the house. This leaves hands and arms free for balance or to use crutches.

- Use a long-handled "reacher" to turn on lights or grab things that are beyond arm's length. Hospital personnel may provide one of these or suggest where to buy one.

What Are Possible Complications of Hip Replacement Surgery?

According the American Academy of Orthopaedic Surgeons, approximately 120,000 hip replacement operations are performed each year in the United States and less than 10 percent require further surgery. New technology and advances in surgical techniques have greatly reduced the risks involved with hip replacements.

The most common problem that may happen soon after hip replacement surgery is hip dislocation. Because the artificial ball and socket are smaller than the normal ones, the ball can become dislodged from the socket if the hip is placed in certain positions. The most dangerous position usually is pulling the knees up to the chest.

The most common later complication of hip replacement surgery is an inflammatory reaction to tiny particles that gradually wear off of the artificial joint surfaces and are absorbed by the surrounding tissues. The inflammation may trigger the action of special cells that eat away some of the bone, causing the implant to loosen. To treat this complication, the doctor may use anti-inflammatory medications or recommend revision surgery (replacement of an artificial joint). Medical scientists are experimenting with new materials that last longer and cause less inflammation.

Less common complications of hip replacement surgery include infection, blood clots, and heterotopic bone formation (bone growth beyond the normal edges of bone).

When Is Revision Surgery Necessary?

Hip replacement is one of the most successful orthopaedic surgeries performed-more than 90 percent of people who have hip replacement surgery will never need revision surgery. However, because more younger people are having hip replacements, and wearing away of the joint surface becomes a problem after 15 to 20 years, revision surgery is becoming more common. Revision surgery is more difficult than first-time hip replacement surgery, and the outcome is generally not as good, so it is important to explore all available options before having additional surgery.

Doctors consider revision surgery for two reasons: if medication and lifestyle changes do not relieve pain and disability; or if x-rays of the hip show that damage has occurred to the artificial hip that must be corrected before it is too late for a successful revision. This surgery is usually considered only when bone loss, wearing of the joint surfaces, or joint loosening shows up on an x-ray. Other possible reasons for revision surgery include fracture, dislocation of the artificial parts, and infection.

What Types of Exercise Are Most Suitable for Someone With a Total Hip Replacement?

Proper exercise can reduce joint pain and stiffness and increase flexibility and muscle strength. People who have an artificial hip should talk to their doctor or physical therapist about developing an appropriate exercise program. Most exercise programs begin with safe range-of-motion activities and muscle strengthening exercises. The doctor or therapist will decide when the patient can move on to more demanding activities. Many doctors recommend avoiding high-impact activities, such as basketball, jogging, and tennis. These activities can damage the new hip or cause loosening of its parts. Some recommended exercises are cross-country skiing, swimming, walking, and stationary bicycling. These exercises can increase muscle strength and cardiovascular fitness without injuring the new hip.

What Hip Replacement Research Is Being Done?

To help avoid unsuccessful surgery, researchers are studying the types of patients most likely to benefit from a hip replacement. Researchers also are developing new surgical techniques, materials, and designs of prostheses, and studying ways to reduce the inflammatory response of the body to the prosthesis. Other areas of research address recovery and rehabilitation programs, such as home health and outpatient programs.

Where Can People Find More Information About Hip Replacement Surgery?

American Academy of Orthopaedic Surgeons
6300 North River Road
Rosemont, IL 60018-4262

847/823-7186
800/346-AAOS
Fax: 847/823-8125
World Wide Web address: http://www.aaos.org

The Hip Society
c/o Richard B. Welch, M.D.
One Shrader Street, Suite 650
San Francisco, CA 94117
415/221-0665
Fax: 415/221-4023

The Society maintains a list of physicians who are specialists in problems of the hip and provides physician referrals by geographic area.

Acknowledgments

The NIAMS gratefully acknowledges the assistance of Charles A. Engh, M.D., of the Anderson Orthopaedic Research Institute, in Arlington, Virginia; James Panagis, M.D., M.P.H., of the National Institutes of Health; and Clement B. Sledge, M.D., of Brigham and Women's Hospital, in Boston, Massachusetts, in the review of this fact sheet.

The National Arthritis and Musculoskeletal and Skin Diseases Information Clearinghouse (NAMSIC) is a public service sponsored by the NIAMS that provides health information and information sources. The NLWS, a part of the National Institutes of Health (NIH), leads the Federal medical research effort in arthritis and musculoskeletal and skin diseases. The NIAMS sponsors research and research training throughout the United States as well as on the NIH campus in Bethesda, MD, and disseminates health and research information.

Chapter 42

Total Hip Replacement

Introduction

More than 120,000 artificial hip joints are being implanted annually in the United States. Successful replacement of deteriorated, arthritic, and severely injured hips have contributed to enhanced mobility and comfortable, independent living for many people who would otherwise be substantially disabled. New technology involving prosthetic devices for replacement of the hip, along with advances in surgical techniques, have diminished the risks associated with the operation and improved the immediate and long-term outcome of hip replacement surgery.

Questions remain, however, concerning which prosthetic designs and materials are most effective for specific groups of patients and which surgical techniques and rehabilitation approaches yield the best long-term outcomes. Issues also exist regarding the best indications and approaches for revision surgery.

As a follow-up to the National Institutes of Health (NIH) Consensus Development Conference (CDC) on Total Hip Joint Replacement held in 1982, the National Institute of Arthritis and Musculoskeletal and Skin Diseases, together with the Office of Medical Applications of Research of the NIH, convened a second CDC on Total Hip Replacement on September 12-14, 1994. The conference was cosponsored by the National Institute on Aging, the National Institute of Child Health

NIH Publication Volume 12, Number 5. Sept. 1994. NIH Consensus Statement.

and Human Development, and the Office of Research on Women's Health. After 1½ days of presentations by experts in the relevant fields and discussion by a knowledgeable audience, an independent, non-Federal consensus panel composed of specialists from the fields of orthopedic surgery, epidemiology, rehabilitation and physical medicine, biomechanics and biomaterials, geriatrics, rheumatology, as well as a public representative, weighed the scientific evidence and formulated a consensus statement in response to the following six previously stated questions:

1. What are the current indications for total hip replacement?

2. What are the design and surgical considerations relating to a replacement prosthesis?

3. What are the responses of the biological environment?

4. What are the expected outcomes?

5. What are the accepted approaches and outcomes for revision of a total hip replacement?

6. What are the most productive directions for future research?

This consensus statement reflects a synthesis of generally accepted observations and recommendations derived from the scientific presentations as well as a general review of current literature by the consensus panel. This panel also identified areas of limited information where further research would be most productive.

What are the current indications for total hip replacement?

Primary total hip replacement (THR) is most commonly used for hip joint failure caused by osteoarthritis; other indications include, but are not limited to, rheumatoid arthritis, avascular necrosis, traumatic arthritis, certain hip fractures, benign and malignant bone tumors, the arthritis associated with Paget's disease, ankylosing spondylitis, and juvenile rheumatoid arthritis. The aims of THR are relief of pain and improvement in function. Candidates for elective THR should have radiographic evidence of joint damage and moderate to severe persistent pain or disability, or both, that is not substantially relieved by an extended course of nonsurgical management. These measures usually include trials of analgesic and nonsteroidal anti-inflammatory drugs (NSAIDs), physical therapy, the use of walking aids, and reduction in physical activities that provoke discomfort. In certain conditions such as rheumatoid arthritis and Paget's disease, additional disease-specific therapies may be appropriate. The patient's goals and expectations should be ascertained before THR to determine whether they are realistic and attainable by the recommended therapeutic approach. Any discrepancies between the patient's expectations and the likely outcome should be discussed in detail with the patient and family members before surgery.

In the past, patients between 60 and 75 years of age were considered to be among the best candidates for THR. Over the last decade, however, the age range has been broadened to include more elderly patients, many of whom have a higher level of comorbidities, as well as younger patients, whose implants may be exposed to greater mechanical stresses over an extended time course. In patients less than 55 years of age, alternative surgical procedures such as fusion and osteotomy deserve consideration. However, there are no data showing that the outcomes of these procedures are as good or better than those from THR when performed for similar indications. Advanced age alone is not a contraindication for THR; poor outcomes appear to be related to comorbidities rather than to age. There are few contraindications to THR other than active local or systemic infection and other medical conditions that substantially increase the risk of serious perioperative complications or death. Obesity has been considered a relative contraindication because of a reported higher mechanical failure rate in heavier patients; however, the prospect of substantial long-term reduction in pain and disability for heavier patients appears to be similar to that for the population in general.

Thus, although the clinical conditions and circumstances leading to THR are broadly defined, several issues regarding indications remained unresolved. For example, data are insufficient on the associations between potential risk factors (e.g., age, weight, smoking, medications) and outcomes to guide treatment of the individual patient. Moreover, indications are not clear for use of the various surgical approaches and types of prostheses in individual patients. Finally, standardized instruments to measure levels of pain, physical disability, and quality of life as perceived by the patient need to be used to guide clinical decision-making and choice of surgery.

What are the design and surgical considerations relating to a replacement prosthesis?

At the NIH CDC on Total Hip Joint Replacement held in 1982, aseptic loosening was identified as a major problem with THR. It was especially prevalent in young, active patients and after revision surgery. Because it appeared with increasing frequency over time, it was feared that a much larger problem would emerge. Newer fixation (cement and cementless) techniques had been introduced, but their long-term efficacy was unknown. Cobalt-, titanium-, and iron-based alloys, higher molecular weight polyethylene, and autocuring polymethylmethacrylate (PMMA) bone cement were the materials used in most implants. Chemical modifications and altered processing of the alloys had been introduced to deal with the problem of fractured stems.

As of 1994, state of the art pertaining to THR has changed substantially. For example, changes have been made in fixation (cement and cementless), device designs, and some materials. Concerns remain about the in vivo durability of femoral and acetabular components of the implants, but the procedure has a more predictable outcome. The newer cementing techniques have proven to be more successful than the original ones on the femoral side. Improved techniques include the use of a medullary plug, a cement gun, lavage of the canal, pressurization, centralization of the stem, and reduction in porosity in the cement. However, the optimum cement-metal interface has yet to be identified. These newer procedures minimize defects and localized stress concentrations in the cement. Their current success indicates that previously observed aseptic loosening within the first 10 years following implantation was primarily a mechanical process and that steps to reduce stresses in the materials and improve strength of the interfaces are reasonable to reduce loosening. Further optimization of the bone implant interface constitutes an important opportunity for future research.

Another important change in fixation has been the introduction and widespread use of noncemented components that rely on bone growth into porous or onto roughened surfaces for fixation. In the femur, selected cementless components have exhibited clinical success, although with shorter follow-up, similar to that of cemented components installed with the newer cementing techniques. There is evidence that bone changes (osteolysis or bone resorption) can occur as well with some of the cementless components. Numerous reports document resorption, and although it has not usually become symptomatic during early stages of follow-up, concerns nevertheless exist about progressive osteolysis and consequent aseptic loosening or fracture.

On the acetabular side, the cementless components have demonstrated less aseptic loosening compared with the cemented components over the short term, although long-term results are not yet available. The prospective and retrospective studies conducted have been specific to device design and technique, and any general comparison of cemented and noncemented systems should be viewed with caution.

The implants themselves have undergone multiple changes. As a result of improved alloys and designs, fracture of femoral stems is no longer a significant problem. Stem cross-sections have been rounded to avoid high stresses in the cement. There is still controversy over the appropriate length of uncemented stems and the extent and location of porous or roughened regions. Metal backing of cemented acetabular components has not been associated with a high degree of success and is now used infrequently. Metal-backed acetabular components with porous coatings have demonstrated good to excellent results in regard to loosening noted at 5- to 7-year follow-up and continue to be followed. Modular components have been introduced and are widely used, but it is recognized that in vivo disassembly, fretting and corrosion, and wear between components can be a source of debris and may contribute to osteolysis and isolated implant fractures. Given the potential problems, routine use of modular components needs to be evaluated specific to particular applications. There appears to be little justification for modularity or customization of femoral stems below the head-neck junction in primary THR, although the modular stem components for revisions may be useful.

Revision rates for cemented femoral components, using modern techniques, have been reported to be less than 5 percent at 10-year follow-up; revision rates for uncemented acetabular components are approximately 2 percent at 5-year follow-up. To be deemed efficacious, new design features should be shown to have a mechanical failure rate equal to or lower than these figures.

As in 1982, the primary implant materials are cobalt- and titanium-based alloys, PMMA bone cement, and ultra-high molecular weight polyethylene. These continue to demonstrate biocompatibility in bulk, but particles of these materials, particularly the polyethylene, are suspected to have a role in bone resorption and potential implant loosening. Osteolysis that can occur with both cemented and cementless components on both the femoral and acetabular sides is thought to be due to an inflammatory process brought on by particulate matter. The articulating surfaces between the femoral and acetabular components are now recognized as a major source of debris, which has been shown to be important in this pathologic tissue response. Most components for femoral heads have polished cobalt alloy, which articulates with polyethylene sockets. Longitudinal research continues on smoothness and ion implantation of the articulating surfaces, ceramic-polymer, ceramic-ceramic, and alloy-alloy components, although the in vivo data remain limited at this time. Efforts to alter or replace the polyethylene are under way, but no new materials with reduced clinical wear rates are routinely available.

Several factors have been suggested to minimize the production of wear debris. Polyethylene acetabular cups with minimum wall thickness of 6 mm and femoral heads with diameters of 28 mm are important design considerations associated with reduced wear. Where metallic shells are used to contain the polyethylene cup, the interior of the shell should be smooth with a minimum number of openings for screws, and the polyethylene liner should be highly conforming and mechanically stable. Polyethylene of the highest quality is strongly advised for the manufacture of the components. Femoral heads with highly polished cobalt alloy, or polished ceramics as some data suggest, may be advantageous to minimize effects of wear on the polyethylene surface.

Studies also continue on surface modifications of implants to provide direct attachment to bone. For example, several types of calcium phosphate ceramics (CPC) (often called hydroxylapatite) have been added as coatings to THR surfaces to enhance fixation of non-ingrowth implants to bone. Concerns have been expressed about the longer term in vivo fatigue strengths of the substrate to coating interfaces, biodegradation, and the potential for generating ceramic particulates, although so far data addressing implant performance are comparable to those from other device designs at the same follow-up times. Research and development on the enhancement of bone growth into porous biomaterials using CPC has also shown promise, although longitudinal data are incomplete at this time. Long-term data are needed on the benefit-to-risk ratio of clinical outcomes for these types of surface modifications.

Although there are in vitro tests for evaluating implant design features and material characteristics, as well as animal testing regimens, the relevance of these tests to in vivo human performance are often unknown and additional approaches are necessary. Long-term clinical studies are the only accepted method for evaluating the efficacy of the design and materials in human use, particularly with regard to patient-defined outcome measures. Since these take many years and are very expensive, few implant design features are supported by well-designed studies.

Adaptive bone remodeling around the prosthesis continues to be a concern, but there is little evidence that it is a significant clinical problem during the first 10 years of follow-up. Joint forces are known with better confidence than in 1982, but it is still unknown which elements of force, magnitude, and time are relevant to implant failures. Detailed analysis of stress distribution is still limited by imprecise data on joint forces, viscoelastic properties, and failure modes of the materials and tissues.

In 1994, the main problems of concern related to implant design are long-term fixation of the acetabular component, osteolysis due to particulate materials, biologic response to particles of implant materials, and the less favorable results of revision surgery.

What are the responses of the biological environment?

Since the NIH CDC on Total Hip Joint Replacement held in 1982, bone resorption, or osteolysis, has emerged as the major concern with regard to the long-term survival of total hip arthroplasty. Significant resorption and massive osteolysis as well as more limited areas of bone destruction had been associated with cemented components and attributed to cement debris. Subsequent findings confirm that similar problems can be associated with cementless prosthetic implants, and some degree of osteolysis may be present in up to 30-40 percent of cases within 10 years of surgery. Both acetabular and femoral components may be affected. Components may remain well fixed in the presence of significant bone loss, but indications are that once osteolysis appears it tends to progress and may ultimately lead to implant failure. This bone loss is now considered to be a reaction to particulate matter derived from the implanted prosthetic components as well as the cement when used. Because osteolysis is an important contributor to failure of hip arthroplasties and may occur in the absence of clinical symptoms, it is important that patients with implants be followed and evaluated at regular intervals throughout life to ensure timely operative intervention, if necessary.

Quantitatively, the material causing the most tissue reaction appears to be particulate polyethylene. These particles have been recovered in significant quantities from periprosthetic tissues, including sites remote from the source. Particle size varies, but the majority recovered are approximately 0.5 micron, with 90 percent less than 1.0 micron. It has been estimated that the average rate of wear for cobalt alloy-to-polyethylene interface is 0.1-0.2 mm/year. The volume of wear debris may increase with larger femoral head size.

Metallic debris has also been identified in significant quantities. The source may be related to stem-bone fretting, particularly in loose prostheses and in more distal portions of proximally fixed prostheses where significant motion between stem and bone may persist. With the use of modular prostheses, corrosion and/or fretting have been identified in up to 35 percent of some retrieved specimens, and these connections could serve as a source of metallic particles. Fretting and corrosion are not limited to the interface between dissimilar alloys. Interactions have also been identified with cobalt-cobalt and titanium-titanium as well as titanium-cobalt alloy junctions. Reactions at the head-neck junctions have been studied in depth. Corrosion and wear debris products can also form at the interfaces between screws and acetabular shells and at modular collars for adapting proximal femoral stems. Some of the metallic particles generated may be larger than the polyethylene debris. The major effect of these larger metallic debris may relate to promoting third body wear of the polyethylene, with the derivative polyethylene particles of submicron size triggering the cellular response. However, smaller metal particles and ions have been demonstrated to be active in direct stimulation of biologic processes.

The leading hypothesis to explain the development of massive osteolysis is that particulate matter derived from prosthetic components and cement stimulates an inflammatory response. Phagocytosis of the particles by macrophage and foreign-body giant cells (arising from the macrophage) appears to be the initial biologic response to particulate matter. The presence of intracellular particles is associated with the release of cytokines and other mediators of inflammation. These factors initiate a focal bone resorptive process largely mediated by osteoclasts. These osteoclasts do not contain debris particles.

Thus, the long-term threat to component failure from a biologic standpoint appears to be wear-debris-associated periprosthetic osteolysis as a result of osteoclastic activity. This is stimulated by cytokines such as tumor necrosis factor, interleukins, and prostaglandins released by macrophages and possibly other cells including fibroblasts. The critical initiating sequence involves the interaction between small particulate materials and responding cells. The process is affected by the number, size, distribution, and type of particulate material, as well as responsiveness of the ingesting cells.

The debris may be distributed beyond the hip joint. Material has been identified in distant lymph nodes, but no systemic consequences are documented up to this time. Since it is now recognized that both cobalt- and titanium-based alloys release soluble products in patients, long-term surveillance to assess possible systemic and remote side effects after THR is advisable.

Adaptive bone remodeling occurs in the proximal femur in response to an altered mechanical environment following hip replacement. This process is commonly referred to as "stress shielding" or stress transfer. Stem rigidity or elasticity plays a major role. Bone resorption in unstressed areas is a common observation, but it has not been shown to be related to loosening. Nevertheless, it presents an important concern in terms of long-term stability and effect on revision surgery.

Factors influencing adaptive bone remodeling have been considered in determining the location and extent of porous coating on uncemented stems. Finite element analysis suggests that proximally coated porous stems are associated with less cortical bone stress shielding than fully coated stems, but the extent of coating on most currently used prosthetic stems is still greater than that calculated necessary to significantly reduce the stress-shielding effect on the proximal femur. Decreasing porous coating to reduce stress shielding must be weighed against providing sufficient coating to ensure fixation. Efforts to reduce stem stiffness have been shown to lessen proximal cortical atrophy under experimental conditions.

What are the expected outcomes?

The success of THR in most patients is strongly supported by nearly 30 years of follow-up data. There appears to be immediate and substantial improvement in the patient's pain, functional status, and overall health-related quality of life. Promising data suggest that these immediate improvements persist in the long term. Over the last two decades, complications associated with THR have declined significantly. Prophylactic antibiotic therapy has helped to prevent infection. Use of anticoagulants in the perioperative period has reduced deep venous thrombosis and pulmonary emboli. The incidence of mechanical loosening has decreased with the introduction of improved fixation techniques. More than 90 percent of all artificial joints are never revised. Rates of revision are decreasing with improved surgical techniques.

The important questions of today are not whether THR is effective compared with no treatment but rather which technology and methodology used for THR are best for a particular patient. For example, the various total hip designs, fixation methods, and surgical techniques need to be rigorously compared with one another. Surgeon's experience and hospital environment should be investigated for possible independent effects. Various rehabilitation interventions, including long-term therapeutic exercise, should be evaluated for effectiveness. Similarly, little is known about patient-level predictors of outcome, e.g., patient expectations, quality of the individual patient's bone stock, demographic characteristics, comorbidities, obesity, and activity level.

Since length of acute hospital stay has become progressively shorter, more emphasis must be given to determining the role of preadmission educational programs, appropriate physical therapy, and rehabilitation during the acute stay and following discharge. Home health programs when indicated may be more effective than prolonged hospitalization. The benefits of a long-term therapeutic exercise program for patients who have undergone THR have not been clearly demonstrated to improve mobility or hip stability. There appears to be insufficient appreciation for the role of exercise in THR rehabilitation; however, there is evidence that hip weakness persists up to 2 years after surgery in the presence of a normal gait. Multiple studies have demonstrated that weakness in the lower extremities is a major risk factor for falls in the geriatric age group. Thus, further studies are needed to assess the relationship between muscle function following THR, mobility, and risk for falls, as well as the role of therapeutic exercise in improving muscle function, with enhancement of mobility and stability.

Outcome assessment in THR has been limited by the lack of standardized terminology and by the use of various scales that have traditionally relied on the surgeon's assessment of the patient's pain, range of motion, muscle strength, and mobility. Most of these measures have not been adequately characterized in terms of validity, reliability, and responsiveness to change. The traditional assessments have not included patient-oriented evaluation of function or satisfaction. There is no consensus on the standard definitions of endpoints with respect to prosthesis failure. The American Academy of Orthopaedic Surgeons has developed recommendations for data to be collected, and this approach should be endorsed for use in clinical practice. The patient's functional status should be further assessed in follow-up by standardized, patient-reported, disease-specific measures and by at least one global outcome measure. Finally, the radiographic and clinical criteria for prosthesis failure should be defined.

Long-term follow-up is essential to determining outcomes and pathological processes (e.g., failures related to osteolysis and particulate debris). These complications were not emphasized in the 1982 CDC on Total Hip Joint Replacement. The problems have been identified only by long-term follow-up of patients.

Methodological issues that have limited THR outcomes assessment include lack of randomized trials and other well-controlled studies, lack of well-characterized patient cohorts for prospective observational studies, and insufficient sample sizes followed for prolonged periods of time.

THR is performed more than 120,000 times per year in the United States. This represents a 64-percent increase in the number of THR procedures per year in the United States since the 1982 CDC. Analysis of Medicare claims data demonstrates significant variations in the rates of performance of THR with respect to geography, age, gender, and race. The highest rates of THR are in the Midwest and Northwest and the lowest rates in the South and East. A fourfold difference exists between the State with the highest rate of THR (Utah) and the State with the lowest rate (Wyoming). A previous study demonstrated a 50-percent higher rate of THR in Boston, Massachusetts, compared with New Haven, Connecticut. Other procedures such as hip fracture repair have very low variation from one geographical area to another. In today's era of cost-containment and outcomes research, it is important to understand the factors contributing to these wide area variations as well as which rate of THR is most appropriate.

Sixty-two percent of all THR procedures in the United States are performed in women. Furthermore, women have significantly worse preoperative functional status than do men and are 35 percent more likely to report the use of a walking aid at the time of surgery. These differences persist even after adjustment for other demographic and clinical characteristics. These data suggest that, compared with men, women are being operated on at a more advanced stage of the disease. Two-thirds of all THR procedures are performed in individuals who are older than 65 years of age. The rate of THR increases for patients up to 75 years of age and then declines. The highest age-specific incidence rates of THR are between 65 and 74 years of age for men and 75 and 84 years of age for women. Recent comparisons of rates of THR reveal that more are being done in the young and in the oldest patients. Among the older patients, there has been an increase in THR in patients with more comorbidities.

Most THR procedures are performed in whites. The prevalence rate of hip implants (fixation devices and artificial joints) was 4.2 per 1,000 in whites compared with 1.7 per 1,000 in African-Americans. The disparity by race increases markedly with age. These findings were confirmed by an analysis of Medicare claims data that focused solely on THR. Observed differences in the rate of THR by race may reflect a disparity in access or referral for care for African-Americans. Additionally, individuals with higher income were 22 percent more likely to undergo THR than were individuals with low income. Health care providers and patients must be cognizant of the variations in the THR rate. It is important to carefully consider the potential influence of access to care, treatment selection biases, and patient knowledge and preferences on these variations in rates.

In this era of cost-containment and managed care, the ultimate selection of a THR system should be based on individualized patient needs, safety, and efficacy. There is consensus that the THR patient requires periodic follow-up including appropriate x-ray examination throughout life. Periodic follow-up, perhaps at 5-year intervals after the first 5 years, could allow identification of osteolysis and other indicators of impending failure in their earliest forms and permits institution of treatment before catastrophic failure.

What are the accepted approaches and outcomes for revision of a total hip replacement?

As more primary THRs occur on a cumulative basis, as indications extend to more conditions and to older and younger individuals, and as the population ages, the absolute number of revision hip replacements will increase, even if the frequency of failures in primary procedures continues to decrease. Revision surgery is highly complex and costly and requires considerable scientific and technical expertise, an array of expensive technological options, a supportive health care environment, and a skilled health care team. Consequently, issues such as the surgeon's experience, the hospital characteristics, the related health care costs, and appropriateness of current hospital reimbursements associated with revision should be carefully examined.

Currently, the results of revision THR are inferior to those of primary procedures. It remains important to refine the indications for revision and to do so on the basis of the best available outcome data. Not all "failed" primary THRs require revision. The decision to revise, as is true of decisions regarding primary procedures, must consider such circumstances as the presence of disabling pain, stiffness, and functional impairment unrelieved by appropriate medical management and lifestyle changes. In addition, radiographic evidence of bone loss or loosening of one or both components should be present. Indeed, evidence of progressive bone loss alone provides sufficient reason to consider revision in advance of catastrophic failure. Fracture, dislocation, malposition of components, and infection involving the implant are other reasons to consider revision.

A number of options must be considered in planning a revision operation. The selection of specific technology is currently a judgment of the surgeon and depends on the amount and quality of the bone stock, the age and functional demands of the patient, and the reason for failure of the primary procedure. The weight of clinical experience suggests that a loose acetabular component, either cemented or porous coated, can be reliably replaced by a porous-coated component in the presence of adequate bone stock. In one study using this approach, 91 percent of implants were radiographically stable and 9 percent required re-revision (for dislocation and infection rather than aseptic loosening) between 8 and 11 years after revision. In elderly patients with lower functional demands and those with osteogenic bone, cemented implants have also provided satisfactory results. To achieve prosthetic stability in the absence of sufficient bone stock, deficits can be filled with morselized or structural bone grafts (either autografts or allografts obtained from accredited tissue banks), customized metal components, or, under some circumstances, bone cement.

The approach to revision of the femoral component must be based on the nature of the remaining bone stock in the proximal femur, and clinical judgment usually takes into account the age and functional demands of the patient. Under many circumstances, revision of the femoral component with a cemented stem is possible using modern cementing techniques. The re-revision rate for this approach is between 10 and 18 percent at 10- to 11-year follow-up.

An acceptable alternative approach to revision of femoral components when there is substantial residual bone stock has been the use of noncemented implants, particularly the extensively coated components. This approach has resulted in 90-percent stem survivorship at a 9-year follow-up.

Morselized bone graft can be used successfully to fill defects in the femoral canal with or without the use of bone cement, and cortical bone can be augmented with only grafts as necessary. Under exceptional circumstances, it may be necessary to use large structural allografts when the proximal femoral bone stock deficiency is substantial. If this is done, the implant should be cemented into the graft.

Both the diagnosis and the treatment of infected implants remain challenging. The infection rates of the past have been dramatically reduced. Current infection rates of less than 1 percent at one year after primary THR are now being reported. Nonetheless, infection remains a devastating complication, and treatment alternatives remain controversial. Recovery of the infecting organism is essential to the selection of appropriate antibiotics and the planning of surgical approaches. For organisms highly susceptible to multiple antibiotics, one-stage surgical approaches that combine extensive debridement and an ensuing exchange of implants are associated with a 77- to 94-percent success rate. Two-stage revisions that include at least four weeks of appropriate antibiotic treatment following implant removal and wound debridement and a variable period of time before reinsertion determined by the characteristics of the organism have resulted in a success rate greater than 80 percent. In young people, there may be value to a third, intermediate stage in which the bone stock is augmented in anticipation of later reimplantation.

What are the most productive directions for future research?

THR is acknowledged as a highly successful procedure that has provided relief of pain, increased mobility, and improved tolerance for activity for thousands of people. Despite the advances made in the past decade, obvious deficiencies in knowledge remain regarding treatment alternatives, patient characteristics, and environmental issues. To address these concerns most effectively, it is important to identify those avenues of investigation that will lead to decreased morbidity and enhanced quality of life for the population at large affected by debilitating hip disease.

Standardized instruments for assessing outcomes need to be developed, validated, and introduced into clinical use. These may also be useful in developing guidelines for surgery and in making physicians aware of their patients' physical capabilities and expectations.

The issues of age, sex, weight, activity level, and comorbidities have been implicated for their effects on the outcome of THR and need to be studied in relation to the indications for surgery and timing of the procedure.

Serious questions have been raised concerning the disparate rates for THR between racial groups and geographic locations that seem to have no direct relationship to incidence of disease. In-depth analysis of rate differential can lead to an identification of underlying reasons. In this way, the benefits of THR can be extended to an appropriate segment of the population that appears to have limited access.

Materials currently used for the manufacture of THR implants have been improved with regard to design and finish. Wear debris, however, remains a factor that affects the durability of the implants and their fixation. Research is ongoing and support is needed to expand investigations of new materials and to create a better understanding of wear processes that can prolong the life of the implant and reduce the wear and wear products.

One of the necessary approaches for evaluating implant failure modes is an organized, ongoing analysis of in situ prostheses retrieved from cadavers. Such a program should be national in scope and supported by grant monies. As part of this effort, it is anticipated that significant data could be obtained concerning wear processes involving the articular surfaces under circumstances where the implant did not fail. At the same time, this avenue of research would further clarify the device and tissue interactions that are characteristic of the cemented and noncemented types of devices.

Randomized clinical trials are needed to determine the efficacy of implant designs and surgical approaches, including the effect of coatings that encourage appositional or interpositional bone growth for fixation.

The contribution of prehospital, inhospital, and posthospital education and rehabilitation programs to the eventual outcome of the surgical procedure deserves an organized, in-depth study to determine optimum regimen, duration of treatment, and expected outcomes. Clinical data suggest that potential capabilities of the patients are not being fully developed.

The biologic interface between the implant and the host bone has been recognized as a source of potential failure. Basic research efforts into the mechanisms by which these changes occur are providing some clues, but much more needs to be known about specific cellular mechanisms associated with osteolysis, suggested immunologic or inflammatory responses, and the reactions to varying stresses encountered by the bone. In addition, further investigation should be encouraged into the ways by which the local inflammatory response to particulate matter could be modified by regional or systemic interventions.

As the indications for THR are extended into the younger age group, patients with THR will be exposed to more rigorous environmental demands, both occupational and recreational. Investigations are needed into the environmental modifications, activity limitations, or types of physical effort that contribute to extended prosthesis survival. Physical conditioning activities—muscle development, improvement in coordination, and exercises that enhance bone integrity without affecting fixation—need to be studied as they relate to the anticipated lifestyle and occupational objectives of the patient.

Outcomes of revision hip surgery are less reliable and satisfactory than those of primary procedures. Those biologic, biomechanical, and rehabilitation factors that influence these results need to be explored and solutions developed.

Regional or national registries should be established to capture a minimum data set on all THR and revision procedures. The goals of this registry should be to better define the natural history and epidemiology of THR in the U.S. population as a whole and to identify risk factors for poor outcomes that relate to the implant, procedure, and patient characteristics.

Conclusions

- THR is an option for nearly all patients with diseases of the hip that cause chronic discomfort and significant functional impairment.

- In the aggregate, THR is a highly successful treatment for pain and disability. Most patients have an excellent prognosis for long-term improvement in symptoms and physical function.

- Perioperative complications such as infection and deep venous thrombosis have been significantly reduced because of use of prophylactic antibiotics and anticoagulants and early mobilization.

- The predominant mode of long-term prosthetic failure appears to be related to generation of particulate matter, which in turn causes an inflammatory reaction and subsequent bone resorption around the prosthesis.

- Revision of THR is indicated when mechanical failure occurs. The surgery is technically more difficult and the long-term prognosis is generally not as good as for primary THR. The optimal surgical techniques for THR revision vary considerably depending on the conditions encountered. Continued periodic follow-up is necessary to identify early evidence of impending failure so as to permit remedial actions before a catastrophic event.

- Improved methods for evaluating existing technology should be developed and implemented, especially with respect to patient-defined outcomes.

- Future research should focus on refining indications for surgery; defining reasons for differences in procedure rates by age, race, gender, and geographic region; developing surgical techniques, materials, and designs that will be clearly superior to

318

current practices; understanding the inflammatory response to particulate material and how to modify it; determining optimal short- and long-term rehabilitation strategies; and elucidating risk factors that may lead to accelerated prosthetic failure.

Statement Availability

Preparation and distribution of this statement are the responsibility of the Office of Medical Applications of Research of the National Institutes of Health. Free copies of this statement as well as all other available NIH Consensus Statements and NIH Technology Assessment Statements may be obtained from the following resources:

NIH Consensus Program Information Service
P.O. Box 2577
Kensington, MD
20891
Telephone 1-800-NIH-OMAR (644-6627)
Fax (301) 816-2494

NIH Office of Medical Applications of Research
Federal Building,
Room 618
7550 Wisconsin Avenue MSC
9120 Bethesda, MD
20892-9120

Full-text versions of statements are also available online through an electronic bulletin board system and through the Internet.

NIH Information Center BBS (301) 496-6203

World Wide Web http://www.nih.gov

Chapter 43

Questions and Answers About Knee Problems

This chapter contains general information about knee problems. It includes descriptions of the different parts of the knee, including bones, cartilage, muscles, ligaments, and tendons. Individual sections of this chapter describe the symptoms, diagnosis, and treatment of specific types of knee injuries and conditions. Information is also provided on the prevention of knee problems.

How Common Are Knee Problems? What Causes Them?

According to the American Academy of Orthopaedic Surgeons, more than 4.1 million people seek medical care each year for a knee problem.

Some knee problems result from wear of parts of the knee, such as occurs in osteoarthritis. Other problems result from injury, such as a blow to the knee or sudden movements that strain the knee beyond its normal range of movement.

How Can People Prevent Knee Problems?

Some knee problems, such as those resulting from an accident, cannot be foreseen or prevented. However, a person can prevent many knee problems by following these suggestions:

1997; National Institute of Arthritis and Musculoskeletal and Skin Diseases; National Institutes of Health, Public Health Service, Department of Health and Human Services.

- First warm up by walking or riding a stationary bicycle, then do stretches before exercising or participating in sports. Stretching the muscles in the front of the thigh (quadriceps) and back of the thigh (hamstrings) reduces tension on the tendons and relieves pressure on the knee during activity.

- Strengthen the leg muscles by doing specific exercises (for example, by walking up stairs or hills, or by riding a stationary bicycle). A supervised workout with weights is another pathway to strengthening leg muscles that benefit the knee.

- Avoid sudden changes in the intensity of exercise. Increase the force or duration of activity gradually.

- Wear shoes that both fit properly and are in good condition to help maintain balance and leg alignment when walking or running. Knee problems may be caused by flat feet or overpronated feet (feet that roll inward). People can often reduce some these problems by wearing special shoe inserts (orthotics). Maintain appropriate weight to reduce stress on the knee. Obesity increases the risk of degenerative (wearing) conditions such as osteoarthritis of the knee.

What Kinds of Doctors Treat Knee Problems?

Extensive injuries and diseases of the knees are usually treated by an orthopaedic surgeon, a doctor who has been trained in the nonsurgical and surgical treatment of bones, joints, and soft tissues (for example, ligaments, tendons, and muscles). Patients seeking nonsurgical treatment of arthritis of the knee may also consult a rheumatologist (a doctor specializing in the diagnosis and treatment of arthritis and related disorders).

What Are the Major Structures of the Knee? What Do They Do?

The knee joint works like a hinge to bend and straighten the lower leg. It permits a person to sit, stand, and pivot. The knee is composed of the following parts:

Bones and Cartilage

The knee joint is the junction of three bones-the femur (thigh bone or upper leg bone), the tibia (shin bone or larger bone of the lower leg), and the patella (kneecap). The patella is about 2 to 3 inches wide and 3 to 4 inches long. It sits over the other bones at the front of the knee joint and slides when the leg moves. It protects the knee and gives leverage to muscles.

The ends of the three bones in the knee joint are covered with articular cartilage, a tough, elastic material that helps absorb shock and allows the knee joint to move smoothly. Separating the bones of the knee are pads of connective tissue called menisci, which are divided into two crescent-shaped discs positioned between the tibia and femur on the outer and inner sides of each knee. The two menisci in each knee act as shock absorbers, cushioning the lower part of the leg from the weight of the rest of the body, as well as enhancing stability.

Muscles

There are two groups of muscles at the knee. The quadriceps muscle comprises four muscles on the front of the thigh that work to straighten the leg from a bent position. The hamstring muscles, which bend the leg at the knee, run along the back of the thigh from the hip to just below the knee.

Ligaments

Ligaments are strong, elastic bands of tissue that connect bone to bone. They provide strength and stability to the joint. Four ligaments connect the femur and tibia:

- The medial collateral ligament (MCL) provides stability to the inner (medial) aspect of the knee.

- The lateral collateral ligament (LCL) provides stability to the outer (lateral) aspect of the knee.

- The anterior cruciate ligament (ACL), in the center of the knee, limits rotation and the forward movement of the tibia.

- The posterior cruciate ligament (PCL), also in the center of the knee, limits backward movement of the tibia.

Other ligaments are part of the knee capsule, which is a protective, fiber-like structure that wraps around the knee joint. Inside the capsule, the joint is lined with a thin, soft tissue, called synovium.

323

Tendons

Tendons are tough cords of tissue that connect muscle to bone. In the knee, the quadriceps tendon connects the quadriceps muscle to the patella and provides power to extend the leg.

The patellar tendon connects the patella to the tibia. Technically, it is a ligament, but it is commonly called a tendon.

How Are Knee Problems Diagnosed?

Doctors use several methods to diagnose knee problems.

- a Medical history—the patient tells the doctor details about symptoms and about any injury, condition, or general health problem that might be causing the pain.

- Physical examination—the doctor bends, straightens, rotates (turns), or presses on the knee to feel for injury and discover the limits of movement and location of pain.

- Diagnostic tests—the doctor uses one or more tests to determine the nature of a knee problem.

- X-ray (radiography)—an x-ray beam is passed through the knee to produce a two-dimensional picture of the bones.

- Computerized axial tomography (CAT) scan—x rays lasting a fraction of a second are passed through the knee at different angles, detected by a scanner, and analyzed by a computer. This produces a series of clear cross-sectional images ("slices") of the knee tissues on a computer screen. CAT scan images show soft tissues more clearly than normal x-rays. Individual images can be combined by computer to give a three-dimensional view of the knee.

- Bone scan (radionuclide scanning)—a very small amount of radioactive material is injected into the patient's bloodstream and detected by a scanner. This test detects blood flow to the bone and cell activity within the bone, and can show abnormalities in these processes that may aid diagnosis.

- Magnetic resonance imaging (MRI)—energy from a powerful magnet (rather than x-rays) stimulates tissues of the knee to produce signals that are detected by a scanner and analyzed by computer. This creates a series of cross-sectional images of a specific part of the knee. An MRI is particularly sensitive for detecting damage or disease of soft tissues, such as ligaments and muscles. As with a CAT scan, a computer can be used to produce three-dimensional views of the knee during MRI.

- Arthroscopy—the doctor manipulates a small, lighted optic tube (arthroscope) that has been inserted into the joint through a small incision in the knee. Images of the inside of the knee joint are projected onto a television screen.

Cartilage Injuries and Disorders

Chondromalacia

What Is Chondromalacia?

Chondromalacia (pronounced KON-DRO-MAH-LAY-SHE-AH), also called chondromalacia patellae, refers to softening of the articular cartilage of the kneecap. The disorder occurs most often in young adults and may be caused by trauma, overuse, parts out of alignment, or muscle weakness. Instead of gliding smoothly across the lower end of the thigh bone, the kneecap rubs against it, thereby roughening the cartilage underneath the kneecap. The damage may range from a slight abnormality of the surface of the cartilage to a surface that has been worn away completely to the bone. Traumatic chondromalacia occurs when a blow to the knee cap tears off either a small piece of articular cartilage or a large fragment containing a piece of bone (osteochondral fracture).

What Are the Symptoms of Chondromalacia? How Is It Diagnosed?

The most frequent symptom of chondromalacia is a dull pain around or under the kneecap that worsens when walking down stairs or hills. A person may also feel pain when climbing stairs or during other activities when the knee bears weight as it is straightened. The disorder is common in runners and is also seen in skiers, cyclists, and soccer players. A patient's description of symptoms and a follow up x-ray usually help the doctor make a diagnosis. Although arthroscopy can confirm the diagnosis of chondromalacia, it is not performed unless the condition requires extensive treatment.

How Is Chondromalacia Treated?

Many doctors recommend that patients with chondromalacia perform low-impact exercises that strengthen muscles, particularly the inner part of the quadriceps, without injuring joints. Swimming, riding a stationary bicycle, and using a cross-country ski machine are acceptable as long as the knee is not bent more than 90 degrees. Electrical stimulation may also be used to strengthen the muscles. If these treatments fall to improve the condition, the physician may perform arthroscopic surgery to smooth the surface of the articular cartilage and "wash out" cartilage fragments that cause the joint to catch during bending and straightening. In more severe cases of chondromalacia, surgery may be necessary to correct the angle of the kneecap and relieve friction involving the cartilage or to reposition parts that are out of alignment.

Injuries to the Meniscus

What Is the Cause of Injuries to the Meniscus?

The two menisci are easily injured by the force of rotating the knee while bearing weight. A partial or total tear of a meniscus may occur when a person quickly twists or rotates the upper leg while the foot stays still (for example, when dribbling a basketball around an opponent or turning to hit a tennis ball). If the tear is tiny, the meniscus stays connected to the front and back of the knee; if the tear is large, the meniscus may be left hanging by a thread of cartilage. The seriousness of a tear depends on its location and extent.

What Are the Symptoms of Injury?

Generally, when people injure a meniscus, they feel some pain, particularly when the knee is straightened. The pain may be mild, and the person may continue activity. Severe pain may occur if a fragment of the meniscus catches between the femur and tibia. Swelling may occur soon after injury if blood vessels are disrupted, or swelling may occur several hours later if the joint fills with fluid produced by the joint lining (synovium) as a result of inflammation. If the synovium is injured, it may become inflamed and produce fluid to protect itself. This causes swelling of the knee. Sometimes, an injury that occurred in the past but was not treated becomes painful months or years later, particularly if the knee is injured a second time. After any injury the knee may click, lock, or feel weak. Symptoms of meniscal injury may disappear on their own but frequently, symptoms persist or return and require treatment.

How Is Meniscal Injury Diagnosed?

In addition to listening to the patient's description of the onset of pain and swelling, the physician may perform a physical examination and take x-rays of the knee. The examination may include a test in which the doctor flexes (bends) the leg then rotates the leg outward and inward while extending it. Pain or an audible click suggests a meniscal tear. An MRI test may be recommended to confirm the diagnosis. Occasionally, the doctor may use arthroscopy to help diagnose and treat a meniscal tear.

How Is an Injured Meniscus Treated?

If the tear is minor and the pain and other symptoms go away, the doctor may recommend a muscle-strengthening program. Exercises for meniscal problems are best performed with initial guidance from a doctor and physical therapist or exercise therapist. The therapist will make sure that the patient does the exercises properly and without risk of new or repeat injury. The following exercises after injury to the meniscus are designed to build up the quadriceps and hamstring muscles and increase flexibility and strength.

- Warming up the joint by riding a stationary bicycle, then straightening and raising the leg (but avoiding straightening the leg too much).

- Extending the leg while sitting (a weight may be worn on the ankle for this exercise).

- Raising the leg while lying on the stomach.

- Exercising in a pool, including walking as fast as possible in chest-deep water, performing small flutter kicks while holding onto the side of the pool, and raising each leg to 90 degrees in chest-deep water while pressing the back against the side of the pool.

If the tear to a meniscus is more extensive, the doctor may perform either arthroscopic surgery or "open surgery" to see the extent of injury and to repair the tear. The doctor can suture (sew) the meniscus back in place if the patient is relatively young, the injury is in an area with a good blood supply, and the ligaments are intact. Most young athletes are able to return to vigorous sports with meniscus-preserving repair.

If the patient is elderly or the tear is in an area with a poor blood supply, the doctor may cut off a small portion of the meniscus to even the surface. In some cases, the doctor removes the entire meniscus. However, degenerative changes, such as osteoarthritis, are more likely to develop in the knee if the meniscus is removed. Medical researchers are currently investigating a procedure called an allograft, in which the surgeon replaces the meniscus with one from a cadaver. A grafted meniscus is fragile and may shrink and tear easily. Researchers have also attempted to replace a meniscus with an artificial one, but the procedure is even less successful than an allograft.

Recovery after surgery to repair a meniscus takes several weeks longer and post-operative activity is slightly more restricted than when the meniscus is removed. Nevertheless, putting weight on the joint actually fosters recovery. Regardless of the form of surgery, rehabilitation usually includes walking, bending the legs, and doing exercises that stretch and build up the leg muscles. The best results of treatment for meniscal injury are obtained in people who do not show articular cartilage changes and who have an intact anterior cruciate ligament.

Arthritis of the Knee

What Is Arthritis of the Knee?

Arthritis of the knee is most often osteoarthritis, a degenerative disease where cartilage in the joint gradually wears away. In rheumatoid arthritis, which can also affect the knees, the joint becomes inflamed and cartilage may be destroyed.[1] Arthritis not only affects joints, it may also affect supporting structures such as muscles, tendons, and ligaments.

Osteoarthritis may be caused by excess stress on the joint, such as from repeated injury, deformity, or if a person is overweight. It most often affects middle-aged and older people. A young person who develops osteoarthritis may have an inherited form of the disease or may have experienced continuous irritation from an unrepaired torn meniscus or other injury. Rheumatoid arthritis usually affects people at an earlier age than osteoarthritis.

What Are the Signs of Knee Arthritis and How Is It Diagnosed?

A person who has arthritis of the knee may experience pain, swelling, and a decrease in knee motion. A common symptom is morning stiffness that lessens after moving around. Sometimes the knee joint locks or clicks when the knee is bent and straightened, but these signs may also occur in other knee disorders. The doctor may confirm the diagnosis by performing a physical examination and taking x-rays, which typically show a loss of joint space. Blood tests may be helpful for diagnosing rheumatoid arthritis, but other tests may be needed as well. Analysis of fluid from the knee joint may be helpful in diagnosing some kinds of arthritis. The doctor may use arthroscopy to directly visualize damage to cartilage, tendons, and ligaments and to confirm a diagnosis, but arthroscopy is usually done only if a repair procedure is to be performed.

How Is Arthritis of the Knee Treated?

Most often osteoarthritis of the knee is treated with analgesics (pain-reducing medicines), such as aspirin or acetaminophen (Tylenol): nonsteroidal anti-inflammatory drugs (NSAIDs), such as ibuprofen (Motrin, Nuprin, Advil); and exercises to restore joint movement and strengthen the knee. Losing excess weight can also help people with osteoarthritis. Rheumatoid arthritis of the knee may require a treatment plan that includes physical therapy and use of more powerful medications. In people with arthritis of the knee, a seriously damaged joint may need to be surgically replaced with an artificial one. (Note: A new procedure designed to stimulate the growth of cartilage using a patient's own cartilage cells is being used experimentally to repair cartilage injuries at the end of the femur at the knee. It is not a treatment for arthritis.)

Ligament Injuries

Anterior and Posterior Cruciate Ligament Injury

What Are the Causes of Injury to the Cruciate Ligaments?

Injury to the cruciate ligaments of the knee is sometimes referred to as a "sprain." The anterior cruciate ligament is most often stretched, torn, or both by a sudden twisting motion (for example, when the feet are planted one way and the knees are turned another way). The posterior cruciate ligament is most often injured by a direct impact, such as in an automobile accident or football tackle.

What Are the Symptoms of Cruciate Ligament Injury? How Is Injury Diagnosed?

Injury to a cruciate ligament may not cause pain. Rather, the person may hear a popping sound, and the leg may buckle when he or she tries to stand on it. To diagnose an injury, the doctor may perform several tests to see if the parts of the knee stay in proper position when pressure is applied in different directions. A thorough examination is essential to the diagnosis. An MRI is very accurate in detecting a complete tear, but arthroscopy may be the only reliable means of detecting a partial tear.

How Are Cruciate Ligament Tears Treated?

For an incomplete tear, the doctor may recommend that the patient begin an exercise program to strengthen surrounding muscles. The doctor may also prescribe a protective knee brace for the patient to wear during activity. For a completely torn anterior cruciate ligament in an active athlete and motivated patient, the doctor is likely to recommend surgery. The surgeon may reattach the torn ends of the ligament or reconstruct the torn ligament by using a piece (graft) of healthy ligament from the patient (autograft) or from a cadaver (allograft). Although repair using synthetic ligaments has been tried experimentally, the procedure has not yielded as good results as use of human tissue. One of the most important elements in a patient's successful recovery after cruciate ligament surgery is following an exercise and rehabilitation program for 4 to 6 months that may involve the use of special exercise equipment at a rehabilitation or sports center. Successful surgery and rehabilitation will allow the patient to return to a normal full lifestyle.

Medial and Lateral Collateral Ligament Injury

What Is the Most Common Cause of Injury to the Medial Collateral Ligament?

The medial collateral ligament is more easily injured than the lateral collateral ligament. It is most often caused by a blow to the outer side of the knee, which often happens in contact sports like football or hockey, that stretches and tears the ligament on the inner side of the knee.

What Are the Symptoms of Collateral Ligament Injury? How Is Injury Diagnosed?

When injury to the medial collateral ligament occurs, a person may feel a pop and the knee may buckle sideways. Pain and swelling are common. A thorough examination is essential to determine the nature and extent of injury. To diagnose a collateral ligament injury, the doctor exerts pressure on the side of the knee to determine the degree of pain and looseness of the joint. An MRI is helpful in diagnosing injuries to these ligaments.

How Are Collateral Ligament Injuries Treated?

Most sprains of the collateral ligaments will heal if the patient follows a prescribed exercise program. In addition to exercise, the doctor may recommend that the patient apply ice packs to reduce pain and swelling and wear a small sleeve-type brace to protect and sta-bilize the knee. A sprain may take 2 to 4 weeks to heal. A severely sprained or torn collateral ligament may be accompanied by a torn anterior cruciate ligament, which usually requires surgical repair.

Tendon Injuries and Disorders

Tendinitis and Ruptured Tendons

What Are the Causes of Tendinitis and Ruptured Tendons?

Knee tendon injuries range from tendinitis (inflammation of a ten-don) to a ruptured (torn) tendon. If a person overuses a tendon dur-ing certain activities such as dancing, cycling, or running, the tendon stretches like a worn-out rubber band and becomes inflamed. Move-ments such as trying to break a fall may cause excessive contraction of the quadriceps muscles and tear the quadriceps tendon above the patella or the patellar tendon below the patella. This type of injury is most likely to happen in older people whose tendons tend to be weaker. Tendinitis of the patellar tendon is sometimes called jumper's knee. This is because in sports requiring jumping, such as basketball, the muscle contraction and force of hitting the ground after a jump strain the tendon. The tendon may become inflamed or tear after re-peated stress.

What Are the Symptoms of Tendon Injuries? How Are Injuries Diag-nosed?

People with tendinitis often have tenderness at the point where the patellar tendon meets the bone. They also may feel pain during faster movements, such as running, hurried walking, or jumping. A complete rupture of the quadriceps or patellar tendon is not only pain-ful but also makes it difficult for a person to bend, extend, or lift the leg against gravity. If there is not much swelling, the doctor will be able to feel a defect in the tendon near the tear during a physical examination.

An x-ray will show that the patella is lower in position than normal in a quadriceps tendon tear and higher than normal in a patellar tendon tear. The doctor may use an MRI to confirm a partial or total tear.

How Are Knee Tendon Injuries Treated?

Initially, the doctor may ask a patient with tendinitis to rest, elevate, and apply ice to the knee and to take medicines such as aspirin or ibuprofen to relieve pain and decrease inflammation and swelling. If the quadriceps or patellar tendon is completely ruptured, a surgeon will reattach the ends. After surgery, the patient will wear a cast for 3 to 6 weeks and use crutches. If the tear is only partial, the doctor might-apply a cast without performing surgery.

A partial or complete tear of a tendon requires an exercise program as part of rehabilitation that is similar to but less vigorous than that prescribed for ligament injuries. The goals of exercise are to restore the ability to bend and straighten the knee and to strengthen the leg to prevent a repeat knee injury. A rehabilitation program may last 6 months, although the patient can return to many activities before then.

Osgood-Schlatter Disease

What Are the Causes of Osgood-Schlatter Disease?

Osgood-Schlatter disease is caused by repetitive stress or tension on a part of the growth area of the upper tibia (the apophysis). It is characterized by inflammation of the patellar tendon and surrounding soft tissues at the point where the tendon attaches to the tibia. The disease may also be associated with an avulsion injury, in which the tendon is stretched so much that it tears away from the tibia and takes a fragment of bone with it. The disease most commonly affects active young people, particularly boys between the ages of 10 and 15, who play games or sports that include frequent running and jumping.

What Are the Symptoms of Osgood-Schlatter Disease? How Is It Diagnosed?

People with this disease experience pain just below the knee joint that usually worsens with activity and is relieved by rest. A bony bump that is particularly painful when pressed may appear on the upper edge of the tibia (below the knee cap). Usually, motion of the knee is not affected. Pain may last a few months and may recur until a child's growth is completed.

Osgood-Schlatter disease is most often diagnosed by the symptoms. An x-ray may be normal, or show an avulsion injury, or, more typically, show that the apophysis is in fragments.

How Is Osgood-Schlatter Disease Treated?

Usually, the disease disappears without treatment. Applying ice to the knee when pain first begins helps relieve inflammation and is sometimes used along with stretching and strengthening exercises. The doctor may advise the patient to limit participation in vigorous sports. Children who wish to continue participating in moderate or less stressful sports may need to wear knee pads for protection and apply ice to the knee after activity. If a great deal of pain is felt during sports activities, participation may be limited until any remaining discomfort is tolerable.

Iliotibial Band Syndrome

What Causes Iliotibial Band Syndrome?

This is an overuse inflammatory condition due to friction (rubbing) of a band of a tendon over the outer bone (lateral condyle) of the knee. Although iliotibial band syndrome may be caused by direct injury to the knee, it is most often caused by the stress of long-term overuse, such as sometimes occurs in sports training.

What Are the Symptoms of Iliotibial Band Syndrome and How Is It Diagnosed?

A person with this syndrome feels an ache or burning sensation at the side of the knee during activity. Pain may be localized at the side of the knee or radiate up the side of the thigh. A person may also feel a snap when the knee is bent and then straightened. Swelling is usually absent and knee motion is normal. The diagnosis of this disorder is usually based on the patient's symptoms, such as pain at the lateral condyle, and exclusion of other conditions with similar symptoms.

How Is Iliotibial Band Syndrome Treated?

Usually, iliotibial band syndrome disappears if the person reduces activity and performs stretching exercises followed by muscle-strengthening exercises. In rare cases when the syndrome doesn't disappear, surgery may be necessary to split the tendon so it is not stretched too tightly over the bone.

Other Knee Injuries

Osteochondritis Dissecans

What Is Osteochondritis Dissecans?

Osteochondritis dissecans results from a loss of the blood supply to an area of bone underneath a joint surface and usually involves the knee. The affected bone and its covering of cartilage gradually loosen and cause pain. A person with this disruption of the joint may eventually develop osteoarthritis. This disorder usually arises spontaneously in an active adolescent or a young adult. It may be due to a slight blockage of a small artery or to an unrecognized injury or tiny fracture that damages the overlying cartilage.

The bone undergoes avascular necrosis (degeneration from lack of a blood supply).[2] The involvement of several joints or the appearance of osteochondritis dissecans in several family members may indicate that the disorder is inherited.

What Are the Symptoms of Osteochondritis Dissecans? How Is It Diagnosed?

If spontaneous healing doesn't occur, cartilage eventually separates from the diseased bone and a fragment breaks loose into the knee joint, causing locking of the joint, weakness, and sharp pain. An x-ray, MRI, or arthroscopy can determine the condition of the cartilage and be used to diagnose osteochondritis dissecans.

How Is Osteochondritis Dissecans Treated?

If cartilage fragments have not broken loose, a surgeon may fix them in place with pins or screws that are sunk into the cartilage to stimulate a new blood supply. If fragments are loose, the surgeon may scrape down the cavity to reach fresh bone and add a bone graft and fix the fragments in position. Fragments that cannot be mended are removed, and the cavity is drilled or scraped to stimulate new growth of cartilage. Research is currently being done to assess the use of cartilage cell transplants and other tissues to treat this disorder.

Plica Syndrome

Plica (pronounced PLI-KAH) syndrome occurs when plicae (bands of remnant synovial tissue) are irritated by overuse or injury. Synovial

plicae are remnants of tissue pouches found in the early stages of fetal development. As the fetus develops, these pouches normally combine to form one large synovial cavity. If this process is incomplete,
plicae remain as four folds or bands of synovial tissue within the knee.
Injury, chronic overuse, or inflammatory conditions are associated
with development of this syndrome.

What Are the Symptoms of Plica Syndrome? How Is It Diagnosed?

People with this syndrome are likely to experience pain and swelling, a clicking sensation, and locking and weakness of the knee. Because the symptoms are similar to symptoms of some other knee
problems, plica syndrome is often misdiagnosed. Diagnosis usually
depends on the exclusion of other conditions that cause similar symptoms.

How Is Plica Syndrome Treated?

The goal of treatment is to reduce inflammation of the synovium
and thickening of the plicae. The doctor usually prescribes medicine
such as ibuprofen to reduce inflammation. The patient is also advised
to reduce activity, apply ice and compression wraps (elastic bandage)
to the knee, and do strengthening exercises. If this treatment program
fails to relieve symptoms within 3 months, the doctor may recommend
arthroscopic or open surgery to remove the plicae. A cortisone injection into the region of the plica folds helps about half of the patients
treated. The doctor can also use arthroscopy to confirm the diagnosis
and treat the problem.

Other Sources of Information on Knee Problems

American Academy of Orthopaedic Surgeons
6300 N. River Road
Rosemont, IL 60018-4262
847/823-7186
800/346-2267
World Wide Web address: http://www.aaos.org

The academy publishes several. brochures on the knee, including
"Knee Arthroscopy" and *"Total Knee Replacement,"* which doctors can
obtain and give to their patients. Single copies of two other pamphlets,
"Arthroscopy" and *"Total Joint Replacement,"* are available free to the
public if a self-addressed, stamped envelope is provided.

American Physical Therapy Association
1111 N. Fairfax Street
Alexandria, VA 22314
800/999-APTA (2782)
World Wide Web address: http://www.apta.org

The association has published a free brochure titled *"Taking Care of the Knees."*

Arthritis Foundation
1330 Peach Tree Street
Atlanta, GA 30309
404/872-7100
800/283-7800 or call your local chapter (listed in the local telephone directory)
World Wide Web address: http://www.arthritis.org

The Foundation has several free brochures about coping with arthritis, taking nonsteroid and steroid medicines, and exercise. A free brochure on protecting your joints is titled *"Using Your Joints Wisely."* The foundation also provides doctor referrals.

American College of Rheumatology/Association of Rheumatology Health Professionals
60 Executive Park South, Suite 150
Atlanta, GA 30329
404/633-3777
Fax: 404/633-1870
World Wide Web address: http://www.rheumatology.org

This national professional organization can provide referrals to rheumatologists and allied health professionals, such as physical therapists. One-page fact sheets are available on various forms of arthritis. Lists of specialists by geographic area and fact sheets are also available on ACR's web site.

National Arthritis and Musculoskeletal and Skin Diseases Information Clearinghouse (NAMSIC)
National Institutes of Health
1 AMS Circle
Bethesda, MD 20892-3675
301/495-4484
TTY: 301/ 565-2966

Automated faxback system: 301/881-2731
World Wide Web address: http://www.nih.gov/niams

The Clearinghouse has additional information about some of the knee problems described in this chapter, including osteoarthritis and avascular necrosis, as well as information about total knee replacement and arthritis and exercise. Single copies of fact sheets and information packages on these topics are available free upon request.

Acknowledgments

The NIAMS gratefully acknowledges the assistance of Frank A Pettrone, M.D., of Arlington/Vienna, Virginia, W Norman Scott, M.D., of Beth Israel Medical Center in New York, New York, and James Panagis, M.D., M.P.H., and John H. Klippel, M.D., of the National Institutes of Health, in the preparation and review of this fact sheet.

The National Arthritis and Musculoskeletal and Skin Diseases Information Clearinghouse (NAMSIC) is a public service sponsored by the NIAMS that provides health information and information sources. The NIAMS, a part of the National Institutes of Health (NIH), leads the Federal medical research effort in arthritis and musculoskeletal and skin diseases. The NIAMS sponsors research and research training throughout the United States as well as on the NIH campus in Bethesda, MD, and disseminates health and research information.

1. The National Arthritis and Musculoskeletal and Skin Diseases Information Clearinghouse has separate information packages on osteoarthritis, rheumatoid arthritis, and knee replacement. Single copies are free.

2. A fact sheet and information package on avascular necrosis are available from the National Arthritis and Musculoskeletal and Skin Diseases Information Clearinghouse.

*   Brand names included in this fact sheet are provided as examples only, and their inclusion does not mean that these products are endorsed by the National Institutes of Health or any other Government agency. Also, if a particular brand name is not mentioned, this does not mean or imply that the product is unsatisfactory.

Chapter 44

New Ways to Heal Broken Bones

Jacqueline Wallace, of Phoenix, sat enjoying the December 1993 holidays at her son's home in Gaithersburg, Md. But when she stood up and took a step, her holiday took a turn for the worse. Wallace fell and fractured her hip. "My foot dragged a little, not exactly a stumble," Wallace says. "I don't know whether the bone broke because I fell, or I fell because the bone broke."

Despite her 84 years and weak heart, Wallace had a lot going for her after her fall: modern medical practice and determination to walk again. Surgery to implant an artificial hip joint took under 45 minutes. Spinal anesthesia and sedation were administered instead of general anesthesia because they are thought to pose less risk. And her physical therapy began the day after the operation. "I fussed," she says. "I was afraid it was going to hurt or I'd fall. But they said if you want to go home, you have to do this. And I did. It was more scary than painful."

Wallace's fracture was one of 1.5 million—including 336,000 hip fractures—reported in 1993, the latest year for which the National Center for Health Statistics has figures. Besides surgical repair, treatments for broken bones include bone manipulation to reduce the fracture, use of a cast, and bone stimulation. Central to fracture healing is bone biology. Many treatments, some on the horizon, are designed to improve the natural course of healing.

FDA Consumer magazine, April 1996; Food and Drug Administration.

Bones at Work

For skeletal growth and maintenance, the body's 206 dynamic, living bones renew themselves lifelong through a continual breakdown, build-up process known as remodeling. This process is also involved in the remodeling of fractures, says Martin Yahiro, M.D., a Baltimore orthopedist in private practice and a consultant on fracture treatment devices to the Food and Drug Administration's Center for Devices and Radiological Health.

In remodeling, complex chemical signals prompt cells called osteoclasts to break down and remove (resorb) old bone, and others called osteoblasts to deposit new bone. Many elements influence remodeling. Among them: weight-bearing, vitamin D, growth factors, prostaglandins, and various hormones, including estrogen, thyroid, parathyroid, and calcitonin.

As 80 percent of the mature skeleton, compact cortical bone supports the body, providing extra thickness mid-shaft in long bones to prevent their bending. Cancellous bone, whose porous structure with small cavities resembles a sponge, predominates in the pelvis and the 33 vertebrae from the neck to the tailbone. A fibrous membrane called the periosteum covers bone. For healing and health, living bone must have a steady supply of nutrients. Blood vessels permeate bone to provide this lifeline. Blood-forming elements fill the long bone inner canals.

When a Bone Breaks

Fracture breaks continuity of bone and of important attached soft tissue—including blood vessels, which spill their contents into surrounding tissue.

Even before treatment, the body automatically seeks to repair the injury. Inflammatory cells rush to destroy, dilute or isolate invaders and injured tissue. Tiny new blood vessels called capillaries begin growing into the site. Cells proliferate. The injured person usually must endure pain, swelling, and increased heat at the breakage site for one to three days.

New tissue bonds the fractured bone ends with a soft callus, a mass of connective tissue and exudate (matter escaped through blood vessel walls). Remodeling begins. Within a few months, a hard callus replaces the soft one. Remodeling restores the inner canal.

Once restoration is complete, which may take years, the healed area is brand new, without a scar. Usually thicker, the new bone may even be stronger than the old, Yahiro says, adding that if the bone should break again, it's unlikely to be at the same place. And children's bones have a healing boost: They're growing. "The growing skeleton is just geared to make bone," Yahiro says. "A very young child's wrist bones grow a millimeter a month, to rapidly correct misalignment or length defects. An adult may take six to eight weeks to heal a wrist fracture, a 5-year-old only three."

When the ends of a fractured bone, such as an arm bone, form an abnormal angle, the doctor must decide whether to push the ends together (manipulation) to reduce the fracture, possibly under anesthesia. Simple x-rays aid evaluation. "If it's a large angle, we'd want to reduce that fracture," Yahiro says. "But if it's a small angle, especially in a young child whose growth will correct it, we'd probably just put the limb in a cast."

Surgery for Joint Fractures

Joint fractures usually require surgery, Yahiro says. "We try to restore the joint to perfect, like putting a jigsaw puzzle back together." An artificial joint can be used to replace a fractured head of the long bone in the hip, like Wallace had, or in the shoulder.

Total hip joint replacements are mainly made of titanium or cobalt-chrome alloys or other metals. Each replacement has a stem that goes into the thigh bone inner canal, a ball for the head, and a plastic cup socket—the latter usually only used if the joint is badly arthritic. Yahiro often uses bipolar joints—a big ball atop a smaller one. All these joint replacements are approved by FDA. Approved replacements for fractures in shoulder joints also consist of a ball and stem.

Andrew Bender, M.D., the orthopedist who implanted Wallace's partial replacement, says this simple model has been in use 30 to 40 years. "It has different size balls, one size stem, so it's not an exact fit. But it gives what we call a three-point fixation for some immediate tightness. The stem has holes for bone to grow through and across for more permanence." Bender pressed in Wallace's device without cement, a snug fit. He cements only if the fit is very, very loose. "Modern day hip replacement without cement is relatively quick, both sides. She had only one side done and good bone, so it didn't take long."

If a replacement fails, it usually does so within 5 to 10 years. Simple models tend not to fail in the very old, Yahiro says. "A person in a chair or bed most of the time won't put demands on the joint that, say, Bo Jackson does." (Jackson had a hip replacement in 1992 due to a football injury.)

For higher demand, there are more precisely fitted models. A robot that drills a more precise hole for the stem, to possibly keep the joint intact longer, is under investigation for use in cementless hip joint replacements. (See "Robots in the Operating Room," July-August 1993 *FDA Consumer*.)

An external fixator—a pin-and-rod frame—can keep the joint from being compressed by other bones, to heal before a load, or stress, is put on it again. Pins are inserted on one side of the limb through the skin, muscle and bone, out the other side, and attached to the external rod, forming the frame. About 30 percent of patients get infected at the pin site, so meticulous hygiene is crucial. "It's a race," says Kenneth McDermott, who reviews the devices for the Center for Devices and Radiological Health. "The pin goes through the skin, and infection can go right down the pin."

Internal fixation devices pose less risk of infection. These metal plates, rods, wires, screws, nails, pins, staples, and anchors may sometimes be left in. A tiny pin may not be felt, but plates or screws may cause irritation or pain. The decision whether to remove the device in a second surgery is made on a case-by-case basis.

Surgery to remove a screw in the very old may be too risky. For a 20-year-old, benefits of a second surgery may outweigh risks. In the ankle, plates and screws are customarily removed. Yahiro says, "The bones are so superficial, the device often rubs on the shoe."

McDermott gives another reason for removing a plate or screw: "It can take the load off the bone, causing the bone to resorb and weaken." Fixators and internal fixation devices are used also for some mid-bone fractures.

Grafts

The surgeon may graft bone to replace a missing segment that had to be surgically removed due to infection. For a small segment, tissue can be taken from the patient's own bone (autologous graft).

Cadaver bone (allograft) may be used, especially for a large segment. Though dead tissue, cadaver bone provides a scaffold for living bone to grow into and remodel the graft. For healing to occur—and sometimes it doesn't—the body must put blood vessels into the graft to nurture the new living bone as it replaces the dead tissue. Healing takes longer than with an autologous graft. Another option is a substitute bone graft, fashioned with help from nonhuman substances. FDA recently approved two such grafts:

- *Pro Osteon Implant 500 Coralline Hydroxyapatite Bone Void Filler(1992)*—Fills holes near the ends of long bones in adults. It derives from marine coral, whose spongy calcium structure resembles human cancellous bone.

- *Collagraft Bone Graft Matrix(1993)*—Treats long-bone fractures and other injury-caused areas of missing bone of 30 milliliters (1.8 cubic inches) or less. The product—consisting of purified cow collagen and a chemical, hydroxyapatite-tricalcium phosphate—is mixed with the patient's marrow into a paste and put into the area of missing bone to encourage new bone growth. It's not for use in certain patients, such as those with osteomyelitis (bone inflammation) at the fracture site, severe allergies, or allergy to cow collagen, and those being desensitized to meat products, as the treatment injections may contain cow collagen.

When these substitute grafts are placed next to healthy bone, the body remodels them in the same way it remodels human grafts. But according to Center for Devices and Radiological Health reviewer Nadine Rosile, "The substitute grafts aren't strong enough for use without a fixation device to stabilize the fracture."

A bone filler paste now under investigation, however, is as strong as bone within 12 hours, according to a report of a study of patients whose wrist fractures were injected with the paste. The report, in the March 24, 1995, issue of Science, stated that the paste stabilized the bone during healing and was eventually remodeled. The patients had greater grip strength at six months than historical controls (other patients in the past who had not been treated with the paste) had at two years, the report stated.

Also under investigation are injections of growth factor proteins, such as morphogenic protein and transforming growth factor-beta, found naturally in the body in very small amounts.

"The proteins turn on cells to produce bone," Yahiro says. "Animal studies show growth with injections similar to that with autologous grafts." The hope, he says, is that injected fractures, even with large areas of missing bone, will heal faster and be stronger, without grafts.

Healing Helpers

FDA has approved seven electrical bone growth stimulators, mainly for fractures at the middle of long bones, such as the shinbone (tibia), that have not healed over at least nine months. Although exactly how the stimulators heal is unknown, manufacturers' studies showed the devices did in fact affect cellular processes. Yahiro explains that loading (stressing) a bone produces in it a small electrical field called piezo electric force, believed to stimulate new bone formation. "It's believed that electrical stimulation does something like that on a large scale," he says.

For direct stimulation, an electrode is implanted at the fracture, linked through the skin to a generator. For indirect stimulation, electric coils outside the limb on the non-fracture side induce an electrical field at the fracture side.

In 1994, FDA approved the first ultrasound bone growth stimulator. The Sonic Accelerated Fracture Healing System (SAFHS) is for adults with small fractures in the lower leg or lower forearm. A cast or splint is used. It is the first stimulator for the treatment of fractures occurring within seven days before treatment. Studies suggest that mechanical forces of the ultrasound waves transform into electrical impulses as they travel through the tissues.

The SAFHS consists of a portable generator cabled to a small, square treatment module that emits ultrasound pulses at about the same low intensity as sonogram fetal monitors. In some instances, the patient may use the unit at home. Recommended treatment is 20 minutes once a day until the fracture heals. The SAFHS is not for patients who need additional fixation or surgery, are pregnant or breast-feeding, have bone disease or circulatory problems, or take medicines that may adversely affect remodeling.

In studies, all treated patients—and especially older people— healed faster than those using a placebo. In those age 50 and older, arms healed 40 days faster, and legs 85 days faster. Six years' follow-up did not suggest long-term adverse effects.

Stimulation, grafts, manipulation, joint replacements, casts. Whatever the treatment, fracture healing is monitored by x-rays and physical examination to answer such questions as: Does it hurt or move when pushed on? On x-ray, does the fracture look healed? On x-ray, are the bones aligned?

For Wallace, healing is now complete. She is indeed walking again, using a cane as she did before the replacement surgery. "If I don't use the cane, my leg aches," she says. "I'm still careful to use my good leg stepping up a curb, and my bad leg stepping down, like I learned in therapy."

Boning Up

The most important influences on fracture healing are nutrition and overall health, including bone health, before the injury, says orthopedist

Martin Yahiro, M.D., a consultant to FDA. "That's why it's so important all your life to do weight-bearing exercise such as walking and get enough calcium and vitamin D, so you lay down as much bone as possible during growth and keep as much as you can later on."

The Recommended Dietary Allowance (RDA) for calcium is 1,200 milligrams a day for people ages 11 to 24 and for pregnant or breast-feeding women. For men and women older than 25 who no longer have to meet the greater demands of growth, the calcium RDA is 800 milligrams a day.

In general, genes decide bone shape and size. But mechanical stress by muscle, body weight, and physical activity influence bone shape and density—and health—throughout life.

Simply put, loaded (stressed) bone strengthens, and unloaded bone weakens. As examples, astronauts' bones weaken in outer space with no gravity pull on them, and the shaft of the humerus (long upper arm bone) in a professional tennis player's dominant arm gets denser and thicker from the extra load. The body increases its bone mass until, usually, the mid-30s, after which a gradual loss begins.

Age-related bone loss can lead to osteoporosis, a condition of thin, weakened bone that fractures easily. The condition affects many post-menopausal women, because bone loss increases with menopause due to lower estrogen levels.

In announcing its recent approval of Fosamax and Miacalcin Nasal Spray for osteoporosis, FDA advised that patients also exercise and get adequate calcium and vitamin D. Drugs approved by FDA to prevent or treat osteoporosis are:

- estrogen—Premarin
- Ogen
- Estrace tablets
- Estraderm patch
- estrogen packaged with progestin hormone tablets—Prempro
- Premphase
- alendronate—Fosamax
- calcitonin—Miacalcin Nasal Spray
- Calcimar Injection
- Miacalcin Injection
- Cibacalcin for injection.

—by Dixie Farley

Dixie Farley is a staff writer for FDA Consumer.

Chapter 45

Stroke Recovery

What Is a Stroke?

A stroke is a type of brain injury. Symptoms depend on the part of the brain that is affected. People who survive a stroke often have weakness on one side of the body or trouble with moving, talking, or thinking.

Most strokes are ischemic (is-KEE-mic) strokes. These are caused by reduced blood flow to the brain when blood vessels are blocked by a clot or become too narrow for blood to get through. Brain cells in the area die from lack of oxygen. In another type of stroke, called hemorrhagic (hem-or-AJ-ic) stroke, the blood vessel isn't blocked; it bursts, and blood leaks into the brain, causing damage.

Strokes are more common in older people. Almost three-fourths of all strokes occur in people 65 years of age or over. However, a person of any age can have a stroke.

A person may also have a transient ischemic attack (TIA). This has the same symptoms as a stroke, but only lasts for a few hours or a day and does not cause permanent brain damage. A TIA is not a stroke but it is an important warning signal. The person needs treatment to help prevent an actual stroke in the future.

A stroke may be frightening to both the patient and family. It helps to remember that stroke survivors usually have at least some spontaneous recovery or natural healing and often recover further with rehabilitation.

1995 Agency for Health Care Policy and Research (AHCPR); publication No. 95-0664.

Purpose of This Text

This article is about stroke rehabilitation. Its goal is to help the person who has had a stroke achieve the best possible recovery. Its purpose is to help people who have had strokes and their families get the most out of rehabilitation.

Note that this article sometimes uses the terms "stroke survivor" and "person" instead of "patient" to refer to someone who has had a stroke. This is because people who have had a stroke are patients for only a short time, first in the acute care hospital and then perhaps in a rehabilitation program. For the rest of their lives, they are people who happen to have had a stroke. The article also uses the word "family" to include those people who are closest to the stroke survivor, whether or not they are relatives.

Rehabilitation works best when stroke survivors and their families work together as a team. For this reason, both stroke survivors and family members are encouraged to read all parts of this article.

Recovering from Stroke

The process of recovering from a stroke usually includes treatment, spontaneous recovery, rehabilitation, and the return to community living. Because stroke survivors often have complex rehabilitation needs, progress and recovery are different for each person.

Treatment for stroke begins in a hospital with "acute care." This first step includes helping the patient survive, preventing another stroke, and taking care of any other medical problems.

Spontaneous recovery happens naturally to most people. Soon after the stroke, some abilities that have been lost usually start to come back. This process is quickest during the first few weeks, but it sometimes continues for a long time.

Rehabilitation is another part of treatment. It helps the person keep abilities and gain back lost abilities to become more independent. It usually begins while the patient is still in acute care. For many patients, it continues afterward, either as a formal rehabilitation program or as individual rehabilitation services. Many decisions about rehabilitation are made by the patient, family, and hospital staff before discharge from acute care.

The last stage in stroke recovery begins with the person's return to **community living** after acute care or rehabilitation. This stage can last for a lifetime as the stroke survivor and family learn to live with the effects of the stroke. This may include doing common tasks in new ways or making up for damage to or limits of one part of the body by greater activity of another. For example, a stroke survivor can wear shoes with Velcro closures instead of laces or may learn to write with the opposite hand.

How Stroke Affects People

Effects on the Body, Mind, and Feelings

Each stroke is different depending on the part of the brain injured, how bad the injury is, and the person's general health. Some of the effects of stroke are:

- Weakness (hemiparesis—hem-ee-par-EE-sis) or paralysis (hemiplegia—hem-ee-PLEE-ja) on one side of the body. This may affect the whole side or just the arm or the leg. The weakness or paralysis is on the side of the body opposite the side of the brain injured by the stroke. For example, if the stroke injured the left side of the brain, the weakness or paralysis will be on the right side of the body.

- Problems with balance or coordination. These can make it hard for the person to sit, stand, or walk, even if muscles are strong enough.

- Problems using language (aphasia and dysarthria). A person with aphasia (a-FAY-zha) may have trouble understanding speech or writing. Or, the person may understand but may not be able to think of the words to speak or write. A person with dysarthria (dis-AR-three-a) knows the right words but has trouble saying them clearly.

- Being unaware of or ignoring things on one side of the body (bodily neglect or inattention). Often, the person will not turn to look toward the weaker side or even eat food from the half of the plate on that side.

- Pain, numbness, or odd sensations. These can make it hard for the person to relax and feel comfortable.

- Problems with memory, thinking, attention, or learning (cognitive problems). A person may have trouble with many mental activities or just a few. For example, the person may have trouble following directions, may get confused if something in a room is moved, or may not be able to keep track of the date or time.

- Being unaware of the effects of the stroke. The person may show poor judgment by trying to do things that are unsafe as a result of the stroke.

- Trouble swallowing (dysphagia—dis-FAY-ja). This can make it hard for the person to get enough food. Also, care must sometimes be taken to prevent the person from breathing in food (aspiration—as-per-AY-shun) while trying to swallow it.

- Problems with bowel or bladder control. These problems can be helped with the use of portable urinals, bedpans, and other toileting devices.

- Getting tired very quickly. Becoming tired very quickly may limit the person's participation and performance in a rehabilitation program.

- Sudden bursts of emotion, such as laughing, crying, or anger. These emotions may indicate that the person needs help, understanding, and support in adjusting to the effects of the stroke.

- Depression. This is common in people who have had strokes. It can begin soon after the stroke or many weeks later, and family members often notice it first.

Depression after Stroke

It is normal for a stroke survivor to feel sad over the problems caused by stroke. However, some people experience a major depressive disorder, which should be diagnosed and treated as soon as possible. A person with a major depressive disorder has a number of symptoms nearly every day, all day, for at least 2 weeks. These always include at least one of the following:

- Feeling sad, blue, or down in the dumps.
- Loss of interest in things that the person used to enjoy.

A person may also have other physical or psychological symptoms, including:

- Feeling slowed down or restless and unable to sit still.
- Feeling worthless or guilty.
- Increase or decrease in appetite or weight.

350

- Problems concentrating, thinking, remembering, or making decisions.
- Trouble sleeping or sleeping too much.
- Loss of energy or feeling tired all of the time.
- Headaches.
- Other aches and pains.
- Digestive problems.
- Sexual problems.
- Feeling pessimistic or hopeless.
- Being anxious or worried.
- Thoughts of death or suicide.

If a stroke survivor has symptoms of depression, especially thoughts of death or suicide, professional help is needed right away. Once the depression is properly treated, these thoughts will go away. Depression can be treated with medication, psychotherapy, or both. If it is not treated, it can cause needless suffering and also makes it harder to recover from the stroke.

Disabilities after Stroke

A "disability" is difficulty doing something that is a normal part of daily life. People who have had a stroke may have trouble with many activities that were easy before, such as walking, talking, and taking care of "activities of daily living" (ADLs). These include basic tasks such as bathing, dressing, eating, and using the toilet, as well as more complex tasks called "instrumental activities of daily living" (IADLs), such as housekeeping, using the telephone, driving, and writing checks.

Some disabilities are obvious right after the stroke. Others may not be noticed until the person is back home and is trying to do something for the first time since the stroke.

What Happens during Acute Care

The main purposes of acute care are to:

- Make sure the patient's condition is caused by a stroke and not by some other medical problem.

- Determine the type and location of the stroke and how serious it is. Prevent or treat complications such as bowel or bladder problems or pressure ulcers (bed sores).

- Prevent another stroke.

351

- Encourage the patient to move and perform self-care tasks, such as eating and getting out of bed, as early as medically possible. This is the first step in rehabilitation.

Stroke survivors and family members may find the hospital experience confusing. Hospital staff are there to help, and it is important to ask questions and talk about concerns.

Before acute care ends, the patient and family with the hospital staff decide what the next step will be. For many patients, the next step will be to continue rehabilitation.

Preventing Another Stroke

People who have had a stroke have an increased risk of another stroke, especially during the first year after the original stroke. The risk of another stroke goes up with older age, high blood pressure (hypertension), high cholesterol, diabetes, obesity, having had a transient ischemic attack (TIA), heart disease, cigarette smoking, heavy alcohol use, and drug abuse. While some risk factors for stroke (such as age) cannot be changed, the risk factors for the others can be reduced through use of medicines or changes in lifestyle.

Patients and families should ask for guidance from their doctor or nurse about preventing another stroke. They need to work together to make healthy changes in the patient's lifestyle. Patients and families should also learn the warning signs of a TIA (such as weakness on one side of the body and slurred speech) and see a doctor **immediately** if these happen.

Deciding about Rehabilitation

Some people do not need rehabilitation after a stroke because the stroke was mild or they have fully recovered. Others may be too disabled to participate. However, many patients can be helped by rehabilitation. Hospital staff will help the patient and family decide about rehabilitation and choose the right services or program.

Types of Rehabilitation Programs

There are several kinds of rehabilitation programs:

- **Hospital programs**. These programs can be provided by special rehabilitation hospitals or by rehabilitation units in acute care hospitals. Complete rehabilitation services are available. The patient stays in the hospital during rehabilitation. An organized team of specially trained professionals provides the therapy. Hospital programs are usually more intense than other programs and require more effort from the patient.

- **Nursing facility (nursing home) programs**. As in hospital programs, the person stays at the facility during rehabilitation. Nursing facility programs are very different from each other, so it is important to get specific information about each one. Some provide a complete range of rehabilitation services; others provide only limited services.

- **Outpatient programs**. Outpatient programs allow a patient who lives at home to get a full range of services by visiting a hospital outpatient department, outpatient rehabilitation facility, or day hospital program.

- **Home-based programs**. The patient can live at home and receive rehabilitation services from visiting professionals. An important advantage of home programs is that patients learn skills in the same place where they will use them.

Individual Rehabilitation Services

Many stroke survivors do not need a complete range of rehabilitation services. Instead, they may need an individual type of service, such as regular physical therapy or speech therapy. These services are available from outpatient and home care programs.

Paying for Rehabilitation

Medicare and many health insurance policies will help pay for rehabilitation. Medicare is the Federal health insurance program for Americans 65 years of age or over and for certain Americans with disabilities. It has two parts: hospital insurance (known as Part A) and supplementary medical insurance (known as Part B). Part A helps pay for home health care, hospice care, inpatient hospital care, and inpatient care in a skilled nursing facility. Part B helps pay for doctors' services, outpatient hospital services, durable medical equipment, and a number of other medical services and supplies not covered by Part A. Social Security Administration offices across the country take applications for Medicare and provide general information about the program.

In some cases, Medicare will help pay for outpatient services from a Medicare-participating comprehensive outpatient rehabilitation facility. Covered services include physicians' services; physical, speech, occupational, and respiratory therapies; counseling; and other related services. A stroke survivor must be referred by a physician who certifies that skilled rehabilitation services are needed.

Medicaid is a Federal program that is operated by the States, and each State decides who is eligible and the scope of health services offered. Medicaid provides health care coverage for some low-income people who cannot afford it. This includes people who are eligible because they are older, blind, or disabled, or certain people in families with dependent children.

These programs have certain restrictions and limitations, and coverage may stop as soon as the patient stops making progress. Therefore, it is important for patients and families to find out exactly what their insurance will cover. The hospital's social service department can answer questions about insurance coverage and can help with financial planning.

Choosing a Rehabilitation Program

The doctor and other hospital staff will provide information and advice about rehabilitation programs, but the patient and family make the final choice. Hospital staff know the patient's disabilities and medical condition. They should also be familiar with the rehabilitation programs in the community and should be able to answer questions about them. The patient and family may have a preference about whether the patient lives at home or at a rehabilitation facility. They may have reasons for preferring one program over another. Their concerns are important and should be discussed with hospital staff.

Things to Consider When Choosing a Rehabilitation Program

- Does the program provide the services the patient needs?
- Does it match the patient's abilities or is it too demanding or not demanding enough?
- What kind of standing does it have in the community for the quality of the program?
- Is it certified and does its staff have good credentials?

- Is it located where family members can easily visit?

- Does it actively involve the patient and family members in rehabilitation decisions?

- Does it encourage family members to participate in some rehabilitation sessions and practice with the patient?

- How well are its costs covered by insurance or Medicare?

- If it is an outpatient or home program, is there someone living at home who can provide care?

- If it is an outpatient program, is transportation available?

A person may start rehabilitation in one program and later transfer to another. For example, some patients who get tired quickly may start out in a less intense rehabilitation program. After they build up their strength, they are able to transfer to a more intense program.

When Rehabilitation Is Not Recommended

Some families and patients may be disappointed if the doctor does not recommend rehabilitation. However, a person may be unconscious or too disabled to benefit. For example, a person who is unable to learn may be better helped by maintenance care at home or in a nursing facility. A person who is, at first, too weak for rehabilitation may benefit from a gradual recovery period at home or in a nursing facility. This person can consider rehabilitation at a later time. It is important to remember that:

- Hospital staff are responsible for helping plan the best way to care for the patient after discharge from acute care. They can also provide or arrange for needed social services and family education.

- This is not the only chance to participate in rehabilitation. People who are too disabled at first may recover enough to enter rehabilitation later.

What Happens during Rehabilitation

In hospital or nursing facility rehabilitation programs, the patient may spend several hours a day in activities such as physical therapy, occupational therapy, speech therapy, recreational therapy, group activities, and patient and family education. It is important to maintain skills that help recovery. Part of the time is spent relearning skills (such as walking and speaking) that the person had before the stroke. Part of it is spent learning new ways to do things that can no longer be done the old way (for example, using one hand for tasks that usually need both hands).

Setting Rehabilitation Goals

The goals of rehabilitation depend on the effects of the stroke, what the patient was able to do before the stroke, and the patient's wishes. Working together, goals are set by the patient, family, and rehabilitation program staff. Sometimes, a person may need to repeat steps in striving to reach goals.

If goals are too high, the patient will not be able to reach them. If they are too low, the patient may not get all the services that would help. If they do not match the patient's interests, the patient may not want to work at them. Therefore, it is important for goals to be realistic. To help achieve realistic goals, the patient and family should tell program staff about things that the patient wants to be able to do.

Rehabilitation Goals

* Being able to walk, at least with a walker or cane, is a realistic goal for most stroke survivors.

* Being able to take care of oneself with some special equipment is a realistic goal for most.

* Being able to drive a car is a realistic goal for some.

* Having a job can be a realistic goal for some people who were working before the stroke. For some, the old job may not be possible but another job or a volunteer activity may be.

Reaching treatment goals does not mean the end of recovery. It just means that the stroke survivor and family are ready to continue recovery on their own.

Rehabilitation Specialists

Because every stroke is different, treatment will be different for each person. Rehabilitation is provided by several types of specially trained professionals. A person may work with any or all of these:

- **Physician**. All patients in stroke rehabilitation have a physician in charge of their care. Several kinds of doctors with rehabilitation experience may have this role. These include family physicians and internists (primary care doctors), geriatricians (specialists in working with older patients), neurologists (specialists in the brain and nervous system), and physiatrists (specialists in physical medicine and rehabilitation).

- **Rehabilitation nurse**. Rehabilitation nurses specialize in nursing care for people with disabilities. They provide direct care, educate patients and families, and help the doctor to coordinate care.

- **Physical therapist**. Physical therapists evaluate and treat problems with moving, balance, and coordination. They provide training and exercises to improve walking, getting in and out of a bed or chair, and moving around without losing balance. They teach family members how to help with exercises for the patient and how to help the patient move or walk, if needed.

- **Occupational therapist**. Occupational therapists provide exercises and practice to help patients do things they could do before the stroke such as eating, bathing, dressing, writing, or cooking. The old way of doing an activity sometimes is no longer possible, so the therapist teaches a new technique.

- **Speech-language pathologist**. Speech-language pathologists help patients get back language skills and learn other ways to communicate. Teaching families how to improve communication is very important. Speech-language pathologists also work with patients who have swallowing problems (dysphagia).

- **Social worker**. Social workers help patients and families make decisions about rehabilitation and plan the return to the home or a new living place. They help the family answer questions about insurance and other financial issues and can arrange for a variety of support services. They may also provide or arrange for patient and family counseling to help cope with any emotional problems.

- **Psychologist**. Psychologists are concerned with the mental and emotional health of patients. They use interviews and tests to identify and understand problems. They may also treat thinking or memory problems or may provide advice to other professionals about patients with these problems.

357

- **Therapeutic recreation specialist**. These therapists help patients return to activities that they enjoyed before the stroke such as playing cards, gardening, bowling, or community activities. Recreational therapy helps the rehabilitation process and encourages the patient to practice skills.

- **Other professionals**. Other professionals may also help with the patient's treatment. An orthotist may make special braces to support weak ankles and feet. A urologist may help with bladder problems. Other physician specialists may help with medical or emotional problems. Dietitians make sure that the patient has a healthy diet during rehabilitation. They also educate the family about proper diet after the patient leaves the program. Vocational counselors may help patients go back to work or school.

Rehabilitation professionals, the patient, and the family are vitally important partners in rehabilitation. They must all work together for rehabilitation to succeed.

Rehabilitation Team

In many programs, a special rehabilitation team with a team leader is organized for each patient. The patient, family, and rehabilitation professionals are all members. The team has regular meetings to discuss the progress of treatment. Using a team approach often helps everyone work together to meet goals.

Getting the Most Out of Rehabilitation

What the Patient Can Do

If you are a stroke survivor in rehabilitation, keep in mind that you are the most important person in your treatment. You should have a major say in decisions about your care. This is hard for many stroke patients. You may sometimes feel tempted to sit back and let the program staff take charge. If you need extra time to think or have trouble talking, you may find that others are going ahead and making decisions without waiting. Try not to let this happen.

- Make sure others understand that you want to help make decisions about your care.

- Bring your questions and concerns to program staff.

- State your wishes and opinions on matters that affect you.

- Speak up if you feel that anyone is "talking down" to you; or, if people start talking about you as if you are not there.

- Remember that you have the right to see your medical records.

To be a partner in your care, you need to be well informed about your treatment and how well you are doing. It may help to record important information about your treatment and progress and write down any questions you have.

If you have speech problems, making your wishes known is hard. The speech-language pathologist can help you to communicate with other staff members, and family members may also help to communicate your ideas and needs.

Most patients find that rehabilitation is hard work. They need to maintain abilities at the same time they are working to regain abilities. It is normal to feel tired and discouraged at times because things that used to be easy before the stroke are now difficult. The important thing is to notice the progress you make and take pride in each achievement.

How the Family Can Help

If you are a family member of a stroke survivor, here are some things you can do:

- Support the patient's efforts to participate in rehabilitation decisions.

- Visit and talk with the patient. You can relax together while playing cards, watching television, listening to the radio, or playing a board game.

- If the patient has trouble communicating (aphasia), ask the speech-language pathologist how you can help.

- Participate in education offered for stroke survivors and their families. Learn as much as you can and how you can help.

- Ask to attend some of the rehabilitation sessions. This is a good way to learn how rehabilitation works and how to help.

- Encourage and help the patient to practice skills learned in rehabilitation.

- Make sure that the program staff suggests activities that fit the patient's needs and interests.

- Find out what the patient can do alone, what the patient can do with help, and what the patient can't do. Then avoid doing things for the patient that the patient is able to do. Each time the patient does them, his or her ability and confidence will grow.

- Take care of yourself by eating well, getting enough rest, and taking time to do things that you enjoy.

To gain more control over the rehabilitation process, keep important information where you can find it. One suggestion is to keep a notebook with the patient.

Discharge Planning

Discharge planning begins early during rehabilitation. It involves the patient, family, and rehabilitation staff. The purpose of discharge planning is to help maintain the benefits of rehabilitation after the patient has been discharged from the program. Patients are usually discharged from rehabilitation soon after their goals have been reached.

Some of the things discharge planning can include are to:

- Make sure that the stroke survivor has a safe place to live after discharge.

- Decide what care, assistance, or special equipment will be needed.

- Arrange for more rehabilitation services or for other services in the home (such as visits by a home health aide).

- Choose the health care provider who will monitor the person's health and medical needs.

- Determine the caregivers that will work as a partner with the patient to provide daily care and assistance at home, and teach them the skills they will need.

- Help the stroke survivor explore employment opportunities, volunteer activities, and driving a car (if able and interested).

- Discuss any sexual concerns the stroke survivor or husband/wife may have. Many people who have had strokes enjoy active sex lives.

Preparing a Living Place

Many stroke survivors can return to their own homes after rehabilitation. Others need to live in a place with professional staff such as a nursing home or assisted living facility. An assisted living facility can provide residential living with a full range of services and staff. The choice usually depends on the person's needs for care and whether caregivers are available in the home. The stroke survivor needs a living place that supports continuing recovery.

It is important to choose a living place that is safe. If the person needs a new place to live, a social worker can help find the best place.

During discharge planning, program staff will ask about the home and may also visit it. They may suggest changes to make it safer. These might include changing rooms around so that a stroke survivor can stay on one floor, moving scatter rugs or small pieces of furniture that could cause falls, and putting grab bars and seats in tubs and showers.

It is a good idea for the stroke survivor to go home for a trial visit before discharge. This will help identify problems that need to be discussed or corrected before the patient returns.

Deciding about Special Equipment

Even after rehabilitation, some stroke survivors have trouble walking, balancing, or performing certain activities of daily living. Special equipment can sometimes help. Here are some examples:

- **Cane**. Many people who have had strokes use a cane when walking. For people with balancing problems, special canes with three or four "feet" are available.

- **Walker**. A walker provides more support than a cane. Several designs are available for people who can only use one hand and for different problems with walking or balance.

- **Ankle-foot orthotic devices (braces).** Braces help a person to walk by keeping the ankle and foot in the correct position and providing support for the knee.

- **Wheelchair**. Some people will need a wheelchair. Wheelchairs come in many different designs. They can be customized to fit the user's needs and abilities. Find out which features are most important for the stroke survivor.

- **Aids for bathing, dressing, and eating**. Some of these are safety devices such as grab bars and nonskid tub and floor mats. Others make it easier to do things with one hand. Examples are Velcro fasteners on clothes and placemats that won't slide on the table.

- **Communication aids**. These range from small computers to homemade communication boards. The stroke survivor, family, and rehabilitation program staff should decide together what special equipment is needed. Program staff can help in making the best choices. Medicare or health insurance will often help pay for the equipment.

Preparing Caregivers

Caregivers who help stroke survivors at home are usually family members such as a husband or wife or an adult son or daughter. They may also be friends or even professional home health aides. Usually, one person is the main caregiver, while others help from time to time. An important part of discharge planning is to make sure that caregivers understand the safety, physical, and emotional needs of the stroke survivor, and that they will be available to provide needed care.

Since every stroke is different, people have different needs for help from caregivers. Here are some of the things caregivers may do:

- Keep notes on discharge plans and instructions and ask about anything that is not clear.

- Help to make sure that the stroke survivor takes all prescribed medicines and follows suggestions from program staff about diet, exercise, rest, and other health practices.

- Encourage and help the person to practice skills learned in rehabilitation.

- Help the person solve problems and discover new ways to do things.

- Help the person with activities performed before the stroke. These could include using tools, buttoning a shirt, household tasks, and leisure or social activities.

- Help with personal care, if the person cannot manage alone.

- Help with communication, if the person has speech problems. Include the stroke survivor in conversations even when the person cannot actively participate.

- Arrange for needed community services.
- Stand up for the rights of the stroke survivor.

If you expect to be a caregiver, think carefully about this role ahead of time. Are you prepared to work with the patient on stroke recovery? Talk it over with other people who will share the caregiving job with you. What are the stroke survivor's needs? Who can best help meet each of them? Who will be the main caregiver? Does caregiving need to be scheduled around the caregivers' jobs or other activities? There is time during discharge planning to talk with program staff about caregiving and to develop a workable plan.

Going Home

Adjusting to the Change

Going home to the old home or a new one is a big adjustment. For the stroke survivor, it may be hard to transfer the skills learned during rehabilitation to a new location. Also, more problems caused by the stroke may appear as the person tries to go back to old activities. During this time, the stroke survivor and family learn how the stroke will affect daily life and can make the necessary adjustments.

These adjustments are a physical and emotional challenge for the main caregiver as well as the stroke survivor. The caregiver has many new responsibilities and may not have time for some favorite activities. The caregiver needs support, understanding, and some time to rest. Caregiving that falls too heavily on one person can be very stressful. Even when family members and friends are nearby and willing to help, conflicts over caregiving can cause stress.

A stroke is always stressful for the family, but it is especially hard if one family member is the only caregiver. Much time may be required to meet the needs of the stroke survivor. Therefore, the caregiver needs as much support as possible from others. Working together eases the stress on everyone.

Tips for Reducing Stress

The following tips for reducing stress are for both caregivers and stroke survivors.

- Take stroke recovery and caregiving one day at a time and be hopeful.

- Remember that adjusting to the effects of stroke takes time. Appreciate each small gain as you discover better ways of doing things.

- Caregiving is learned. Expect that knowledge and skills will grow with experience.

- Experiment. Until you find what works for you, try new ways of doing activities of daily living, communicating with each other, scheduling the day, and organizing your social life.

- Plan for "breaks" so that you are not together all the time. This is a good way for family and friends to help on occasion. You can also plan activities that get both of you out of the house.

- Ask family members and friends to help in specific ways and commit to certain times to help. This gives others a chance to help in useful ways.

- Read about the experiences of other people in similar situations. Your public library has life stories by people who have had a stroke as well as books for caregivers.

- Join or start a support group for stroke survivors or caregivers. You can work on problems together and develop new friendships.

- Be kind to each other. If you sometimes feel irritated, this is natural and you don't need to blame yourself. But don't "take it out" on the other person. It often helps to talk about these feelings with a friend, rehabilitation professional, or support group.

- Plan and enjoy new experiences and don't look back. Avoid comparing life as it is now with how it was before the stroke.

Follow-up Appointments

After a stroke survivor returns to the community, regular follow-up appointments are usually scheduled with the doctor and sometimes with rehabilitation professionals. The purpose of follow-up is to check on the stroke survivor's medical condition and ability to use the skills learned in rehabilitation. It is also important to check on how well the stroke survivor and family are adjusting. The stroke survivor and caregiver can be prepared for these visits with a list of questions or concerns.

Where To Get Help

Many kinds of help are available for people who have had strokes and their families and caregivers. Some of the most important are:

- **Information about stroke**. A good place to start is with the books and pamphlets available from national organizations that provide information on this subject. Many of their materials are available free of charge. A list of these organizations follows.

- **Local stroke clubs or other support groups**. These are groups where stroke survivors and family members can share their experiences, help each other solve problems, and expand their social lives.

- **Home health services**. These are available from the Visiting Nurses Association (VNA), public health departments, hospital home care departments, and private home health agencies. Services may include nursing care, rehabilitation therapies, personal care (for example, help with bathing or dressing), respite care (staying with the stroke survivor so that the caregiver can take a vacation or short break), homemaker services, and other kinds of help.

- **Meals on Wheels**. Hot meals are delivered to the homes of people who cannot easily shop and cook.

- **Adult day care**. People who cannot be completely independent sometimes spend the day at an adult day care center. There they get meals, participate in social activities, and may also get some health care and rehabilitation services.

- **Friendly Visitor (or other companion services)**. A paid or volunteer companion makes regular visits or phone calls to a person with disabilities.

- **Transportation services**. Most public transportation systems have buses that a person in a wheelchair can board. Some organizations and communities provide vans to take wheelchair users and others on errands such as shopping or doctor's visits.

Many communities have service organizations that can help. Some free services may be available or fees may be on a "sliding scale" based on income. It takes some work to find out what services and payment arrangements are available. A good way to start is to ask the social workers in the hospital or rehabilitation program where the stroke survivor was treated. Also, talk to the local United Way or places of worship. Another good place to look is the Yellow Pages of the telephone book, under "Health Services," "Home Health Care," "Senior Citizen Services," or "Social Service Organizations." Just asking friends may turn up useful information. The more you ask, the more you will learn.

Additional Resources

ACTION
1100 Vermont Avenue, NW
Washington, DC 20525
(202) 606-4855
(call for telephone number of regional office) Sponsors older American volunteer programs.

Administration on Aging
330 Independence Avenue, SW
Washington, DC 20201
Toll-free (800) 677-1116
(call for list of community services for older Americans in your area)

AHA Stroke Connection (formerly the Courage Stroke Network)
American Heart Association
7272 Greenville Avenue
Dallas, TX 75231
Toll-free (800) 553-6321
(or check telephone book for local AHA office)
Provides prevention, diagnosis, treatment, and rehabilitation information to stroke survivors and their families.

American Dietetic Association/National Center for Nutrition and Dietetics
216 West Jackson Boulevard
Chicago, IL 60606
Toll-free (800) 366-1655
(Consumer Nutrition Hotline) Consumers may speak to a registered dietitian for answers to nutrition questions, or obtain a referral to a local registered dietitian.

American Self-Help Clearinghouse
St. Clares-Riverside Medical Center
Denville, NJ 07834
(201) 625-7101
(call for name and telephone number of State or local clearinghouse)
Provides information and assistance on local self-help groups.

National Aphasia Association
P.O. Box 1887
Murray Hill Station
New York, NY 10156
Toll-free (800) 922-4622
Provides information on the partial or total loss of the ability to speak or comprehend speech, resulting from stroke or other causes.

National Easter Seal Society
230 West Monroe Street, Suite 1800
Chicago, IL 60606
(312) 726-6200
(or check telephone book for local Easter Seal Society) Provides information and services to help people with disabilities.

National Stroke Association
8480 East Orchard Road, Suite 1000
Englewood, CO 80111
(303) 771-1700
Toll-free (800) STROKES (787-6537)

Rosalynn Carter Institute
Georgia Southwestern College
600 Simmons Street
Americus, GA 31709
Provides information on caregiving. Reading lists, video products, and other caregiver resources are available by writing to the address listed above.

Stroke Clubs International
805 12th Street
Galveston, TX 77550
(409) 762-1022
(call for the name of a stroke club located in your area) Maintains list of over 800 stroke clubs throughout the United States.

The Well Spouse Foundation
P.O. Box 801
New York, NY 10023
(212) 724-7209 Toll-free (800) 838-0879
Provides support for the husbands, wives, and partners of people who are chronically ill or disabled.

Medicare Information
Consumer Information Center
Department 59 Pueblo, CO 81009
By writing to this address, you can receive a free copy of The Medicare Handbook (updated and published annually). This handbook provides information about Medicare benefits, health insurance to supplement Medicare, and limits to Medicare coverage. It is also available in Spanish.

For Further Information

Information in this booklet is based on *Post-Stroke Rehabilitation. Clinical Practice Guideline*, Number 16. It was developed by a non-Federal panel sponsored by the Agency for Health Care Policy and Research (AHCPR), an agency of the Public Health Service. Other guidelines on common health problems are available, and more are being developed.

Four other patient guides are available from AHCPR that may be of interest to stroke survivors and their caregivers:

- *Preventing Pressure Ulcers: Patient Guide* gives detailed information about how to prevent pressure sores (AHCPR Publication No. 92-0048).

- *Treating Pressure Sores: Patient Guide* gives detailed information about treating pressure sores (AHCPR Publication No. 95-0654).

- *Urinary Incontinence in Adults: Patient Guide* describes why people lose urine when they don't want to and how that can be treated (AHCPR Publication No. 92-0040).

- *Depression Is a Treatable Illness: Patient Guide* discusses major depressive disorder, which most often can be successfully treated with the help of a health professional (AHCPR Publication No. 93-0053).

For more information about these and other guidelines, or to get more copies of this booklet, call toll-free: 800-358-9295 or write to:

Agency for Health Care Policy and Research Publications Clearinghouse
P.O. Box 8547
Silver Spring, MD 20907

U.S. Department of Health and Human Services Public Health Service Agency for Health Care Policy and Research
Executive Office Center, Suite 501
2101 East Jefferson Street
Rockville, MD 20852
AHCPR Publication No. 95-0664 May 1995

Chapter 46

Recovering from Heart Problems through Cardiac Rehabilitation

Purpose of This Chapter

Cardiac rehabilitation are (rehab) services are designed to help patients with heart disease recover faster and return to full and productive lives. Cardiac rehab includes exercise, education, counseling, and learning ways to live a healthier life. Together with medical and surgical treatments, cardiac rehab can help you feel better and live a healthier life.

You can benefit from cardiac rehab if you:

- Have heart disease, such as angina or heart failure, or have had a heart attack.
- Have had coronary bypass surgery or a balloon catheter (PTCA) procedure on your heart.
- Have had a heart transplant.

Cardiac rehab can make a difference. It is a safe and effective way to help you:

- Feel better faster.
- Get stronger.
- Reduce stress.

1995 U.S. Department of Health and Human Services, Public Health Service, Agency for Health Care Policy and Research, Executive Office Center, Suite 501, 2101 East Jefferson Street, Rockville, MD 20852, AHCPR Publication No. 96-0674, October 1995.

- Reduce the risks of future heart problems.
- Live longer.

Almost everyone with heart disease can benefit from some type of cardiac rehab. No one is too old or too young. Women benefit from cardiac rehab as much as men.

This booklet can help you learn how to lower your risk for future heart problems. You will also learn tips for finding a cardiac rehab plan that is right for you. Most important, you will learn what you can do to be healthier.

Risk Factors for Coronary Disease

The controllable risk factors for coronary disease are shown below. There are some risk factors that you cannot change, such as older age or a family history of heart disease. But you can change or control the ones shown below. Cardiac rehab can help you do this.

Coronary Disease Risk Factors You Can Control

- Smoking
- High blood pressure
- High blood cholesterol
- Sedentary lifestyle
- Overweight
- Diabetes
- Stress

The Cardiac Rehab Team

Cardiac rehab services can involve many health care providers. Your team may include:

- Doctors (your family doctor, a heart specialist, and perhaps a surgeon).
- Nurses.
- Exercise specialists.
- Physical and occupational therapists.
- Dietitians.
- Psychologists or other behavior therapists.

Sometimes a primary care provider, such as your family doctor or nurse practitioner, works alone playing many roles or refers patients to other health care specialists as needed. But the most important member of your cardiac rehab team is you. No one else can make you exercise. Or quit smoking. Or eat a more healthful diet.

To be an active member of the cardiac rehab team:

- Learn about your heart condition.
- Learn what you can do to help your heart.
- Follow the treatment plan.
- Feel free to ask questions.
- Report symptoms or problems.

Family members and friends can make a difference. They may want to learn more about heart problems so their help can be even more valuable. For example, family members may have to learn to let you do things for yourself. Or they may want to learn about preparing heart-healthy meals. Your family and friends can give you emotional support as you adjust to a new, healthier lifestyle.

You may also want the support of other people who have heart disease. Ask your cardiac rehab team if they know of a support group you can join, or get in touch with one of the organizations listed at the end of this chapter.

How Do I Get Started?

Cardiac rehab often begins in the hospital after a heart attack, heart surgery, or other heart treatment. It continues in an outpatient setting after you leave the hospital. Once you learn the habits of heart-healthy living, stick with them for life.

In an outpatient setting. Outpatient rehab may be located at the hospital, in a medical or professional center, in a community facility such as the YMCA, or at your place of work. You may even have cardiac rehab at home. You will be advised to increase the amount of exercise you do. You will also receive education and encouragement to control your risk factors.

For life. After you have learned the skills of heart-healthy living, you should continue to use them for life.

You need your doctor's approval to get started in cardiac rehab. Tell your doctor or nurse that you're interested in cardiac rehab and ask which rehab services or plans are best for you.

How Does Cardiac Rehab Work?

Cardiac rehab has two major parts:

1. **Exercise training** to help you learn how to exercise safely, strengthen your muscles, and improve your stamina. Your exercise plan will be based on your individual ability, needs, and interests.

2. **Education, counseling, and training** to help you understand your heart condition and find ways to reduce your risk of future heart problems. The cardiac rehab team will help you learn how to cope with the stress of adjusting to a new lifestyle and to deal with your fears about the future.

Cardiac rehab often takes place in groups. However, each patient's plan is based on his or her specific risk factors and special needs.

Cardiac rehab helps you recognize and change unhealthy habits you may have and establish new, healthier ones. Your rehab may last 6 weeks, 6 months, or even longer. It is important that you complete the recommended rehab plan.

Is It Safe for Me?

Cardiac rehab is safe. Studies show that serious health problems caused by cardiac rehab exercise are rare. The cardiac rehab team is trained to handle emergencies. Your health care provider can help you choose a plan that is safe for you. Many patients can safely exercise without supervision once they learn their own exercise plan.

Checking how your heart reacts and adapts to exercise is an important part of cardiac rehab. You may be connected to an EKG transmitter while you exercise. If your cardiac rehab is done at home, you may be connected to an EKG machine by telephone, or you may phone the cardiac rehab team to let them know how you are doing. In some settings, you check your own pulse rate or estimate how hard you are exercising.

What's in It for Me?

The goals of cardiac rehab are different for each patient. In helping set your personal goals, your health care team will look at your general health, your personal heart problem, your risks for future heart problems, your doctor's recommendations, and of course, your own preferences.

Cardiac rehab can reduce your symptoms and your chances of having more heart problems. And it has many other benefits:

- Exercise tones your muscles and improves your energy level and spirits. It helps both your heart and your body gets stronger and work better. Exercise also can get you back to work and other activities faster.

- A healthy diet can lower blood cholesterol, control weight, and help prevent or control high blood pressure and other problems such as diabetes. Plus, you will feel better and have more energy.

- Cardiac rehab can help you quit smoking. Kicking the habit means less risk of lung cancer, emphysema, and bronchitis, as well as less risk of heart attack, stroke, and other heart and blood vessel problems. It means more energy, and it means better health for your loved ones.

- You can learn to manage stress instead of letting it manage you. You will feel better and improve your heart health.

Make a habit of the heart-healthy lifestyle you learn In cardiac rehab. Your life depends on it!

How Do I Find a Plan That's Right for Me?

Your doctor or nurse may recommend a cardiac rehab plan or help you to arrange for exercise training, education, counseling, and other services. Many hospitals and outpatient health care centers offer cardiac rehab— so do some local schools and community centers. You can also check the Yellow Pages of your telephone book.

When choosing a cardiac rehab plan, ask about:

- **Time.** Is it offered when you can get there without causing added stress? Cardiac rehab services offered at the workplace are sometimes an option.

- **Place.** Is it easy to get to? Keep in mind that traffic problems can add to your stress. Is there parking? Public transportation?

- **Setting.** Is it an individual or group plan? Is it home-based or in a facility? Think about whether you want to be in a group with professional supervision.

- **Services.** Does it offer a wide range of services? More importantly, does it include the areas you need help with, such as quitting smoking?

- **Cost.** Is it affordable? Is it covered by insurance? Your insurance may cover all or part of the cost of some cardiac rehab services but not others. Find out what will be covered and for how long. Consider what you can afford and for how long.

Cardiac rehab has life-long favorable effects, so choose a plan that will serve your needs. For example, if you smoke, look for a plan that will help you quit. Choose a plan that includes activities you enjoy, such as regular walking in a shopping mall or park. Before you sign up, visit and ask any questions you may have.

How Can I Get the Most Out of Cardiac Rehab?

Studies show that controlling your risk factors for heart disease can help you lead a healthier life. So make sure your cardiac rehab plan works for you. Here's how:

- **Plan.** Work with your health care team to design or change your services to meet your needs.

- **Communicate.** Ask questions. If you don't understand the answers, keep asking until you do. Report changes in your feelings or symptoms.

- **Take charge of your recovery.** No one else can do it for you. Your new lifestyle is healthy for your heart, so stick with it—for life.

To gain more control over your cardiac rehab, remember your goals and keep important information where you can find it. You may want to have a special calendar just for your rehab activities or keep a notebook.

Where Can I Get More Information and Support?

For additional information about heart disease and ways you can help yourself through cardiac rehab, contact:

American Association of Cardiovascular and Pulmonary Rehabilitation (national program directory) (608) 831-6989

American Heart Association (patient education materials) 800-AHA-USAI (800-242-8721)

Mended Hearts, Inc. (patient support group) (214) 706-1442, http://www.mendedhearts.org

National Heart, Lung, and Blood Institute (patient education materials) (301) 251-1222

For Further Information

The information in this booklet is based on the Clinical Practice Guideline on Cardiac Rehabilitation. The guideline was developed by a non-Federal panel of experts sponsored by the Agency for Health Care Policy and Research (AHCPR), a U.S. Government agency. Additional support came from the National Heart, Lung, and Blood Institute. Other guidelines on common health problems are available from AHCPR, and more are being developed.

Three other patient guides available from AHCPR may be of interest to people participating in cardiac rehab:

Managing Unstable Angina (AHCPR Publication No. 94-0604).

Living With Heart Disease: Is It Heart Failure? (AHCPR Publication No. 940614).

Depression Is a Treatable Illness (AHCPR Publication No. 93-0553).

For more information about these and other guidelines, or to get more copies of this booklet, call toll free: 800-358-9295, or write to:

Agency for Health Care Policy and Research Publications Clearinghouse P.O. Box 8547 Silver Spring, MD 20907, 800-358-9295

These and other guidelines are available online through a free electronic service from the National Library of Medicine called HSTAT.

Copies of this brochure and other consumer brochures are free through InstantFAX, which operates all day every day. If you have a fax machine equipped with a touchtone telephone, dial (301) 594-2800, push 1, and then press the start button for instructions and a list of publications.

Chapter 47

The Best Way to Recover from Heart Disease

According to the Agency for Health Care Policy and Research (AHCPR), two-thirds of those with heart disease are not getting cardiac rehabilitation, one of the most effective means of prolonging life and controlling cardiac symptoms. Cardiac rehabilitation programs include exercise training, along with classes in good nutrition and the causes of heart disease. Programs often begin in the hospital, as patients recuperate from a heart attack, bypass surgery, or angioplasty, and then continue in an outpatient setting for three to six months. But new AHCPR guidelines make it clear that nearly all patients with heart disease should consider such a program, whether or not they've been hospitalized. Completing a rehabilitation program may either decrease the need for other treatments, or increase their effectiveness should they be required.

During the past three decades, the eligibility criteria for admission to cardiac rehabilitation have broadened, In the 1960s, most patients were middle-aged men who had survived a heart attack and were free of sever complications such as unstable angina, uncontrolled hypertension, or advanced congestive heart failure (CHF). As little as 10 years ago, most experts advised patients with CHF to avoid all but the mildest exertion. Such thinking is outdated. Patients with heart disease — including women and the elderly — are now advised to be as active as possible. And studies show that those who participate in supervised programs are more likely to make lasting lifestyle changes and to lead longer, more comfortable lives than those who go it alone.

The number of people who can benefit from the recommendations specified in the AHCPR guidelines is staggering. Some 13.5 million Americans have heart disease, and each year nearly 1 million people survive heart attacks. Seven million patients have unstable angina, and about 650,000 have bypass Surgery or angioplasty. Heart failure is the most common discharge diagnosis for hospitalized Medicare patients, and the fourth most common diagnosis among all patients hospitalized in the United States. Most heart patients are candidates for rehabilitation—but a doctor's recommendation is required first. The AHCPR guidelines urge all heart patients to ask about rehabilitation, and they encourage doctors to prescribe it when appropriate.

What to Expect

Participating in a comprehensive cardiac rehabilitation program increases stamina and strength, and lessens symptoms such as chest pain, fatigue, and shortness of breath. It may also help patients lower cholesterol levels, lessen the need for cholesterol-lowering drugs, and reduce the stress and depression that often accompany heart disease. The most successful programs have two major components:

Exercise Training

During rehabilitation, most patients generally do some form of aerobic activity (such as walking or cycling), plus resistance exercise (weight lifting). Patients are encouraged to do as much as they can, based on their cardiac limitations. The type, intensity, and duration of the recommended activities depend on a baseline or starting heart rate established by comparing the results of a standard electrocardiogram (ECG), taken when the heart is at rest, with an ECG taken when the heart is working (an exercise stress test).

Over time, muscles become stronger, and the heart becomes more efficient. Thus, patients can accomplish more work at lower heart rates with fewer symptoms. Studies show that patients who exercise after having a heart attack are 25% less likely to die of a second heart attack than those who do not.

Education

Classes include dietary counseling, such as tips on how to choose healthy foods and prepare tasty, low-fat meals; support for smokers trying to quit (as many as 25% of cigarette smokers who participate in a supervised program are able to break the habit); stress reduction workshops; and information about the causes of heart disease and the importance of lifestyle changes. The curriculum focuses on practical, realistic suggestions designed to help patients adopt and maintain healthy behaviors.

Tailoring a Plan

Exercise training and education are most effective when implemented together. Doctors, nurses, exercise specialists, physical and occupational therapists, dietitians, psychologists, and social workers all contribute their expertise in designing a customized plan that will be safe and effective. The program generally calls for three or four group exercise sessions a week, each lasting about 30 to 60 minutes, for eight to 12 weeks.

The aerobic portion of the program might consist of a 10 minute warm-up that includes some stretching and light jogging or cycling; 20 to 30 minutes of more-intensive walking, jogging, cycling, or swimming; and a five minute cool-down period with stretching and easy activities similar to those done in the warm-up. Weight training usually involves about 10 different exercises using light weights or machines. Patients begin with a few repetitions and slowly increase the number to as many as three sets of twelve repetitions each. The amount of weight is also gradually increased.

The greatest benefit accrues to those who exercise at least three times a week, 20 to 40 minutes at a time, at 70 to 85% of their maximum safe heart rate (which is determined through exercise testing). However, patients who are frail, disabled, or severely ill can benefit from less-intensive workouts. Less exertion is also appropriate for patients with pacemakers and for those taking drugs to slow heart rate (such as beta-blockers).

Classes about diet, smoking cessation, weight control, and stress management may be held on the same day as exercise training or scheduled for a non-exercise day.

The cost of a comprehensive program ranges from $800 to $1,800. Insurance coverage varies, but many plans, including Medicare, cover at least a portion of the expense. Rehabilitation centers can be freestanding, but most are based at hospitals, which frequently have arrangements with community centers and sometimes, local gyms or YM/YWCAs. Your doctor can provide a referral, and a list of selected centers is available from the American Association of Cardiovascular and Pulmonary

Rehabilitation (call 608-831-6989), or the American Heart Association (call 800-242-8721 for the phone number of a local chapter).

Are There Any Risks?

Cardiac rehabilitation is considered safe and rarely causes health problems because participants are so carefully followed. After an assessment and orientation, exercise sessions can be monitored at the rehabilitation center or at home, depending on the health and transportation needs of the individual patient. Continued attendance is usually preferred for patients with severe coronary disease and certain arrhythmias, and those who smoke or are overweight.

But patients who are stable and well motivated can often exercise on their own as long as they check in with rehabilitation staff according to a predetermined schedule. Some patients take their pulse before, during, and after exercise, then report these findings to the rehabilitation staff over the phone. It's even possible to be connected via the phone to an ECG located at the center.

To ensure success, work with your health care team in designing services that meet your needs and goals. Ask questions, and be sure to report any changes in symptoms. Whatever type of heart disease you have, following through on rehabilitation will enhance recovery, slow disease progression, and bolster the success of virtually all medical or surgical treatments.

For More Information

Agency for Health Care Policy and Research.
Publications Clearinghouse
PO Box 8547
Silver Spring, MD 20907-8547
800-358-9295
http://www.ahcpr.gov/info

> *"Cardiac Rehabilitation: Exercise Training, Education, Counseling, and Behavioral Interventions"* (pub. # 96-0672).
>
> *"Cardiac Rehabilitation Guideline."*
>
> *"Recovering From Heart Problems Through Cardiac Rehabilitation"* (pub. # 96-0674).

Johns Hopkins Cardiac Rehabilitation Home Page. Available on the Internet at www.jhbmc.jhu.edu.

Chapter 48

Cardiac Rehab: Still a Good Idea?

Cardiac rehabilitation presents issues and choices that typify the larger health care debate: Are rehabilitation programs of genuine value to an increasingly diverse group of patients, or do other alternatives offer comparable, better, or more cost-effective care?

Not surprisingly, the answer is complex and heralds a move away from traditional exercise-based programs to a more comprehensive array of services, including preventive and psychosocial interventions, for a wider range of patients. Meanwhile, primary care physicians should be prepared to take on an expanded role in supporting and coordinating care, with greater involvement in risk factor reduction and cardiac assessment and referral.

The goals of cardiac rehab are to improve functional and psychological status, reduce risk, and maximize quality of life while reintegrating the patient with the family, community, and workplace. The relative value of specific interventions—supervised exercise training, nutritional and behavioral counseling, targeted risk factor reduction, and pharmacotheraphy—is the focus of current research.

Answers to the following questions will help you determine what your patients can gain from cardiac rehab. They'll also acquaint you with existing alternatives and the increasing role you may play in preventive cardiology.[a]

© 1994 Medical Economics Publishing, from *Patient Care*, October 30, 1994 Vol. 28 No.17 p24(12); by Ezra A. Amsterdam, Roger J. Cadiux, Robert F. Debusk, Albert Oberman, reprinted with permission.

What Are the Known Benefits of Cardiac Rehab?

Comprehensive cardiac rehabilitation, with both exercise and nonexercise components, improves functional and physical work capacity, reduces anxiety and depression, increases sense of well-being, promotes an understanding of disease and its treatment, and helps patients return to their customary routines. These benefits are most often seen after an acute myocardial infarction (MI) or surgical procedure but are increasingly available to patients with other cardiovascular conditions.

The benefits of traditional programs are close medical supervision, trained staff to assist with exercises, patient education, psychosocial services, and social support. However, only a small percentage of eligible patients make use of these services due to issues such as cost and convenience. Home-based programs have the potential to offer some of the same advantages at a lower cost and with more convenience.

Does Cardiac Rehab Increase Survival?

Despite several small trials and meta-analyses, the effects of cardiac rehab in prolonging life and preventing recurrence following MI are unproven. Two meta-analyses do suggest a survival benefit for exercise-based programs in the years immediately following MI, especially in middle-aged men at moderate to high risk.

Since most studies in the meta-analyses included both an exercise and a nonexercise component, it was not possible to determine the effects of exercise alone. Nor was it possible to determine the independent effects of increased surveillance of patients once they were randomized to rehabilitation. Thus, while the two meta-analyses yield consistent results with regard to survival, the mechanisms responsible for the benefits are not clearly defined.

How Important Is Exercise Training?

Exercise remains a key component of cardiac rehab by virtue of its ability to increase cardiovascular functional capacity and decrease myocardial oxygen demand for a given level of activity. It can also provide a framework within which other risk factors can be modified an effort to improve well being and reduce post-MI mortality.

Most of the metabolic benefits of exercise occur through more efficient oxygen consumption in the peripheral muscles. This results in reduced myocardial oxygen consumption and reduced cardiac workload, measured by lower heart rate and blood pressure, for a given amount of work. The net effect is that patients are able to engage in more physical exertion without cardiac signs or symptoms such as angina.

Patients who experience an uncomplicated acute MI now have a much shorter hospital stay and a much better prognosis and functional capacity due to more aggressive inpatient management (for example, with thrombolytic therapy and revascularization) than they did in the 1970s and 1980s, when the early studies were published. Some feel this reduces the significance of exercise training in improving post-MI survival. All patients about to be discharged after an MI should be advised about safe levels of general activity.

How Does Exercise Improve the Risk Factor Profile?

Physical inactivity is an independent risk factor for heart disease and is related to cardiovascular mortality. Exercise training reduces serum triglycerides and levels of very-low-density lipoprotein (VLDL) cholesterol, and in combination with weight loss it may raise high-density lipoprotein (HDL) cholesterol. In a study of 237 outpatients, improvements occurred in low-density lipoprotein (LDL) and HDL cholesterol, triglycerides, bodymass index, and percentage body fat following exercise-based cardiac rehab.[b] Exercise training also has an independent, modest blood-pressure-lowering effect in certain hypertensive patients, increases insulin sensitivity, and promotes weight loss.

In combination with other therapies, exercise can modify medication requirements for control of lipids or blood pressure. A combination of diet and exercise often reduces lipids by 10-20%, beyond which pharmacotherapy may be needed. The physiologic benefits of exercise may also improve dosing requirements or medication choices for treatment of angina. In addition, exercise may help to ease depression, a key feature in rehabilitation for many cardiac patients.

Which Exercise Programs Are Best?

Improvements in functional capacity through aerobic training can generally be accomplished over three months of supervised exercise training at moderate intensity. The usual prescription is to exercise at 70-85% of maximal heart rate, three times per week, for 20-40 minutes per session. Benefits can be obtained at even lower levels of intensity, at heart rates not exceeding 130 beats per minute (see "New trends in exercise for all").

Despite the potential for cardiovascular complications, supervised programs usually carry a low risk if patients are properly selected and surveillance is adequate. Any exercise program should have a five-minute warm-up and cool-down period. Patients should remain in the rehab unit for observation during the cool-down.

The goal for most cardiac patients is to reduce the heart's mechanical effort (heart rate and blood pressure) at submaximal work levels, such as those required for routine activities. Whether exercise training can be pursued at home or in a structured, supervised setting depends on the patient's physical condition, level of education, motivation, and understanding, and on the safety and convenience of the home environment.

Prior treadmill testing is required of all candidates for home-based exercise programs in order to detect arrhythmias or other problems. Patients can probably exercise safely at home if they have an exercise capacity of at least 5-7 metabolic equivalents (METs), can monitor themselves for warning signs and symptoms, are able to take their own carotid and radial pulses and blood pressure, and have some understanding of exercise physiology and heart disease. A MET is the energy expended in a resting state, burning 3-4 ml of oxygen per kilogram of body weight per minute.

Another component of exercise training is circuit weight training with repetitive lifting of light weights. Free weights may also be used (3-10 lb. in each hand). Weight training improves functional capacity by increasing strength and fitness and improving joint stability and muscle tone. Increased strength should also help to attenuate the heart rate and blood pressure responses to lifting any given workload.

Who Is a Candidate For a Rehab Program?

Cardiac rehab traditionally has been prescribed for patients recovering from acute MI or coronary artery bypass grafting (CABG). Other potential candidates include those who have undergone percutaneous transluminal coronary angioplasty (PTCA), valve surgery, or heart transplantation, and those with congestive heart failure who are stable on medical therapy. Patients at high risk for coronary disease—those with hypertension, dyslipidemia, diabetes, and people who smoke or have other cardiovascular risk factors—may benefit from exercise.

Some patients with cardiomyopathy, severe left ventricular dysfunction, or severe heart failure may improve their functional capacity through exercise. In patients with heart failure, however, improving the prognosis requires a combination of digitalis, diuretics, and angiotensin-converting enzyme inhibitors.

Patients with the most to gain from exercise training have the lowest functional capacity to begin with and tend to be the most sedentary. Most surgical patients are in this category. Comprehensive cardiac rehab can be especially worthwhile for heart transplant patients by addressing the psychological and physiologic effects of chronic illness and disability as well as the physical and metabolic effects of long-term corticosteroid therapy.

The exercise prescription should be based on the results of prior exercise testing. This immediately disqualifies from training anyone who is not eligible for testing. The maximum heart rate during exercise training must be 5-10 beats per minute lower than the heart rate during testing at which abnormalities became evident.

Some Absolute Contraindications to Exercise Training

- Unstable angina pectods
- Dangerous arrhythmias
- Overt cardiac failure
- Severe obstruction of the left ventricular outflow tract
- Dissecting aneurysm
- Myocarditis or pedcarditis (acute)
- Serious systemic disease
- Thrombophlebitis
- Recent systemic or pulmonary embolus
- Severe hypertension
- Overt psychoneurotic disorders
- Uncontrolled diabetes mellitus
- Severe orthopedic limitations

Don't discount elderly patients as candidates for cardiac rehabilitation. Exercise at low to moderate levels can be safe for older patients if the cardiovascular changes of aging, cardiac dysfunction, and co-existing morbidity are taken into account. Improvements in exercise capacity, weight control, glucose tolerance, and lipid levels can be similar to those achieved by younger patients in cardiac rehab programs.[c]

How Should I Handle the Emotional Aspects of Rehab?

Patients in cardiac rehab programs usually have an array of concerns that begin in the acute phase of illness and extend into long-term cardiac care. Fears about dying, diminished authority within the family, altered lifestyle, perceptions of altered body image, and worries about resuming sexual activity are common and need to be addressed, even if the patient does not ask about them directly. First speak to the patient alone, but be sure to talk with both patient and partner before discharge or early in the postdischarge phase.

For the majority of patients who have just suffered an MI, the biggest fear is that of dying, even though their actual risk of death may be low. Giving patients actual percentages may greatly reduce anxiety since in many cases the perceived risk is far greater than the actual risk.

For patients at high risk, focus on what's being done to reduce the risk, such as revascularization for ischemia or treatment with afterload-reducing agents for heart failure. Patients can benefit from a greater understanding of their physical capabilities and limits.

Some may fear that their status within the family is less secure than before. Family members eager to relieve the patient of worry and responsibility may inadvertently reinforce feelings of insecurity and diminished authority. When combined with other losses, such as loss of health and wellness, this can diminish feelings of self-esteem. Let family members know that the patient needs to be involved in making decisions, performing tasks, and taking control of life again.

Fears that sexual activity will precipitate another heart attack are common and begin almost immediately for both the patient and spouse. Even when patients do not ask directly about sex—and most will not—you can prompt them to voice their concerns in the context of a general discussion. Also consider the effects that any prescribed medications may have on sexual activity.

How Should Psychiatric Difficulties Be Handled?

Psychiatric problems are not uncommon in hospitalized patients following acute MI, especially in the coronary care unit. Anxiety, depression, and delirium may surface in the immediate post-MI period but often go unrecognized and untreated (see "Post-MI delirium, depression, and anxiety").

Denial is also common following acute MI, especially since patients may not have been aware of their coronary risk to begin with. In the acute period, denial may serve to reduce anxiety about future events, but if it extends into the rehab period it may hinder compliance and efforts to change behavior. For patients who have undergone PTCA or CABG, it is important to convey that the procedure is not a cure and that compliance is essential to prevent future problems.

Personality traits may also affect compliance and recovery. Compulsive patients may do best if they are given some measure of control over their own care. Likewise, a patient's anger and hostility may alert you to behavioral coronary risk factors. Some patients will not be compliant unless they are in a structured setting, such as a formal rehab program, and may be totally nonfunctional without one.

Given the link between suppressed anger and hostility and the development of coronary disease, patients who exhibit extreme competitiveness and hostility throughout rehab—especially observable in group exercise—may need counseling to reduce their added risk. Identifying sources of stress is a key component and requires looking beyond obvious sources such as overinvolvement with work. Ask about potential sources of stress at home.

Refer to a psychiatrist when your best efforts at treating anxiety, depression, or delirium in the post-MI patient are not having the desired effect. Also consider a referral if your patient becomes psychotic or has active or passive suicidal ideation, or if a personality trait evolves into a disorder that interferes with acceptance of treatment.

Such feelings can be preceded by a depression or may arise spontaneously because patients feel that life as they know it is over. Isolation is also a factor. During the first three years after MI, the risk of death for patients who are depressed and lack social support is four times that of patients who have lower levels of isolation and life stress.[d]

What Should a Comprehensive Rehab Program Provide?

A good program should offer a wide range of services aimed at restoring optimal physical, psychological, occupational, and recreational status. In addition to exercise training, this includes risk reduction through lipid management, dietary intervention, and behavioral counseling. Efforts should focus on interventions for which genuine benefit has been observed, such as reducing LDL cholesterol and quitting smoking.

Lipid management may be approached through dietary means, although pharmacotherapy is likely to become more important now that the National Cholesterol Education Program has revised its guidelines to emphasize lipid management in patients with atherosclerosis or coronary heart disease. Even if medical therapy is needed, the approach should focus on restoring overall health status.

Don't underestimate the value of peer support in group rehab settings. The opportunity to talk with other patients and to learn how they have handled similar problems seems to be of great value. Groups may also provide motivation, since social support is an extremely powerful influence on exercise behavior in the training and maintenance periods.

Some programs offer vocational rehabilitation, although no evidence exists that such programs speed the return to work. State vocational rehabilitation departments can assist in providing care, guidance, and placement. The main determinants for returning to work, however, are probably psychosocial and economic rather than medical: Patients are more likely to return to work if the job has a high salary and high prestige. The patient's perception of illness may also count more than actual physical status. Your own assessment and advice can play an important role in reassuring patients about when to go back to work.

How Can I Tell If a Program Is Any Good?

Among the requirements of a good outpatient facility are direct professional supervision by a qualified staff, adequate equipment, and emergency support including personnel, procedures, and capabilities for cardiopulmonary resuscitation (CPR) and advanced cardiac life support. The staff should include a physician/medical director, certified program director, nurse, exercise physiologist, nutritionist, and behavioral psychiatrist or psychologist. The staff-to-patient ratio should not exceed 1 to 5 in an immediate posthospital exercise program and 1 to 15 in a maintenance program that does not involve continuous ECG monitoring.

In addition to exercise training, a comprehensive cardiac rehab program should offer smoking cessation counseling, lipid management, and nutritional, psychological, and behavioral counseling. It should also provide patient education about risk factors, cardiac signs and symptoms, and self-monitoring during exercise training. Services must be individualized based on the goals of treatment, severity of the patient's underlying condition, associated medical problems, and cardiopulmonary reserve capacity.

In evaluating a program, ask: What specific services are offered? What is the record with regard to morbidity and mortality? What are the staff's credentials—are they certified in the provision of cardiac rehab services? Is the physician actually in attendance on a regular basis? Does the physical educator have at least a master's degree in exercise physiology or a medical background? How is communication handled between the rehab program and the referring physician? Will you receive regular reports on your patient's care and progress?

A good program should function as a resource to help you meet specific management goals. Assure yourself that the program is suitable for your patient and that you feel comfortable with the referral.

How Expensive—and Reimbursable—Is Cardiac Rehab?

Typical costs for cardiac rehab vary widely depending on what services are included and how long patients are enrolled. In the San Francisco Bay area, for example, cardiac rehab for three months, emphasizing exercise training and to a lesser degree smoking cessation and lipid management, costs $1,800 - $2,700. In nearby Sacramento, costs are $9,000 for two years of a comprehensive program designed to reverse coronary disease. Profit margins of rehab programs are said to be small, and many programs just break even.

Coverage by insurance carriers and through managed care plans is even more difficult to pinpoint since it varies by type of plan, individual need, diagnosis, and physician approval. The typical period of coverage for outpatient cardiac rehabilitation is 12 weeks. Coverage for other types of interventions such as smoking cessation, nutritional counseling, weight reduction, and lipid-lowering pharmacotherapy varies widely.

Is Cardiac Rehab a Worthwhile Investment?

The worth of cardiac rehab may be measured by the extent to which it saves lives, saves money, prevents reinfarction and rehospitalization, and improves quality of life. Good data are hard to come by. The survival benefits following MI, based on meta-analyses of older studies, may be outweighed by the more recently available benefits of early thrombolytic therapy and mechanical revascularization.[e] Reduced rehospitalization rates may be difficult to prove given already improved reinfarction rates.

So what's more expensive—rehab or no rehab? Twelve weeks of comprehensive cardiac rehab cost a fraction of what one hospitalization costs for MI, PTCA, or CABG. At least one study shows that participation in comprehensive cardiac rehab may lower cardiac rehospitalization costs in the three years following a coronary event.[f] In 580 patients following MI or CABG, the 230 patients who underwent rehab had a lower incidence of hospitalizations and lower charges per hospitalization than the 350 non-rehab patients. This study was not randomized, raising the possibility that patients going into rehab had healthier behaviors to begin with.

Beyond cost-effectiveness and survival, comprehensive cardiac rehab addresses a spectrum of health and wellness issues. Based on available evidence, comprehensive rehab is probably a good investment to modify risk factors and improve functional status in most eligible patients. Whether this is best accomplished in an outpatient facility or at home is an open question.

How Feasible Is a Home Rehab Program?

If a patient is eligible for group rehab but no program is available, a home program should include appropriate exercise training, risk factor modification, and pharmacotherapy. This approach requires a greater effort by the physician to provide ongoing reinforcement, education, and referral. You may need the support of community resources or those available through a large group practice.

To exercise safely at home, patients can pursue a walking program after they have undergone a treadmill test to detect silent ischemia, arrhythmias, and other problems. Prescribe a level of exercise that is even lower than that determined by the treadmill test. A good approach is to start with 5-10 minutes of walking per day, gradually increasing over a period of weeks to 30-60 minutes of brisk walking almost daily.

Safety can be monitored through periodic treadmill testing and primary care visits, self-monitoring of signs and symptoms, and regular phone contact. Use of a Holter monitor or transtelephonic ECG transmission is also an option. Family members should receive instruction in CPR.

Despite the convenience of home, compliance can still be a problem for patients who are not in a supervised setting. A case-management approach, in which trained nurse practitioners use regular phone contact to help patients comply with structured home rehab, has recently been described for post-MI patients (see "One Approach to Rehab at Home").

Coronary regression programs are another intervention that may be of value in selected patients. These programs have been shown to reduce coronary event rates through the use of cholesterol-lowering drugs, nonpharmacologic behavioral interventions such as diet, smoking cessation, and exercise, or a combination approach. While the reversal of coronary disease is minimal (less than 5% reduction in the diameter of stenosis), rates of infarction, unstable angina and the need for PTCA or CABG decrease over a relatively short period of time. Control of lipids, either dietary or pharmacologic, may be a key factor in reducing coronary risk.

[a] See also "Postdischarge decisions in acute MI," *Patient Care* October 30, 1993.

[b] Lavie CJ, Milani RV: Factors predicting improvements in lipid values following cardiac rehabilitation and exercise training. *Arch Intern Med* 1993;153:982-988.

[c] Lavie CJ, Milani RV, Littman AB: Benefits of cardiac rehabilitation and exercise training in secondary coronary prevention in the elderly. *J Am Coll Cardiol* 1993;22:678-683.

[d] Frasure-Smith N, Lesperance F, Talajic M: Depression following myocardial infarction: Impact on six-month survival. *JAMA* 1993;270:1819-1825.

[e] See "Rising to the challenge of acute MI," Patient Care July 15, 1994.

[f] Ades PA, Huang D, Weaver SO: Cardiac rehabilitation participation predicts lower rehospitalization costs. *Am Heart J* 1992;123:916-921.

Cardiac Rehab and Post-MI Survival

Two meta-analyses suggest that exercise-based cardiac rehabilitation programs improve survival following myocardial infarction (MI), especially in middle-aged men at moderate to high risk.

Study 1

This meta-analysis combined the results of 10 randomized, controlled clinical trials of cardiac rehab following MI, including exercise and risk factor management.[g] It included 2,202 patients randomized to exercise-based cardiac rehab, mostly men under 71, and 2,145 controls.

The risks for all-cause mortality and cardiovascular mortality were significantly lower in the rehab group, with no significant difference in the risk of nonfatal recurrent MI. The reduction was 24% for total mortality and 25% for cardiovascular mortality.

Study 2

This overview includes 22 controlled, randomized trials of post-Ml cardiac rehab with structured exercise and nonexercise components.[h]

The studies evaluated 2,310 patients randomized to rehab (mostly men aged 40-59) and 2,244 patients in a comparison group.

After three years, odds ratios were significantly lower in the rehab group for total and cardiovascular mortality and fatal reinfarction. The odds ratio for sudden death in the rehab group was significantly lower at one year. For nonfatal reinfarction, there were no significant differences between the two groups after one, two, or three years.

Exercise-based cardiac rehab reduced three-year mortality from all causes by 20% and mortality from reinfarction by 25%. The odds ratios for cardiovascular mortality and for sudden death were substantially lower in the exercise-plus-other-interventions group than in the exercise-only trials.

[g] Oldridge NB, Guyatt GH, Fisher ME, et al: Cardiac rehabilitation after myocardial infarction: Combined experience of randomized clinical trials. *JAMA* 1988; 260:945-950.

[h] O'Connor GT, Buring JE, Yusuf S, et al: An overview of randomized trials of rehabilitation with exercise after myocardial infarction. *Circulation* 1989; 80:234-244.

New Trends in Exercise For All

Exercise prescriptions are changing not only for cardiac patients but the general population as well. Until recently, the maintenance threshold for noncardiac patients was 20-30 minutes of continuous aerobic exercise at least three times per week at an intensity of at least 60% maximal functional capacity (70% maximal heart rate). More recently, the emphasis has shifted toward even lower exercise intensities (as low as 55% of maximal heart rate) and longer durations, which are thought to confer general cardiovascular health benefits with a low risk of orthopedic injury.

Even low-intensity activities, performed daily, may reduce the risk of cardiovascular disease. Current recommendations from the American College of Sports Medicine, for example, favor brisk walking over jogging as a regular form of aerobic exercise.

To improve overall fitness, patients can begin exercising at around 50% of their maximum heart rate for several months. They can then build toward the upper limit of their target heart rate zone (75% of maximal heart rate). It is not necessary to exercise beyond 75% of the maximal heart rate to stay in shape. For patients taking antihypertensive agents that reduce the heart rate, other methods of monitoring might be needed, such as the Borg Scale for rating perceived exertion, which correlates closely with peak oxygen uptake.

Above all, patients should exercise at a comfortable pace that enables them to carry on a conversation comfortably. The exercise prescription should be tailored to the patient's functional capacity, health status, exercise goals, and response to conditioning.

Post-MI Delirium, Depression, and Anxiety

Delirium and depression in patients who have just had a myocardial infarction (MI) occur more often than is recognized and affect not only the acute presentation but also rehabilitation and recovery. By conservative estimates, 10% of patients in the coronary care unit (CCU) experience acute delirium, including hallucinations and delusions. Probably many more are subacutely delirious, appearing hyperalert, anxious, and disoriented.

Delirium is linked to such factors as fear, depression, medication, and changes in body image. The CCU environment also plays a role: Overstimulation, sensory monotony, disrupted sleep or wakefulness, impaired communication, lack of privacy, and the illness or death of others intensify the subacute state.

Untreated, delirium hinders the patient's ability to absorb instructions and information and exacerbates already-reduced cognitive functioning in the period after MI or bypass surgery. Measures to ease disorientation include reducing overstimulation and environmental confusion; allowing patients time to put on glasses or hearing aids or to insert dentures; enhancing privacy; encouraging family members to bring a familiar item from home; and addressing patients by name.

Depression is also common (60%) in MI patients in the CCU, although only a small percentage develop a major depressive disorder from a combination of stress and predisposing factors. Severe depression in post-MI patients must be adequately treated. It is not only debilitating but carries a threefold to fourfold increase in risk of mortality over the first six months in post-MI patients with untreated major depression.[i]

Consider a psychiatric consultation for depression when the reactive sadness of an adjustment disorder begins to take on characteristics of a major depressive disorder. Symptoms such as loss of appetite, consistent weight loss, problems falling or staying asleep, feelings of hopelessness and helplessness, loss of sexual desire or interest, early-morning anxiety that improves later in the day, and diurnal variations are more likely to occur during outpatient rehab, several weeks after the acute event.

Anxiety occurs in 80% of post-Ml patients in the CCU. Many can probably benefit from treatment of severe anxiety at the time they are admitted. Left untreated, anxiety will become even more difficult to manage since the drug of choice—a low-dose, high-potency anxiolytic such as a benzodiazepine—may exacerbate symptoms once anxiety has progressed to the point where the patient is hyperalert, potentially hostile, and disoriented.

When treating post-MI patients, stay away from highly anticholinergic medications such as tricyclic antidepressants because of their adverse cardiac effects. While benzodiazepines are recommended for immediate treatment of anxiety, newer antidepressants like selective serotonin reuptake inhibitors are the drugs of choice for treating post-MI patients who are depressed.[j] Use a high-potency, low-dose antipsychotic drugs such as haloperidol (Haldol) or thiothixene (Navane) so you can reduce the anticholinergic load while effectively treating delirium.

[i] See also "The new psychopharmaceuticals," *Patient Care*, January 30, 1994.

[j] Frasure-Smith N, Lesperance F, Talajic M: Depression following myocardial infarction: Impact on six-month survival. *JAMA*, 1993;270:1819-1825.

Women and Cardiac Rehab

Until recently, the study of women recovering from acute cardiac events has been neglected, despite the fact that heart disease is the leading cause of death in women. Following myocardial infarction (MI), women have higher rates of morbidity and mortality than men. This is only partially attributable to their older age at the time of MI and more frequent history of diabetes. Women also may be more psychologically disabled by MI and take longer to recover.[k]

Older women are not enrolled in cardiac rehab as often as older men, even when they have similar clinical profiles. Women also have been found to comply less with exercise regimens, even in supervised group programs. Competing responsibilities, comorbid conditions, greater degree of pain, and fear of exercise are potential contributory factors.

The good news is that several studies show an equal or greater degree of improvement in maximum exercise capacity for women in cardiac rehab compared with men. Even older women have been shown to have similar improvements in functional capacity to those of older men.

A review of existing literature (16 publications) on psychosocial factors and recovery in women looks specifically at return to work, reporting of symptoms, resumption of sexual activity, and compliance with rehab programs following MI or cardiac surgery.[l] The data suggest that women, following MI or surgery, experience more anxiety and depression, report more cardiac symptoms and functional impairment, have more fears about resuming sexual activity, experience more symptoms during sex, return to work outside the home less often but are quicker to resume domestic responsibilities, are referred less often to rehab, enroll less frequently, and have poorer attendance than men.

That women perceive themselves to be more disabled by cardiac disease, have more fear and depression, and report more symptoms could be related to poorer prognosis, older age, less aggressive treatment, and greater pain. At this time, data are insufficient to draw conclusions.

In the meantime, women can gain more from cardiac rehab than their enrollment record shows. Greater efforts can be directed toward recognizing and treating factors that inhibit recovery and investigating the sources of anxiety, depression, and reporting of cardiac symptoms. This is especially important in light of poorer outcomes.

[k] For more on the topic, see "What's unique about CHD in women?" *Patient Care* November 15, 1993.

[l] Low KG: Recovery from myocardial infarction and coronary artery bypass surgery in women: Psychosocial factors. *Journal of Women's Health* 1993:2:133-139.

One Approach to Rehab at Home

To help patients comply with a structured, home-based program of cardiac rehabilitation, a recent study used nurse case managers to provide ongoing counseling on coronary risk factor modification.[m] Directed by a physician, the case managers initiated and maintained interventions for smoking cessation, exercise training, and diet-plus-drug management for hyperlipidemia. The program began in the hospital and was continued after discharge largely through nurse-initiated telephone and mail contact.

In a randomized trial, 585 patients were assigned either to this special intervention or to usual care in the first year following acute myocardial infarction (MI). Usual care consisted primarily of in-hospital counseling on smoking cessation and nutrition. The exercise component of the special intervention, which began three weeks post-MI, included 30 minutes of home-based daily exercise (walking, jogging, bicycling, or swimming) for five days a week, at a maximal heart rate calculated on the basis of tread-mill testing.

At one year, the smoking cessation rate and functional capacity were higher and plasma cholesterol levels were lower in patients assigned to the case-management system. The rate of smoking cessation was 70% in the intervention group and 53% in the usual care group. Mean plasma low-density lipoprotein cholesterol dropped to 107 mg/dL in the study group—approaching the level at which coronary regression has been noted—compared with 132 mg/dL in the usual care group.

The lack of peer support was compensated for by the support of the nurse case managers through their regular phone contact—approximately five hours per patient in the first year. These phone contacts facilitated psychosocial adjustment and provided counseling on dietary and other life-style changes. A psychiatrist, cardiologist, lipid specialist, nutritionist, and nurse coordinator were available by phone to consult with the case managers on difficult management problems.

[m] DeBusk RF, Miller NH, Superko R, et al: A case-management system for coronary risk factor modification after acute myocardial infarction. *Ann Intern Med* 1994:120:721-729.

References for Amsterdam EA, Cadieux RJ, DeBusk RF, Oberman A: Cardiac rehab: Still a good idea? (JN Travalino, ed) *Patient Care* October 30, 1994, pp 24-40.

1. Ades PA, Huang D, Weaver SO: Cardiac rehabilitation participation predicts lower rehospitalization costs. *Am Heart J* 1992;123:916-921.

2. Ades PA, Waldmann ML, Polk DM, et al: Referral patterns and exercise response in the rehabilitation of female coronary patients aged [greater than or equal to] 62 years. *Am J Cardiol* 1992;69:1422-1425.

3. American College of Sports Medicine: *Guidelines for Exercise Testing and Prescription*, ed 4. Philadelphia, Lea & Febiger, 1991.

4. Balady GJ, Fletcher BJ, Retcher E, et al: Cardiac rehabilitation programs. *Circulation* 1994, in press.

5. Cannistra LB, Balady GJ, O'Malley CJ, et al: Comparison of the clinical profile and outcome of women and men in cardiac rehabilitation. *Am J Cardiol* 1992;69:1274-1279.

6. DeBusk RF, Miller NH, Superko R, et al: A case-management system for coronary risk factor modification after acute myocardial infarction. *Ann Intern Med* 1994;120:721-729.

7. Dennis C: Rehabilitation of patients with coronary artery disease, in Braunwald E (ed): *Heart Disease: A Textbook of Cardiovascular Medicine, ed 4*. Philadelphia, WB Saunders Co, 1992.

8. Fletcher GF (ed): *Cardiology Clinics: Exercise Testing and Cardiac Rehabilitation*. Philadelphia, WB Saunders Go, 1993.

9. Fletcher GF, Blair SN, Blumenthal J, et al: Statement on exercise: Benefits and recommendations for physical activity programs for all Americans. A statement for health professionals by the Committee on Exercise and Cardiac Rehabilitation of the Council on Clinical Cardiology, American Heart Association. *Circulation* 1992;86(1):340-344.

10. Frasure-Smith N, Lesperance F, Talajic M: Depression following myocardial infarction: Impact on six-month survival. *JAMA* 1993;270:1819-1825.

11. Greenland P: Efficacy of supervised cardiac rehabilitation programs for coronary patients: Update 1986 to 1990. *J Cardiopulmonary Rehabilitation* 1991;11:197-203.

12. Laslett L, Paumer L, Amsterdam EA: Exercise training in coronary artery disease. *Cardiol Clin* 1987;5:211-225.

13. Lavie CJ, Milani RV: Factors predicting improvements in lipid values following cardiac rehabilitation and exercise training. *Arch Intern Med* 1993;153:982-988.

14. Lavie CJ, Milani RV, Littman AB: Benefits of cardiac rehabilitation and exercise training in secondary coronary prevention in the elderly. *J Am Coll Cardiol* 1993;22:678-683.

15. Levy JK: Standard and alternative adjunctive treatments in cardiac rehabilitation. *Texas Heart Institute Journal* 1993;20:198-212.

16. Low KG: Recovery from myocardial infarction and coronary artery bypass surgery in women: Psychosocial factors. *Journal of Women's Health* 1993;2:133-139.

17. Oberman A: Does cardiac rehabilitation increase long-term survival after myocardial infarction? *Circulation* 1989;80:416-418.

18. O'Connor GT, Buring JE, Yusuf S, et al: An overview of randomized trials of rehabilitation with exercise after myocardial infarction. *Circulation* 1989;80:234-244.

19. Oldridge N, Guyatt G, Jones N, et al: Effects on quality of life with comprehensive after myocardial infarction. *Am J Cardiol* 1991;67:1084-1089.

20. Oldridge NB, Guyatt GH, Fischert ME, et al: Cardiac rehabilitation after myocardial infarction: Combined experience of randomized clinical trials. *JAMA* 1988;260:945-950.

21. Squires RW, Gau GT, Miller TD, et al: Cardiovascular rehabilitation: Status 1990. *Mayo Clin Proc* 1990;65:731-755.

22. Wenger NK: Guidelines for exercise training of elderly patients with coronary artery disease. *South Med* 1994;87:S66-S69.

Chapter 49

Traumatic Brain Injury: Cognitive and Communication Disorders

What Is Traumatic Brain Injury?

Traumatic brain injury is sudden physical damage to the brain. The damage may be caused by the head forcefully hitting an object such as the dashboard of a car (closed head injury) or by something passing through the skull and piercing the brain, as in a gunshot wound (penetrating head injury). The major causes of head trauma are motor vehicle accidents. Other causes include falls, sports injuries, violent crimes, and child abuse.

The physical, behavioral, or mental changes that may result from head trauma depend on the areas of the brain that are injured. Most injuries cause focal brain damage, damage confined to a small area of the brain. The focal damage is most often at the point where the head hits an object or where an object, such as a bullet, enters the brain.

In addition to focal damage, closed head injuries frequently cause diffuse brain injuries or damage to several other areas of the brain. The diffuse damage occurs when the impact of the injury causes the brain to move back and forth against the inside of the bony skull. The frontal and temporal lobes of the brain, the major speech and language areas, often receive the most damage in this way because they sit in pockets of the skull that allow more room for the brain to shift and sustain injury. Because these major speech and language areas often receive damage, communication difficulties

1998 National Institute on Deafness and Other Communication Disorders.

frequently occur following closed head injuries. Other problems may include voice, swallowing, walking, balance, and coordination difficulties, as well as changes in the ability to smell and in memory and cognitive (or thinking) skills.

Who Suffers From Head Trauma?

Head trauma can affect anyone at any age. Males who are between 15 and 24 years of age have been more vulnerable because of their high-risk lifestyles. Young children and individuals over 75 years of age are also more susceptible to head injury. Falls around the home are the leading cause of injury for infants, toddlers, and elderly people. Violent shaking of an infant or toddler is another significant cause. The leading causes for adolescents and adults are automobile and motorcycle accidents, but injuries that occur during violent crimes are also a major source.

Approximately 200,000 Americans die each year from their injuries. An additional half million or more are hospitalized. About 10 percent of the surviving individuals have mild to moderate problems that threaten their ability to live independently. Another 200,000 have serious problems that may require institutionalization or some other form of close supervision.

What Are the Cognitive and Communication Problems That Result From Traumatic Brain Injury?

Cognitive and communication problems that result from traumatic brain injuries vary from person to person. These problems depend on many factors which include an individual's personality, preinjury abilities, and the severity of the brain damage.

The effects of the brain damage are generally greatest immediately following the injury. However, some effects from traumatic brain injury may be misleading. The newly injured brain often suffers temporary damage from swelling and a form of "bruising" called contusions. These types of damage are usually not permanent and the functions of those areas of the brain return once the swelling or bruising goes away. Therefore, it is difficult to predict accurately the extent of long-term problems in the first weeks following traumatic brain injury.

Focal damage, however, may result in long-term, permanent difficulties. Improvements can occur as other areas of the brain learn to take over the function of the damaged areas. Children's brains are much more capable of this flexibility than are the brains of adults. For this reason, children who suffer brain trauma might progress better than adults with similar damage.

In moderate to severe injuries, the swelling may cause pressure on a lower part of the brain called the brainstem, which controls consciousness or wakefulness. Many individuals who suffer these types of injuries are in an unconscious state called a coma. A person in a coma may be completely unresponsive to any type of stimulation such as loud noises, pain, or smells. Others may move, make noise, or respond to pain but be unaware of their surroundings. These people are unable to communicate. Some people recover from a coma, becoming alert and able to communicate.

In conscious individuals, cognitive impairments often include having problems concentrating for varying periods of time, having trouble organizing thoughts, and becoming easily confused or forgetful. Some individuals will experience difficulty learning new information. Still others will be unable to interpret the actions of others and therefore have great problems in social situations. For these individuals, what they say or what they do is often inappropriate for the situation. Many will experience difficulty solving problems, making decisions, and planning. Judgment is often affected.

Language problems also vary. Problems often include word-finding difficulty, poor sentence formation, and lengthy and often faulty descriptions or explanations. These are to cover for a lack of understanding or inability to think of a word. For example, when asking for help finding a belt while dressing, an individual may ask for "the circular cow thing that I used yesterday and before." Many have difficulty understanding multiple meanings in jokes, sarcasm, and adages or figurative expressions such as, "A rolling stone gathers no moss" or "Take a flying leap." Individuals with traumatic brain injuries are often unaware of their errors and can become frustrated or angry and place the blame for communication difficulties on the person to whom they are speaking. Reading and writing abilities are often worse than those for speaking and understanding spoken words. Simple and complex mathematical abilities are often affected.

The speech produced by a person who has traumatic brain injury may be slow, slurred, and difficult or impossible to understand if the areas of the brain that control the muscles of the speech mechanism are damaged. This type of speech problem is called dysarthria. These individuals may also experience problems swallowing. This is called dysphagia. Others may have what is called apraxia of speech, a condition in which strength and coordination of the speech muscles are unimpaired but the individual experiences difficulty saying words correctly in a consistent way. For example, someone may repeatedly stumble on the word "tomorrow" when asked to repeat it, but then be able to say it in a statement such as, "I'll try to say it again tomorrow."

How Are the Cognitive and Communication Problems Assessed?

The assessment of cognitive and communication problems is a continual, ongoing process that involves a number of professionals. Immediately following the injury, a neurologist (a physician who specializes in nervous system disorders) or another physician may conduct an informal, bedside evaluation of attention, memory, and the ability to understand and speak. Once the person's physical condition has stabilized, a speech-language pathologist may evaluate cognitive and communication skills, and a neuropsychologist may evaluate other cognitive and behavioral abilities. Occupational therapists also assess cognitive skills related to the individual's ability to perform "activities of daily living" (ADL) such as dressing or preparing meals. An audiologist should assess hearing. All assessments continue at frequent intervals during the rehabilitative process so that progress can be documented and treatment plans updated. The rehabilitative process may last for several months to a year.

How Are the Cognitive and Communication Problems Treated?

The cognitive and communication problems of traumatic brain injury are best treated early, often beginning while the individual is still in the hospital. This early therapy will frequently center on increasing skills of alertness and attention. They will focus on improving orientation to person, place, time, and situation, and stimulating speech understanding. The therapist will provide oral-motor exercises in cases where the individual has speech and swallowing problems.

Longer term rehabilitation may be performed individually, in groups, or both, depending upon the needs of the individual. This therapy often occurs in a rehabilitation facility designed specifically for the treatment of individuals with traumatic brain injury. This type of setting allows for intensive therapy by speech-language pathologists, physical therapists, occupational therapists, and neuropsychologists at a time when the individual can best benefit from such intensive therapy. Other individuals may receive therapy at home by visiting therapists or on an outpatient basis at a hospital, medical center, or rehabilitation facility.

The goal of rehabilitation is to help the individual progress to the most independent level of functioning possible. For some, ability to express needs verbally in simple terms may be a goal. For others, the goal may be to express needs by pointing to pictures. For still others, the goal of therapy may be to improve the ability to define words or describe consequences of actions or events.

Therapy will focus on regaining lost skills as well as learning ways to compensate for abilities that have been permanently changed because of the brain injury. Most individuals respond best to programs tailored to their backgrounds and interests. The most effective therapy programs involve family members who can best provide this information. Computer-assisted programs have been successful with some individuals.

What Research Is Being Done for the Cognitive and Communication Problems Caused by Traumatic Brain Injury?

Researchers are studying many issues related to the special cognitive and communication problems experienced by individuals who have traumatic brain injuries. Scientists are designing new evaluation tools to assess the special problems that children who have suffered traumatic brain injuries encounter. Because the brain of a child is vastly different from the brain of an adult, scientists are also examining the effects of various treatment methods that have been developed specifically for children. These new strategies include the use of computer programs. In addition, research is examining the effects of some medications on the recovery of speech, language, and cognitive abilities following traumatic brain injury.

Where Can I Get Additional Information?

American Academy of Neurology
1080 Montreal Avenue
St. Paul, MN 55116
(612) 695-1940 (Voice)
www.aan.com (Internet)

American Speech-Language Hearing Association
10801 Rockville Pike
Rockville, MD 20852
(301) 987-5700 (Voice)
(301) 897-0157 (TTY)
(800) 498-2071 (Toll-free)
(301) 571-0457 (Fax)
www.asha.org (Internet)

Brain Injury Association, Inc.
105 North Alfred Street
Alexandria, VA 22314
(703) 236-6000 (Voice)
(800) 444-6443 (Toll-free)
(703) 236-6001 (Fax)
www.biausa.org (Internet)

National Center for Neurogenic Communication Disorders
Speech and Hearing Sciences
Building 71
The University of Arizona
Tucson, AZ 85721
(520) 621-1472 (Voice)
(800) 926-2444 (Toll-free)
(520) 621-2226 (Fax)
w3.arizona.edu/~cnet/homepage.html (Internet)

National Institute of Child Health and Human Development (NICHD)
31 Center Drive
National Institutes of Health
Bldg. 31, Rm. 2A32, MSC 2425
Bethesda, MD 20892-2425
(301) 496-5133 (Voice)
(301) 496-7101 (Fax)
www.nih.gov/nichd (Internet)

National Institute of Mental Health (NIMH)
National Institutes of Health
5600 Fishers Lane
Parklawn Bldg., Rm. 7C02, MCS 8030
Rockville, MD 20892-8030
(301) 443-4513 (Voice)

(301) 443-4279 (Fax)
www.nimh.nih.gov (Internet)

National Institute of Neurological Disorders and Stroke (NINDS)
National Institutes of Health
31 Center Drive
Bldg. 31, Rm. 8A16
Bethesda, MD 20892
(301) 496-5751 (Voice)
(301) 402-2186 (Fax)
(800) 352-9424 (Toll-free)
www.ninds.nih.gov (Internet)

National Institute on Aging (NIA)
National Institutes of Health
NIA Information Office
P.O. Box 8057
Gaithersburg, MD 20898-8057
(800) 222-2225 (Toll-free/Voice)
(800) 222-4225 (Toll-free/TTY)
www.nih.gov/nia (Internet)

Chapter 50

Recognizing Communication Disorders

What Are Communication Disorders?

Communication disorders can be grouped into two main categories:

1. People with Hearing Disorders do not hear sounds clearly. Such disorders may range from hearing speech sounds faintly, or in a distorted way, to profound deafness.

2. Speech and Language Disorders affect the way people talk and understand. These disorders may range from simple sound substitutions to the inability to use speech and language at all.

What Are the Signs of a Communication Disorder?

Hearing: Hearing loss might be suspected when a person does not always hear sounds such as telephone or doorbell ringing, turns his or her ear toward the source of sound, frequently asks the speaker to repeat, turns the TV or radio up too loud, or shows obvious signs of confusion or misunderstanding of speech.

Speech and Language Disorders might be present when a person's speech or language is different from that of others of the same age, sex, or ethnic group; when a person's speech and/or language is hard to understand; when a person is overly concerned about his or her own speech; or when a person frequently avoids communicating with others.

Are Communication Disorders Serious Problems?

Yes. The ability to communicate is our most human characteristic. Human communication is essential to learning, working, and social interaction. Impaired communication can affect every aspect of a person's life.

Common Communication Disorders

Hearing

Conductive: sound is not conducted efficiently through the outer and/or middle ear, causing speech and other sounds to be heard less clearly or to sound muffled. This kind of hearing loss can often be medically or surgically corrected.

Sensorineural: caused by damage in the inner ear or nerve pathways to the brain. Certain sounds are heard less distinctly than others, causing distortion and reduced understanding of speech. Although this kind of hearing loss is usually not medically correctable, people with sensorineural hearing loss can often be helped by using a hearing aid or other amplification device.

Mixed: a combination of conductive and sensorineural hearing loss.

Language

Delayed Language: a noticeable slowness in the development of the vocabulary and grammar necessary for expressing and understanding thoughts and ideas.

Aphasia: the loss of speech and language abilities resulting from stroke or head injury.

Speech Disorders

Stuttering: an interruption in the rhythm of speech characterized by hesitations, repetitions, or prolongations of sounds, syllables, words, or phrases, for example, cow . . . boy, tuh-tuh-tuh-table, ssssun.

Articulation Disorders: difficulties with the way sounds are formed and strung together usually characterized by substituting one sound for another (wabbit for rabbit), omitting a sound (han for hand), or distorting a sound (shlip for sip).

Voice Disorders: inappropriate pitch (too high, too low, never changing or interrupted by breaks); loudness (too loud or not loud enough); or quality (harsh, hoarse, breathy, or nasal).

What Causes Communication Disorders?

Hearing: Some of the causes of hearing loss are chronic ear infections, heredity, birth defects, health problems at birth, certain drugs, head injury, viral or bacterial infection, exposure to loud noise, aging, and tumors.

Speech and Language: Some of the causes of speech and language disorders are related to hearing loss, cerebral palsy and other nerve/muscle disorders, severe head injury, stroke, viral diseases, mental retardation, certain drugs, physical impairments such as cleft lip or palate, vocal abuse or misuse, an inadequate speech and language models; frequently, however, the cause is unknown.

What Can You Do if You Suspect a Speech, Language, or Hearing Problem?

A thorough evaluation by a speech-language pathologist or audiologist is needed to determine a person's communication strengths and weaknesses. After this evaluation, the speech-language pathologist or audiologist will be able to provide a plan for meeting individual needs.

What Is a Speech-Language Pathologist?

A speech-language pathologist is a professional educated in the study of human communication, its development, and its disorders. By evaluating the speech and language skills of children and adults, the speech-language pathologist determines if communication problems exist and decides the best way to treat these problems.

What Is an Audiologist?

An audiologist is a professional educated in the study of normal and impaired hearing. The audiologist determines if a person has a hearing impairment, what type of impairment it is, and how the individual can make the best use of remaining hearing. If a person will benefit from using a hearing aid or other listening device, the audiologist can assist with the selection, fitting, and purchase of the most appropriate aid and with training the individual to use the aid effectively.

Where Can You Find Speech-Language Pathology and Audiology Services?

Speech-language pathologists and audiologists provide professional services in many different types of facilities such as:

- public and private schools
- hospitals
- rehabilitation centers
- nursing care facilities
- community clinics
- colleges and universities
- private practice
- state and local health departments
- state and federal governmental agencies

A speech-language pathologist or audiologist will have a master's or doctoral degree and should hold a Certificate of Clinical Competence (CCC) from the American Speech-Language-Hearing Association and/or a license from the state.

For help in locating a qualified audiologist or speech-language pathologist in your area, write or call:

American Speech-Language-Hearing Association
10801 Rockville Pike
Rockville, Maryland 20852
(800)638-8255 (Voice or TTY)
(301)897-5700 (Voice or TTY)
(301)571-0457 Fax
E-mail: irc@asha.org
http://www.asha.org

Chapter 51

Respiratory Disorders and Home Oxygen Therapy

It has been reported that only long-term oxygen therapy (LTOT) is able to improve survival in patients with chronic obstructive pulmonary disease (COPD). Disabling dyspnea in these patients is often the leading cause of physical deconditioning, which in turn worsens exertional dyspnea. This vicious cycle may result in a marked reduction in patients' functional capacity and inability to cope with the activities of daily life (ADL) and consequent reduction in the quality of life (QOL). Rehabilitation programs have been developed with the primary aim of increasing exercise tolerance and improving the QOL of COPD patients.

The "NIH Workshop Summary: Pulmonary Rehabilitation Research" defined pulmonary rehabilitation as "a multidimensional continuum of services directed to persons with pulmonary disease and their families, usually by an interdisciplinary team of specialists, with the goal of achieving and maintaining the individual's maximum level of independence and functioning in the community." Pulmonary rehabilitation programs are designed to manage patients throughout the natural history of their disease, from the onset of symptoms until the final stages (Table 51.1), and should be considered an implementation of standard medical therapy.

Selection Criteria—Who is Likely to Benefit?

The appropriate selection of patients plays a key role in the success of pulmonary rehabilitation (Table 51.2). Appropriate patients for pulmonary rehabilitation programs are those who recognize that their symptoms depend upon their lung disease and are motivated to be active participants in their own care to improve their health status. The only absolute contraindications are a long history of lack of compliance and unwillingness to participate.

Most patients referred for pulmonary rehabilitation have COPD, and the benefit of pulmonary rehabilitation in patients with COPD has been well documented. However, a small number of nonCOPD patients are usually included in pulmonary rehabilitation studies. One study enrolling only patients with respiratory diseases other than COPD reported beneficial effects from pulmonary rehabilitation. Rehabilitation programs are commonly recommended for patients with bronchial asthma, neuromuscular diseases, cystic fibrosis, as well as pre- and post-operatively for abdominal and thoracic surgery and lung transplantation (Table 51.3).

As stated above, the only absolute contraindication for pulmonary rehabilitation programs appears to be the lack of compliance or unwillingness to participate. However, studies on rehabilitation programs report some exclusion criteria. In the study by Goldstein and colleagues subjects determined ineligible suffered from coexisting diseases (41%), were still smoking (7%), lived too far from the hospital (16%) or had language barriers, cognitive impairment, social circumstances, or were too disabled (31%). Whether these conditions should be considered general criteria for exclusion from a therapeutic routine pulmonary rehabilitation program is still a matter of debate, particularly in smoking or disabled patients.

Contraindications should be considered in the context of the specific patient in relation to his/her disease and to the specific therapeutic program chosen. The issues in this consideration should include age, nutritional status, the severity of respiratory impairment and degree of compliance with therapeutic regimens.

Age

Elderly patients with COPD are often undertreated—practitioners may overlook the reversible component of COPD in the elderly, or attribute dyspnea to excessive smoking or to atypical heart failure. Similarly, until a few years ago, patients older than 70 years had been excluded from some pulmonary rehabilitation studies. In fact, several factors do affect the ultimate success of rehabilitation in the elderly, including the presence of other disabling diseases (e.g. cancer or arthritis), long-term medical therapy (for example, with oral steroids for COPD or other systemic diseases), level of education, family support, and personal motivation.

However, advanced age in itself is no longer thought to limit successful management of COPD. On the contrary, many factors suggest that the elderly might be particularly suitable for multidisciplinary pulmonary rehabilitation. Extensive education and training on the appropriate medications and the use of metered-dose inhaler (MDI) and spacers can improve their ability to inhale. Supervised and monitored physical therapy and exercise training may be beneficial in patients with cardiac and musculoskeletal disorders, sensory impairment and reduced cognitive function. Moreover recent literature has highlighted the beneficial effects of regular participation in long-term aerobic exercises in the aged. Improvements in muscle strength, flexibility, percent body fat, mass and aerobic fitness have been shown.

Basic guidelines for frequency, intensity and duration of training appropriate for the elderly have been established. Generally these guidelines suggest low to moderate intensity and low-impact activities. In a randomized, controlled study, high-intensity exercise training has been shown to be a feasible and effective means of counteracting muscle weakness and physical frailty in the very elderly—even in those over 90. Comprehensive programs of pulmonary rehabilitation including education, lower and upper extremity training, breathing retraining and chest physiotherapy, have been shown to improve exercise capacity in patients with COPD who are older than 75.

Nutritional Status

Factors related to nutritional status have an independent influence on the natural history of COPD. In a study by Wilson and associates body weight was directly related to FEV1, whereas mortality appeared to be influenced by body weight independent of FEV1. After adjusting for FEV1, body weight correlated with exercise capacity. Therefore, compromised nutritional state may contribute to a reduced exercise performance in patients with COPD, and a positive association between nutritional state and maximal exercise performance has been found. Patients with different levels of nutritional depletion, as determined by body weight and fat-free mass, may be eligible for pulmonary rehabilitation.

Severity of Respiratory Impairment

The severity of respiratory impairment influences both patient motivation and compliance. Patients with severe disease and minimal respiratory reserve may be physically unable to participate fully or benefit from the program. In contrast, in patients with mild disease and minimal physiologic limitation, the low motivation resulting from the lack of perceived need for rehabilitative therapy may be the main cause for ineffective rehabilitation. The degree of respiratory impairment may be assessed by pulmonary function tests, which offer objective evidence to patients in denial about the severity of their disease and may, therefore, enhance compliance. However, it should be noted that exercise-induced hypoxemia might not be revealed by pulmonary function tests alone. Niederman and colleagues showed that lung function tests did not correlate with changes in 12 mwd, maximal exercise performance, or subjective parameters.

In a study of comprehensive pulmonary rehabilitation programs, equal benefits were seen in patients presenting with a spectrum of disease progression, ranging from mild to very severe. Resting hypercapnia should not be considered an exclusion criteria for pulmonary rehabilitation since studies have shown that pulmonary rehabilitation has resulted in the same improvements in exercise tolerance in hypercapneic and eucapneic patients.

The improvement in the 12-minute walking test (12 minute walking distance, or 12 mwd) observed in patients having completed a 6-week pulmonary rehabilitation program, was evaluated by Zu Wallack and coworkers. No significant relationship between improvement in the 12 mwd and age, sex, oxygen requirement, arterial blood gas levels, and pulmonary function was found. However, the patients with a greater ventilatory reserve showed a greater improvement in their 12 mwd, both in terms of distance and percentage of increase over baseline. Moreover patients with a lower peak of oxygen consumption (V'O2) showed greater percentage of improvement in their 12 mwd. The magnitude of the initial 12 mwd was inversely related to its improvement following pulmonary rehabilitation, both with respect to distance and percentage of increase. We may therefore argue that patients with poor performance on either a 12 mwd or maximal exercise test are not necessarily poor candidates for a pulmonary rehabilitation program.

Compliance with Therapy

Studies on adherence to rehabilitation programs are lacking, but some information may be derived from studies on adherence to medical therapy for COPD requiring changes in daily routines. Turner and associates showed that white race, married status, abstinence from cigarettes and alcohol, high serum theophylline level, more severe dyspnea and reduced FEV1 were good predictors of adherence to home nebulizer therapy. Sociodemographic, physiologic and quality of life variables were associated with adherence to therapy as well. Whether these parameters may be applicable in predicting adherence to rehabilitation programs is not known. In the prospective controlled study of pulmonary rehabilitation by Goldstein and colleagues 29% of the 126 eligible COPD patients refused rehabilitation.

Therapeutic Modalities—The Components of the Pulmonary Rehabilitation Package

Any patient presenting with symptomatic COPD or another pulmonary disease as listed in Table 51.3, should be considered for pulmonary rehabilitation according to the criteria previously discussed. Once a patient has been selected, the key to their success is the individualization of the program. The global outcomes resulting from individual elements of a program are difficult to assess because the possible therapeutic modalities are blended differently for each patient. The components of pulmonary rehabilitation programs are still under discussion. This review will address the rationale for modality selection. Well-accepted therapeutic components of rehabilitation already shown to prolong life (smoking cessation and oxygen therapy) will not be considered in this discussion.

Breathing Control Techniques

Techniques for coordinating the breathing process were once widely used in therapeutic pulmonary rehabilitation programs. Sometimes referred to as "breathing retraining," these techniques include pursing the lips and diaphragmatic breathing. The overall goals of these techniques are to improve the breathing pattern of symptomatic patients with the purpose of relieving dyspnea and improving the efficiency of the respiratory muscles (RM). Objective markers of efficacy are increased expiratory flow rates, reductions in the work of breathing, increased coordination of breathing patterns; and improvements in blood gas values and exercise tolerance. Subjective markers are improvements in dyspnea and a greater sense of well-being.

The outcomes of these maneuvers has only been studied in acute setting. Positive effects of these techniques have been reported in the COPD patient with moderate airflow obstruction and without respiratory insufficiency, and in selected cases of bronchial asthma. Pursed lip breathing results in slower and deeper breaths with significant increase in oxygenation and a shift in ventilatory muscle recruitment from the diaphragm to the accessory muscles of ventilation. During exercise, the shift to pursed lip breathing results in decreased dyspnea. In a study conducted on patients with severe COPD during loaded and unloaded breathing, coordination of chest wall motion, as well as mechanical efficiency, was found to be detrimentally affected by diaphragmatic breathing, while dyspnea sensation was not improved.

Chest Physical Therapy

This term describes a series of techniques designed to facilitate the clearance of heavy secretions from the airways. Techniques of chest physical therapy include postural drainage, chest percussion, pounding the back with cupped hands, vibration, directed cough and the forced expiratory technique.

These maneuvers should lessen the resistance of the airways, thereby improving gas exchange and reducing the incidence of respiratory tract infections. Chest physical therapy is implemented for hospitalized patients with COPD who are at risk of either disease exacerbation or of developing pulmonary complications secondary to surgical interventions. In this latter group, however, a randomized study showed that outcomes of patients with marked atelectasis at extubation undergoing single-handed percussions did not significantly differ from those obtained with early ambulation. In the outpatient setting, chest physical therapy is primarily indicated in diseases determining chronic production of large sputum volumes (>30 mL/day): cystic fibrosis, bronchiectasis, chronic bronchitis.

Lower Extremity Exercise Training

Marked functional limitation often occurs in patients with respiratory disease. Dyspnea begins a vicious cycle in which there is a progressive decrease in physical activity, reduction in muscle mass, and deconditioning, which in turn results in more dyspnea at increasingly lower levels of exertion. The main goal of exercise training is to break this debilitating pattern.

Improvements in exercise tolerance may be achieved through both physiologic and psychologic interventions. Although exercise training programs employing cycling and/or treadmill walking, stair-climbing etc., have been widely and indiscriminately used for the rehabilitative management of individuals with different respiratory diseases, in the case of the COPD patient, they should not be considered until optimal medical control of the disease has been achieved. Motivation, the degree of functional impairment, age, and the results of a pre-enrollment incremental exercise test are also critical factors in the selection of patients for exercise training. Most studies on the efficacy of exercise training relied on hospital programs. A recent European trial confirms that exercise training can be successfully implemented in the home-setting. It seems safe to state that any patient capable of undergoing training will benefit from a program that includes leg exercise. The optimal exercise intensity, duration and maintenance program remain to be determined.

Respiratory Muscle Training

Conditions such as neuromuscular diseases, malnutrition, restrictive lung diseases, and pulmonary hyperinflation may severely affect respiratory muscles. RM training results in increased strength and endurance. There are conflicting results about benefits of RM training on both exercise and ADL performance. A meta analysis reported little evidence of clinically important benefit of RM training in patients with COPD. We therefore propose that RM training is indicated for high spinal cord lesions without diaphragmatic involvement, pre- and post-operative management of abdominal or thoracic surgery patients, and weaning from ventilatory support. More research is needed before final recommendations may be given on the patients, if any, who may benefit from these therapeutic modalities. Although a specific physiologic effect (fiber hypertrophy in rat diaphragm) has been reported with this technique, RM training should not be used in patients with damaged or adapted respiratory muscle fibers.

Training of Upper Extremity Muscle Groups

Many exercise programs focus on lower-extremity training. However, many ADLs, such as bathing, dressing and grooming, require use of the upper extremities. For a given workload, upper-extremity work demands more energy than lower-extremity work and a higher ventilatory demand is needed. For elderly patients, the increased energy and ventilatory demands of simple self-care activities result in marked functional limitation. Because exercise training must be specific to the muscles involved in performing the task, it is important that upper-extremity exercises tailored to the patient's needs be included in the program.

A critical review of the literature suggests that exercise conditioning comprehensive of leg and arm training improves exercise performance. Moreover, COPD patients showed greater improvements in dyspnea and quality of life (QOL) resulting from the inclusion of arm exercise in their training than from general exercise programs. Upper extremity muscle group programs are indicated for patients with dyspnea on exertion, patients with long-term deconditioning (post-surgical, and specifically post-lung transplantation), or patients with cystic fibrosis.

Occupational Therapy

Chronic pulmonary diseases are the primary cause of disability and loss of time from work. The goal of occupational therapy is the patient's restoration to occupational or recreation activities with less energy expenditure and fewer symptoms. Patients below retirement age or those wishing to cultivate specific hobbies may undergo this type of treatment.

Education

Education may be defined as a learning process that improves patients' ability to cope and make informed decisions regarding their own care. All patients with COPD should be educated on oxygen therapy, smoking cessation, nutrition, exercise and health preservation, and the importance of compliance with medications. The focus of educational programs are patients with chronic pulmonary diseases and their families. There has been particular emphasis on development of educational programs for patients with bronchial asthma, cystic fibrosis and COPD. Education alone is of little benefit compared with education in adjunct to an exercise program. Therefore although more research is needed to assess its value, education should not be considered as an alternative to exercise training in the rehabilitation programs.

Psychosocial Support

Anxiety, depression and lack of self-esteem often coexist in patients with chronic pulmonary disease. Anxiety and depression are the two most commonly reported emotional sequelae of asthma. Male COPD patients show both psychophysiologic disturbances and depression. Anxiety and depression are also commonly reported in patients with respiratory insufficiency. Psychological problems may result in decreased participation in social activities and are commonly reflected in the sexual sphere.

These problems are likely to improve as the patient becomes involved in a pulmonary rehabilitation program resulting in desensitization to dyspnea (defined here as the reduction or abolition of the sensation to a given dyspneic stimulus), reduced fear, and regaining of self-control. Rehabilitation sessions including education, exercise breathing techniques, and relaxation techniques have been shown to be more effective in reducing anxiety than have a similar number of psychotherapy sessions. Patients with dyspnea-associated distress and anxiety may benefit from exercise training as well.

Nutritional Programs

Reduced body weight in COPD patients is a risk factor independent of the deterioration of airflow. Malnutrition, obesity, and weight loss are associated with respiratory disease and may lead to RM dysfunction, an increased incidence of respiratory infections, reduced control of ventilation, and alterations in lung parenchymal structure. Nutritional supplementation may also result in increased CO_2 production and increased respiratory drive. Nutritional supplementation and/or correction is indicated in COPD patients with malnutrition and/or obesity, cystic fibrosis and bronchiectasis, before and after lung transplantation, interstitial lung diseases, and sleep apnea syndromes.

Proper evaluation of candidates, according to the parameters previously described, is the cornerstone of a successful rehabilitation program. Evaluation by the pulmonary rehabilitation team should include somatic and physiologic issues, as well as the quantification and monitoring of variables that are important determinants of a patient's QOL. One such method of assessment is the so-called "functional approach," which considers the impairment (the physiologic deficit), disability (total effect of impairment on the patient's life), and handicap (the social disadvantages) as part of the comprehensive program of care. The functional approach is not only useful for monitoring the patient's functional status, but it enables the rehabilitation team to set and achieve goals to improve the health-related quality of a patient's life.

Outcomes—Methods of Medical and Physiologic Evaluation

The major aims of medical assessment for pulmonary rehabilitation include confirming the diagnosis, characterizing the severity of primary symptoms, identifying the impact of the diseases on patient life-style, and evaluating the impact of therapy. The first step is to record the patient's medical history and ascertain psychosocial problems and needs. The history should elucidate the functional severity of the patient's lung disease, and reveal other problems that might preclude participation in the program, such as neurologic deficits and lack of compliance to previous medical regimens. Laboratory data should include pulmonary function tests, exercise tests, arterial blood gases, chest radiograph, electrocardiogram, and blood chemistries. Additional diagnostic testing can be planned as needed.

It is important to note that limitation of exercise capacity is not the same as disability. Tests of the effectiveness of the rehabilitation program must recognize the synergistic nature of affective factors, and must be adjusted to suit individual patient capabilities.

Pulmonary Function Tests

Pulmonary function tests are aimed at characterization and quantification of impairment resulting from the patient's lung disease. Dynamic and static lung volume measurements, the most useful references, may be supplemented by other tests such as diffusing capacity, airway resistance, and RM strength and endurance.

Pulmonary function tests have some limitations. The degree of airflow obstruction as estimated by FEV1 and exercise capacity do not correlate well in COPD patients. Several intervening factors (pulmonary vascular disease, diffusion disorder, and generalized muscle weakness) obscure the correlation. Muscle weakness may be the result of malnutrition, detraining, and corticosteroid treatment. Furthermore, it has been reported that baseline lung function cannot predict benefits of pulmonary rehabilitation programs.

Assessment of RM function is mandatory for prescribing and evaluating the results of a pulmonary rehabilitation program in patients with COPD, in pre- and post-operative conditions, and in cases of neuromuscular disease. The most direct approach to this assessment is to measure inspiratory and expiratory pressures at the mouth when the subject performs maximal efforts against a closed airway (maximum inspiratory pressure [MIP] and maximum expiratory pressure [MEP], respectively) according to the technique described by Black and Hyatt. This measurement is especially useful in evaluating the efficacy of a pulmonary rehabilitation program.

Direct testing of inspiratory muscle (IM) endurance is based on the capacity of these muscles to sustain high levels of pressure. The most fundamental test consists of simply determining the level of ventilation that can be sustained for 15 minutes or longer, termed the maximum sustainable ventilatory capacity (MSVC). This is a practical test of the maximal time and submaximal levels of minute ventilation that can be sustained. There is no ventilatory load other than the intrinsic resistive and elastic characteristics of the respiratory system. Currently, the most commonly used endurance test is based on the pressure required to overcome an inspiratory load. The ability to sustain such a breathing effort depends on the force and duration of inspiratory muscle contraction. An alternative test uses an inspiratory threshold load instead of an inspiratory resistive load to test endurance. In this technique, inspiration can be accomplished only by achieving a target pressure sufficient to lift a plunger. Thereafter the inspiratory pressure remains constant for the entire inspiration, and the level of pressure is independent of inspiratory flow rate. The pressure required to inspire is directly proportional to the load. Both devices are of simple construction and are easy-to-use.

Peripheral Muscle Function

Pulmonary rehabilitation programs should not be planned without evaluation of peripheral muscle function.

Chronic inactivity, psychological factors, steroid myopathy, and drug effects may reduce skeletal muscle function in COPD patients. Peripheral muscle force has been reported as an important determinant of exercise capacity in COPD patients who tend to use healthcare services more as ventilatory and peripheral muscle force decreases.

Peak torque of flexor and extensor leg muscles during isokinetic exercise has been used to assess general muscle performance. Isokinetic exercise is a dynamic form of resistive exercise. A correlation between torque values and age, sex, and conditioning state has been identified, but more extensive studies are needed to adequately define it.

Exercise Testing

The exercise test is generally necessary to assess patients' exercise tolerance and to reveal possible blood gas changes that cannot be predicted from the baseline lung function tests. The exercise test is generally used to safely and appropriately grade intensity of subsequent training.

Cardiopulmonary exercise testing has proven effective for the evaluation of exercise tolerance in patients with dyspnea and cardiopulmonary diseases. When compared with a clinical laboratory approach (including history, clinical signs, chest radiograph, eco-doppler evaluation, spirometry, blood gas analysis), this test allowed for the detection of an underestimated circulatory component causing exercise limitation. Graded exercise testing has been shown to be useful in diagnosing patients with chronic unexplained dyspnea. Variables measured and/or monitored during testing should include workload, heart rate, electrocardiogram, arterial oxygenation, and symptoms associated with the activity. Other measurements, such as expired gas analysis to calculate variables (such as oxygen uptake [$V'O_2$]), may be performed depending on the interest and expertise of referring physician, laboratory personnel and program staff. The most effective assessment of exercise focuses on the type that will be employed in training (e.g. treadmill testing for a walking exercise training program); however gains from one type of exercise test can be translated to similar forms of exercise. However, even in patients who are unfamiliar with regular bicycle exercise, and in spite of the greater lactate response generated by cycling compared with treadmill walking, $V'O_2$ max was not different during cycle versus treadmill exercise testing in patients with COPD.

In a study by Vallet and colleagues, patients who exercised at an intensity corresponding to heart rate at the anaerobic threshold showed a significant increase in symptom-limited $V'O_2$ and maximal O_2 pulse, and a significant decrease in minute ventilation, CO_2 production, and venous lactate concentration, compared with patients engaging in the standard protocol. The standard protocol involves the same training schedule—one session of stationary bicycle exercise per day, 5 days per week over a 4 week period—at a level of 50% maximal cardiac frequency.

Measuring the distance covered during a walking test is considered a simple and reproducible way to determine exercise tolerance in patients with chronic lung disease and heart failure. The distance covered in the 12 minute walking test (12 minute walking distance [12 mwd]) was initially proposed as a good determinant of disease severity, and the distance walked was shown to be related to $V'O_2$ peak. The test has been progressively shortened to a 6 mwd, and more recently a "shuttle" 2 mwd test has been proposed. The smallest difference in 6 mwd that was associated with a noticeable difference in patients' subjective comparison ratings of their walking ability was 54 m. The timed walking distance following out-patient pulmonary rehabilitation is an important predictor of survival in patients with advanced pulmonary disease. The 6 mwd has been shown to predict $V'O_2$ max and short-term event-free survival in cases of advanced heart failure.

Blood Gases

Blood gas sampling during exercise adds a significant degree of complexity to testing. Noninvasive techniques, such as transcutaneous oximetry of arterial oxygen saturation, may be useful for continuous monitoring, but should not be relied on for precise assessment of arterial oxygenation because of their limited accuracy.

Measurements of Dyspnea

Pulmonary function tests have been traditionally used both for diagnostic purposes (e.g. to detect airflow obstruction) and to follow the course of the lung disease. This approach is problematic because the severity of dyspnea, which is usually the patient's primary complaint, is only weakly related to physiologic lung function. Furthermore clinical ratings of dyspnea and pulmonary function tests are separate factors or quantities describing different aspects of COPD. General health status in symptomatic patients with COPD is better predicted, and influenced to a greater extent, by dyspnea ratings than by physiologic measurements.

Clinical methods of measuring dyspnea have depended primarily on the use of exertional tasks that evoke breathlessness. Both psychophysical methods and clinical scales have been used to assess breathlessness. Fletcher' scale and the British Medical Research Council (BMRC) scale rate patients based upon the magnitude of the performed task, but there is little provision for the individual patient's effort at performing it. Functional impairment resulting from dyspnea is neglected in these scales. This drawback can be circumvented by using the visual analogue technique, consisting of a line marked with phrases describing levels of exertion at various points along its length. The visual analog scale (VAS) has been used to draw an oxygen cost diagram in which daily activities are ranked by the patient along the line in proportion to their rated oxygen cost. The Borg scale offers a quantitative approach to estimate dyspnea sensation at given exercise loads.

The methods described above provide information when serial measurements are performed within a single patient. However, they are not useful for comparing dyspnea among patients, nor for comparing groups of patients with different conditions, because each patient's subjective scale is different. Mahler has recently proposed a new instrument—the Baseline Dyspnea Index (BDI)—which might be able to account for the components of functional impairment, magnitude of effort and magnitude of task for dyspnea evaluation. BDI is a multidimensional instrument which has proven to be valid and reliable in patients with chronic respiratory disease.

The Future of Qualitative Rating Systems

Patients with different cardiorespiratory conditions experience distinct qualities of breathlessness, and their recall of the experience is reliable and comparable to dyspnea while walking. A questionnaire containing descriptions of the quality of breathlessness has been suggested as a helpful means to establish a specific diagnosis and to identify mechanisms whereby a specific intervention relieves dyspnea.

Because of the lack of correlation between ratings of dyspnea and physiologic measures, techniques such as expiratory flow limitation, as assessed by the negative expiratory pressure technique, have been suggested to be more useful in the evaluation of dyspnea than spirometry measurements, in patients with COPD.

Quality of Life Tests

Most patients with chronic respiratory disease seek medical evaluation when difficulty in breathing interferes with their ability to perform various daily activities and/or adversely affects their quality of life (QOL). An individual's QOL is strongly influenced by factors that healthcare does not directly affect; consequently many researchers use the more restrictive term "Health-related quality of life (HRQL)" to mean the quality of life as it is affected by health status. In general HRQL questionnaires measure the impact of an individual's health on his/her ability to perform and enjoy the activities of daily life. HRQL instruments vary from disease-specific measures of a single symptom (e.g. dyspnea) to a generic global assessment of many facets which may include emotional functioning, social role functioning activities of daily living, and ability to enjoy activities. HRQL measures have adequate, and often excellent, reproducibility. However, physiological measures such as pulmonary function and exercise tolerance do not correlate strongly with measures of HRQL.

There are generic and disease-specific HRQL-measuring instruments that have been used extensively in patients with COPD. The generic HRQL instrument that has predominantly been used in patients with COPD is the "Sickness Impact Profile" (SIP). The "Nottingham Health Profile" is a reproducible and valid instrument in the assessment of chronic diseases. Among the disease-specific

HRQL instruments, the "Chronic Respiratory Disease Questionnaire" (CRQ) developed by Guyatt was shown to be reproducible, valid, and more responsive than other measures of dyspnea. The "St. George's Respiratory Questionnaire (SGRQ)" is divided into 3 components: symptoms, activity, and impact on daily life. In a comparison with SIP, SGRQ was shown to be twice as responsive in patients with respiratory disease as the generic instrument. Other psychosocial measures have been proposed and used in randomized clinical trials of effects of pulmonary rehabilitation in COPD patients. CRQ was used by Wijkstra and colleagues to show that rehabilitation at home for three months followed by once monthly physiotherapy sessions improved QOL measurements over 18 months, although the change in QOL was not associated with a change in exercise tolerance. Poor scores on the SGRQ are associated with hospital re-admissions for COPD and use of resources such as nebulizers, independent of physiologic measures of disease severity.

Occupational Evaluation

Occupational therapy aims to restore and maximize independence, prevent associated disability and maintain health. An occupational therapy assessment includes a subjective interview, observation of functional performance, and the administration and interpretation of specific tests. The following areas are assessed: self-care, home and community skills, vocation, leisure interests, upper extremity muscle strength, range of motion, endurance, coordination, physiologic responses to daily activities, psychosocial status, and cognitive and behavioral problems related to function. To perform these evaluations, the occupational therapist must utilize many tools and techniques. An assessment of the upper extremity function can be done with an arm cranking ergometer, which serves as an isolated task that can be used to test submaximal and maximal cardiorespiratory function. Objective parameters monitored routinely as part of the functional task evaluation include measurement of the rate of perceived exertion and dyspnea, heart rate response, respiratory rate, VO_2 and oxygen saturation.

Simulated Work Testing—A New Technique

Recently new functional rehabilitation techniques have been introduced. Simulated work testing can be used by rehabilitation specialists to evaluate the individual functional ability to perform home, work and leisure activities. This type of testing is typically accomplished by having the individual perform a specified task using the actual tools and equipment at a workstation setup in the laboratory. Work simulator devices are commercially available. Simulation of daily activities with task specific tools has been well tolerated by elderly patients and has been shown to improve physical work capacity. The advantages of such techniques include the generation of mechanical parameters monitored by the dynamometer (work exerted, power output, strength, mechanical fatigue, number of repetitions per time) and the possibility to perform strength or endurance tests with the actual tools used in daily living.

Selection of a functional task for performance should be done after reviewing information collected from the subject. It is important to consider activities that the patients must be able to manage as part of their basic self-care or to consider specific activities the subject has a strong desire to successfully perform. It is also important to remember that before a subject is discharged from the rehabilitation program, the results of the testing should be well documented. Quantitative indicators of physical capacity and tolerable workloads could be obtained by adopting these "functional techniques" with work simulators and metabolic analyzers.

Nutritional Testing

Interactions between nutritional status and lung disease have been the focus of research only in the recent past. The problem of obesity and its implications for RM function have been greatly overlooked. Optimal nutritional status should help to maximize the patient's state of health, RM function and overall sense of well-being and could improve disease outcome.

There is a large body of literature on nutritional assessment in COPD which is poorly standardized. This is because malnutrition is not well-defined. Most of the measures of poor nutrition are be influenced by a chronic negative energy balance. As a result, in western medical practice the terms undernutrition or malnutrition are indiscriminately used whether the clinical condition results from lack of food or from disease. It may therefore be more appropriate to refer to patients as "depleted" rather than undernourished.

It is generally acknowledged that a substantial proportion of patients with COPD are malnourished and that malnutrition contributes to deterioration in the clinical condition. The association between malnutrition and COPD has been recognized for many years. A significant percentage of patients with advanced COPD lose weight and muscle mass, a process which also affects the RMs. Factors related to nutritional status are considered as an independent influence on the course of COPD and in a previous study of ours, patients with a reduced percentage of ideal body weight (%IBW) had a greater probability to need ICU admission.

Measurements of Nutritional Status

The calculation of % IBW by comparing measured body weight to a standard has been a traditional method. Anthropometric parameters may also be useful in defining the prognosis of the disease. Weight standards are an incomplete assessment of nutritional status because they do not detail variations in specific body components. Serial measurements to determine percent of usual body weight are useful to reference the individual to himself.

Schols and associates advocate the use of measures that reflect fat free mass. Fat free mass is a better indicator of body mass depletion than body weight and therefore it may have consequences for planning rehabilitative strategies. These investigators found that normal-weight COPD patients with depletion of free fat mass undergoing rehabilitative programs had greater impairment than underweight patients with relative preservation of fat-free mass.

Lean body mass (LBM) measurement would be a useful outcome parameter. Its determination involves the use of anthropometric measurements as assessed by the size of skinfold, skeletal breadth, and circumference at various body sites. An alternative approach to estimate LBM is bioelectrical impedance analysis. Biochemical assessment of various body fluids, such as blood and urine, has been advocated as a marker of nutritional status. Components measured include albumin, pre-albumin, transferrin and retinol-binding protein, lymphocyte count (for assessment of immunocompetence) and urine metabolites. Visceral proteins are considered to reflect the severity of injury and prognosis in critically ill hospitalized patients, but they often do not accurately reflect nutritional status or adequacy of nutritional support. Other methods to assess nutritional status rely on delayed cutaneous hypersensitivity response which is decreased or completely suppressed in malnutrition.

Psychological Evaluation

In addition to progressive physical disability, high levels of depression and anxiety as well as impaired performance on tests of memory and concentration, have been found in patients with COPD. The

clinical syndromes of depression and anxiety, in turn, further reinforce the patient's social isolation and physical inactivity. It has been
reported that the 4-year mortality in male patients with severe COPD
is influenced by overall psychological distress and difficulty in coping with their disease, which seem to be important prognostic indicators irrespective of lung function or oxygenation. Standardized
neuropsychological tests of memory, concentration, psychomotor
speed, emotional state and cognitive performance have been used to
evaluate functional status and the effect of rehabilitation programs.
One of the most established psychological tests is the Trail-making
Test, which is sensitive to changes in brain function. The Digit Symbol subtest of the Wechsler Adult Intelligence Scale (WAIS) is a timed
test of psychomotor performance, which has been shown to decline
with age. The Digit Span subtest of the WAIS-R (an updated version
of this scale) provides a good measure of concentration and short-term
memory, both of which may be impaired among COPD patients.

Conclusion

The only limitation to a pulmonary rehabilitation program appears
to be unwillingness to participate or poor compliance. Selection criteria merely serve as indication to a specific therapeutic program.
Proper evaluation of candidates is the cornerstone of a successful rehabilitation program.

— by N. Ambrosino, MD, K. Foglio, MD, L. Bianchi, MD,
Salvatore Maugeri Foundation IRCCS, Lung Function
Laboratory, Pulmonary Rehabilitation and Respiratory
Day-Hospital Unit, Rehabilitation Center of Gussago, Italy.

Dr. Ambrosino is Attending Physician in the Pulmonary Department
at the Medical Center of Gussago (BS), Italy. Dr. Foglio is Chief Assistant and Dr. Bianchi is Assistant, at the Lung Function Unit of
Salvatore Maugeri Foundation IRCCS, Gussago, Italy.

Table 51.1 Components of Pulmonary Rehabilitation Programs

- Drug maximization
- Smoking cessation
- Education
- Chest physiotherapy
- Exercise training
- Respiratory muscle training
- Peripheral muscle training
- Occupational therapy
- Long-term oxygen therapy
- Respiratory muscle rest (mechanical ventilation)
- Psychosocial support
- Nutrition

Table 51.2 Factors Influencing the Outcome of Pulmonary Rehabilitation

- Appropriate selection of patients
- Age
- Nutritional status
- Severity of respiratory impairment
- Compliance to therapy

Table 51.3 Indications for Pulmonary Rehabilitation

- Chronic obstructive pulmonary disease
- Bronchial asthma
- Cystic fibrosis
- Bronchiectasis
- Chronic respiratory insufficiency (CRI) from any cause
- Acute respiratory insufficiency in patients with CRI from any cause
- Neuromuscular and chest wall diseases
- Pulmonary fibrosis, pneumoconiosis and other interstitial diseases
- Before and after surgical procedures
- Sleep respiratory disorders
- Lung transplantation

Chapter 52

Burn Rehabilitation

"I'm told I'm lucky to be alive—that only five years ago a person burned as severely as I would have died. Maybe that would have been best." Shortly after his injury and months before his initial hospitalization ended, the young man quoted above was trying desperately to answer the question: *What about the quality of my life as a survivor of a severe burn injury?*

Survival rates for severely burned people have increased dramatically during the past twenty years, so this question deserves careful deliberation. The improvements have been attributed to the application of basic principles of medicine and systematic research into physiological and metabolic problems. For instance, less than ten years ago, it was learned that burn patients were dying of malnutrition because a severely burned body requires an enormous number of calories to maintain body temperature. Now careful attention is given to adequate calorie intake.

The medical aspects of treating burns have improved significantly. By contrast, the systematic application of rehabilitation principles and practices has not kept pace with acute treatment advances, according to Dr. Irving Feller. Concerned about this lag, Dr. Feller of the University of Michigan Burn Center and his colleagues at the National Institute for Burn Medicine (NIBM) began

Rehab Brief, Vol. VI, No.5, May 1983; NIHR Publication No. 0732-2623. Although relatively old, this document is currently circulated by the National Institute of Handicapped Research and offers a useful framework for understanding burn rehabilitation.

a program of research into burn rehabilitation in 1959. In 1977, the Rehabilitation Services Administration awarded a grant to NIBM. The project was later continued by the National Institute of Handicapped Research. *A Comprehensive Rehabilitation Program for Severe Burns: Final Report* summarizes the project work carried out by Dr. Feller and colleagues at NIBM. The report forms the basis of this BRIEF and answers some basic questions for the rehabilitation practitioner who becomes involved only upon referral late in the rehabilitation process.

Who Gets Burned?

Each year approximately two million people who are burned require medical attention. Seventy thousand require hospitalization and nine thousand die of their injuries. The comprehensive literature review and the three studies done by Dr. Feller and colleagues helped to identify and describe the burn population. While burn patients comprise a heterogeneous group with diverse needs, some generalizations about factors that make the occurrence of a burn more likely can be made. More males than females are burned, except for the population over sixty-five. Of adults, those in their twenties are more likely to be burned. The presence of other significant personal and environmental factors likely to contribute to a burn are summarized in Table 52.1. The reader is reminded that only a limited amount of research has been published and summaries and conclusions are only suggestive, not definitive.

What Is a Severe Burn?

The depth of the burn wound and the percentage of the body surface burned determine the severity of the burn. The depth of the wound is commonly classified in three degrees, but it is measured more precisely in terms of the thickness of the burn. A first-degree or superficial burn involves only the epidermis (top layer of the skin). A second-degree or partial thickness burn involves the dermis as well as the epidermis. A third-degree or full-thickness burn involves both layers of skin and the skin appendages—the hair follicles, sweat glands, and sebaceous glands. Generally, anyone with partial and full-thickness burns over twenty percent of the body is considered to be severely burned. Other factors such as age, pre-existing health problems, and body parts burned are considered also.

Table 52.1. Personal and Environmental Factors Affecting the Occurrence of a Burn.

PERSON

Age

Sex

Premorbid Psychopathology
—Behavior problems
—Psychiatric diagnosis/ hospitalization
—Alcoholism-drug abuse
—Suicide
—self-destructive behaviors

Previous Physical Disability
—Neurological disorders
—Cardiovascular disease
—Obesity

Pre-existing Behavior Patterns
—Presence of accident behavior
—Absence or lack of protective behavior

ENVIRONMENT

Socio-Economic Factors
—Unskilled or semi-skilled wage earner
—Crowded housing
—Poor housing

Family Behaviors
—Lack of information about safety, danger, protection
—Presence of accident-prone behaviors

Family Stress
—Poor physical/emotional health
—Pregnancy
—Marital problems
—Conflict with immediate or extended family members

New Environments
—Frequent moves
—Migrants/immigrants
—Isolation

What Is the Rehabilitation Process for People Who Have Been Burned?

Successful rehabilitation requires the simultaneous management of all problems—especially medical and psychological—according to an individualized plan. To help the practitioner understand the complicated process, Dr. Feller and colleagues have divided it into three phases (described later). The medical aspects can more reliably be assigned to phases than the psychological aspects. Psychological reactions to a severe burn, like reactions to any disablement, depend on the nature of the disability and many variables relating to the person and the environment. The nature of the disability is influenced by many factors, too, including the resulting functional impairments, visibility of the scars, number of readmissions for corrective surgery, secondary complications, and cause of the burn (suicide attempt, accident, or inflicted burn). Personal characteristics that influence reactions to burns include sex, activities affected, lifestyle, and personality. The immediate environment is especially influential in determining the outcome or adjustment to a severe burn. Family acceptance and support, income, community resources, and hospital capabilities (burn center vs. general hospital) are a few of the environmental factors. Bearing all of these factors in mind and allowing for individual reactions, the practitioner can nevertheless recognize common reactions in each phase.

The Emergent Phase

From the scene of the accident, the severely burned person is rushed to the hospital where the burns are bathed and assessed. The first objective is to stabilize the body's fluids. Damaged capillaries allow fluids to escape to the surrounding tissues and since the skin no longer can control evaporation, the patient becomes dehydrated and goes into shock. Large volumes of fluids are pumped back into the body during the first twenty-four hours after injury. A great deal of swelling occurs and large incisions are sometimes made to release the pressure caused by the swelling. A second objective is to maintain the body temperature since there may be little skin to regulate heat loss. The body uses excessive calories to maintain the temperature and these must be replaced to prevent malnutrition. A weight loss of one pound per day is common. Debridement, or cutting away loose, dead skin begins. This is a painful process—despite injections of morphine. The burns are then coated with solutions to destroy bacteria and antibiotics are also injected. A range of behaviors from passivity and numbness to extreme agitation may be observed as the individual attempts to assimilate what has happened. This phase lasts from one to five days.

The Acute Phase

As the patient slowly understands what has happened, s/he may begin to feel the isolation required to subdue the possibility of infection. The person may realize that s/he has caught the last glimpse of a human face until this phase of rehabilitation is over. Every visitor—family, friend, or medical staff—must wear cap, gown, gloves, and mask. Only the eyes can be seen, but much can be read from them by a person who may be looking for signs of rejection. Having "things" done to one's body without full understanding of the planned outcome can create confusion and fear. Support and acceptance from staff and family are critical during this phase. Daily visits to the hydrotherapy tank continue where the burned, dead flesh is cut away with small, sharp scalpels designed to lessen the blood loss. The loss is so great that only a small area can be cleaned at any one time. Since the person's own skin will be needed for grafting, the muscle and fat are initially covered by pig skin or the skin of cadavers to allow those tissues to heal before grafting.

The pain increases, and although that is a sign of improvement (the pain receptors in full thickness burns are rejuvenating), it only complicates the emotions of the patient. She may be asking, "If getting better means adding pain to an already intolerable amount, then why get better?" Depression and anxiety are common and the person most likely wants to withdraw from all interaction. Still the physical therapist visits daily to manipulate joints to prevent loss of range of motion. Once a healthy base of tissue develops in the partial and full thickness burns, grafting can proceed. A donor site is chosen from an unburned area of the body and the skin taken can be stretched up to six (rarely, even to ten) times its original size to cover the wounds. Slowly, the grafts can be expected to cover the body and lower the risks of infection.

The Rehabilitation Phase

This phase begins when the burn wound is decreased to less than 20 percent of the total body surface. It is geared toward preventing cosmetic and functional deformities and returning the person to a place in society. The work done by NIBM indicates that social support from family, friends, peers, and personnel in community agencies facilitates the rehabilitation process independent of the severity of the burn injury.

This support network is challenged by the transition from hospital to home. If the burn happened in the home, fear and anxiety of returning to that environment may occur. Nightmares of being on fire are common for those who have been burned by flames. Unresolved issues about the accident and pre-existing disabilities or personal and family problems which may have been factors in causing burn injuries may surface as complications. Discipline is tested when energy levels are low and physical demands are high. Skin care is essential and physical therapy must be continued. Splints and elastic pressure garments to reduce contractures or scarring must be worn twenty-four hours a day by some people. Financial hardship may increase the strain of new procedures and experiences. The result may be frustration and anger. Gradually the medical condition improves and the person can be expected to assume preburn roles and responsibilities. Then, just as progress is being made, it may be interrupted. Twenty to 30 percent of all survivors require at least one readmission to the hospital and sometimes many more. Most surgeries to correct cosmetic deformities and functional limitations are performed within the first several years after injury, but some people will undergo recurrent surgeries for as many as twenty years. This is especially true for children who require release of scar contractures around developing breasts or growing joints.

As a person begins to realize that s/he will never look or be the same as before the injury, anger, remorse, and despair may surface. Some people reminisce with old photographs about "the way things used to be." They may try to believe that surgery will restore them completely. Yet, they know it is not true. Grief and emotional withdrawal are common as the individuals vacillate between reality and false hope. One young man, a year after injury and several corrective surgeries, realized that his appearance had not improved as much as he had hoped. He angrily tore to shreds every picture of himself taken before the injury. After several more months of depression and grieving, he decided to have only enough additional surgeries to correct contractures, and to forego surgeries intended only to improve appearance. He decided the pain was not worth the improvement he could realistically expect. Practitioners should be careful not to hold out false hopes about what the person can expect from surgery. The significance of the injury should be discussed openly and grief should be respected, but the person is usually helped most if encouraged to resume preburn roles, responsibilities, and activities as soon as possible. Slowly, s/he must be helped to accept a life that has been unalterably changed, but also must be helped to recognize that the quality of a changed life is not necessarily lessened. It is encouraging to note that severely burned people often emerge from the whole process with higher self-esteem than before injury. Sometimes, the support found during the rehabilitation process not only helps them accept the results of being burned, but also helps them learn to master other problems.

What Are the Vocational Implications?

Feller and his colleagues found that the majority of those employed pre-burn resume employment and that a quick return to employment is related to successful rehabilitation. Size of full-thickness burns was found to be an important variable in determining time it took to return to work, but other factors also played a role. Employees who did not return to the same jobs took significantly longer than those who did. Married people returned to work faster than single people. Those who had an adequate to good adjustment preburn returned faster. Litigation almost doubled the time it took to return. Skilled workers were more likely to return to previous jobs than laborers. Coverage by Worker's Compensation did not seem to be a factor. For those who were injured at work, fear of objects or situations (e.g., ovens, torches, carburetors), and physical impairments led to job change. Inability to work as long or as hard as before injury also caused job change. On-the-job complaints were most often related to hand, feet, and leg functioning.

Additional common problems that interfere with work or education are:

- **Contractures.** Contractures result when scar tissue forms over or adjacent to a joint or skin fold. The shortened skin causes a loss of range of motion. These may be corrected through continued physical therapy, but may often require surgery.

- **Hypertrophic scars.** This ropey, thick formation of skin is an abnormal configuration of collagen fibers. The scars may be corrected with elastic pressure garments, steroid injection, or partial removal of scar and regrafting. (Keloid formation is a special kind of scarring and is common to dark pigmented skin.)

- **Eye Injuries.** Inability to close the eyes due to badly burned eyelids can be corrected with grafting. Scarring of the corneas

439

often responds to medication, but a corneal transplant may be helpful.

- **Body part loss.** Amputations may be required if burns involve muscle and bone. The loss of the nose and ears is a fairly frequent complication and requires plastic surgery.

- **Neuromuscular problems.** Peripheral neuromuscular problems are evidenced by numbness, tingling, peripheral weakness, impaired hearing, or other nerve deficit signs. Hemiplegia, seizure disorders, aphasia, encephalitis, and meningitis have been found.

- **Loss of sweat glands.** The person must avoid overheating.

- **Hair loss.** A full-thickness burn involves the hair follicles and thus the grafted areas will not grow hair. If the scalp is involved, hair transplants may be desired, if the person works with the public.

- **Loss of sebaceous glands.** Daily lubrication is needed to maintain pliable skin.

- **Delicate skin.** During the first year after grafting, even scratching can break the skin and the skin will sunburn easily.

- **Itching.** Itching is a common complaint.

- **Lack of sensation.** Grafted areas lack the sensation of normal skin.

- **Drug dependency.** Whether a problem before or after injury, drug dependency complicates vocational planning.

Other serious complications are total loss of hearing and brain damage. Electrical burns merit special consideration. All electrical burns are full-thickness burns and usually occur at work. They often appear to involve only small areas where the current entered and exited, but the tissue beneath the skin may be severely damaged. This can lead to amputation and/or serious neuromuscular problems.

While a person with many physical complications may present a challenge to the rehabilitation practitioner, severity of the injury may not be the major factor influencing return to preburn activities. Often a person with relatively few complications will take a long time to return to work and other activities. Evidence exists to show that young adults with no previous work experience represent a supreme challenge regardless of the severity of physical limitations or complications.

What Are the Components of a Model Program for Burn Care?

One of the most important tasks of the project undertaken by NIBM was to identify the components of a model rehabilitation program. Outlined in depth in the Final Report to the National Institute of Handicapped Research, the six components are listed below:

1. The planning and organization of a regionalized burn care system.

2. The development of a program designed to meet the needs of the burn patient population it serves.

3. The process of rehabilitation for the burn patient.

4. The burn rehabilitation team.

5. Education and involvement of the patient, family, and community.

6. Rehabilitation research.

How Can Information Be Shared?

The National Burn Information Exchange (NBIE) was started by NIBM to provide a method to define the natural course of burn trauma by collecting and disseminating information from burn centers throughout the world that can be used to more knowledgeably plan for rehab needs. Presently, over 65,000 cases are on file from over 100 hospitals.

Conclusions

NIBM studies indicate that a person who is treated at a major burn center and is provided with a supportive environment during the rehabilitation process can be expected to achieve social, emotional, and vocational adjustment. Indeed, some report higher self-esteem and life satisfaction than before injury. Thus, the practices demonstrated to be effective in such a supportive environment should be systematically applied to all settings providing burn-related services.

Rehabilitation professionals' roles and responsibilities must be clearly defined. The literature defines the roles of practitioners on the primary care team-surgeon, psychologist, psychiatrist, nurse, social worker, occupational therapist, and physical therapist—but not the roles of professionals in community agencies to which referrals are made. The rehabilitation counselor is particularly important in that return to productive work is recognized as a major factor contributing to overall adjustment. Yet, of the 325 people studied, only 16 per cent could remember being referred to a state vocational rehabilitation agency and only 11 per cent reported contact with an agency. The results of that small study are not definitive, but raise questions as to why rehabilitation counselors are not more involved in the rehabilitation of people who are burned. Improvements may have been made since 1977, but counselors might ask themselves if greater efforts could be made to service this population. Assigning liaison counselors to burn units and burn centers would be one step in the right direction.

Counselors should recognize that while medical and physical facts may differ from other populations, the human reactions are similar to those they've observed with other disabilities. Therefore, the roles and responsibilities of the rehabilitation counselor are not new. They include:

1. Facilitating independence

2. Providing support and counseling

3. Providing vocational guidance and placement

4. Involving and educating the family

5. Recognizing the long-term implications

6. Providing follow-up when possible

Counselors can contribute to the management of psychological stresses during the medical treatment and provide counseling and guidance aimed toward a quick return to preburn activities. The most outstanding medical treatment can be negated by lack of appropriate counseling and guidance. State rehabilitation agencies must see that this doesn't happen.

Sources

Three books developed during the grant are appended to, but not included in the Final Report:

Bowden, M.L. and Feller, Irving, M.D. *Progress in Burn Rehabilitation: A Report of Three Studies*, Ann Arbor, Michigan:
NIBM, 1982.

Bowden, M.L.; Jones, Claudelia A.; and Feller, Irving, M.D.
*Psycho — Social Aspects of a Severe Burn: A Review of the Litera-
ture*. Ann Arbor, Michigan: NIBM, 1979.

Feller, Irving, M.D. et al. *Reconstruction and Rehabilitation of
the Burned Patient*. Ann Arbor, Michigan: NIBM, 1979.

Part Seven

Additional Help
and Information

Chapter 53

Glossary of Head Injury Terms

Hospital Equipment

arterial line: a catheter placed in an artery, used to monitor blood pressure in the arteries and to allow for access to arterial blood for laboratory studies.

catheter: a hollow tube placed into a part of the body for the removal of fluids or to allow fluids to be introduced into the body.

central venous pressure (CVP) line: a catheter that is threaded into the right atrium of the heart. The CVP reading directly reflects the right ventricular filling and diastolic pressure in the right atrium of the heart.

chest tubes: tubes that are placed into the chest to drain fluid from the body.

endotrachial tube: a tube that is inserted into the trachea through either the mouth or nose to ensure an open airway.

Foley catheter: a catheter that has a small inflatable balloon on the end, usually inserted into the bladder. The balloon is inflated to keep the catheter in the bladder so that urine can be continuously drained into an external bag.

halo: a metal ring used with patients who have spinal cord injuries to preserve proper alignment of the neck and spinal columns. This helps keep the patient still and the body aligned during healing.

intracranial pressure monitor: a monitor, inserted through the skull, that measures pressure of the fluid inside the brain and skull.

intravenous (IV) line: a small catheter placed into a vein, which can be used to give a patient fluids, drugs, or blood; also used to monitor venous blood pressure.

intravenous board: a board that is used to hold an extremity immobile so as not to dislodge an IV line.

monitor: any machine that gives a reading of vital body processes, such as cardiac (heart) monitors or intracranial pressure monitors.

nasogastric tube: a tube inserted through the nose into the stomach, through which to feed a patient, to give medications, etc.; used if a patient is unconscious, has severe jaw injury, or is unable to swallow.

respirator/ventilator: machines that either assist a patient with breathing or actually breathe for him or her by forcing oxygen into the lungs.

space boots: large, soft protective shoes used to support muscles and tendons during coma.

Swan-Ganz catheter: a catheter that is threaded into the heart and wedged in a pulmonary arteriole; used to measure pulmonary artery pressure and pulmonary capillary wedge pressure, both good indicators of left ventricular function.

traction: traction devices apply a pulling force to reduce, align, and immobilize fractures; to lessen, prevent, or correct deformity associated with bone injury and muscle disease; and to reduce muscle spasms in fracture of a long bone or in back injury.

transducer: a device that changes input energy of one form into output energy of another. For example, physiological energy such as the heart beating is changed from beats to lines on a strip of paper that can be read.

ventriculostomy: an operation that is performed to drain fluid from a ventricle of the brain to treat hydrocephalus.

Medications

antibiotics: a category of medications used to control the infections to which injured persons are prone.

Baclofen: relieves muscle spasms and muscle tone problems.

BuSpar: used to alleviate anxiety.

Dantrim: relieves muscle spasms, cramping, and tightness of muscles.

Decadron: a cortiosteroid used to reduce inflammation and improve brain functioning through reduction of brain swelling.

Dilantin: used to control or prevent seizures and convulsive disorders.

Haldol: used to calm agitated, combative, anxious, or tense patients, usually during the relatively early stages of post-acute treatment.

imipramine: used as an antidepressant.

Lasix: used to reduce excess water from the body and help reduce intracranial pressure, water in the lungs, or sluggish kidneys.

laxatives: a category of drugs used to encourage bowel movements and to relieve constipation.

Maalox: used to help prevent stomach ulcers or stomach discomforts that hospitalized patients are prone to develop.

Mannitol: removes water from the brain, used to decrease intracranial pressure.

morphine sulfate: used to reduce pain and to reduce bodily reflexes through sedation.

Mysoline: an antiseizure medication, often used if other similar-acting drugs fail to work.

Nembutal: used to reduce intracranial pressure and reduce pain.

Pavulon: used to relax skeletal muscles to help keep the patient from struggling, usually while on a respirator.

phenobarbital: used to control or prevent seizures and convulsive disorders.

Prozac: used as an antidepressant.

Ritalin: used as a brain stem stimulant to help improve attention and concentration.

sleeping medications: a category of drugs used to assist in maintaining regular sleep/wake cycles; examples are Dalmane, Halcion, Restoril.

steroids: a category of drugs used to reduce brain swelling.

Tagamet: used to help prevent stomach ulcers to which hospitalized patients are prone.

Tegretol: antiseizure medication that also effects impulsive behaviors.

Valium: used to reduce anxiety, tension, and muscle activity.

Xanax: antianxiety medication to help reduce tension and muscle activity.

Neurological Tests and Procedures

BEAM (brain electrical activity mapping): a computerized analysis of background EEG activity, much more sensitive than conventional EEG, which is especially helpful in identifying abnormalities of early dementia or suspected brain damage from head injury.

brain stem evoked responses: brain stem response to a specific stimulus recorded electronically.

CT scan (Computerized Tomography): computerized x-ray taken at different levels of the brain to yield a three-dimensional representation of the physical shape of the brain.

electrocardiogram (ECG or EKG): electrical measure of heart activity and heartbeat that is produced on a chart recording.

electroencephalogram (EEG): an evaluation of electrical activity of the brain.

lumbar puncture: a tap into the spinal fluid to assess presence of toxic agents or infections that might be present in the brain.

MRI scan (Magnetic Resonance Imaging): an instrument that develops images from biochemical operations of the brain by using a magnetic field.

neurological examination: an assessment of gross nerve functioning via reflexes and reactions; performed by a neurologist or neurosurgeon.

450

PET scan (Positron Emission Tomography): an instrument that records chemical activity in specific regions of the brain.

Neuropsychological Terms

abstract reasoning: process of generalizing from concrete examples and experiences to larger, broader principles.

acalculia: dysfunction or inability to perform mathematical operations, recognize numbers, or count.

acuity: keenness of sensation.

agnosia: loss of ability to recognize familiar people, places, and objects.

agraphia: loss of ability to express thoughts in writing.

alexia: inability to read or recognize words.

anomia: dysfunction or inability to name objects or recall individual names.

anterograde amnesia: loss of memory for events and periods of time following an injury or traumatic event.

apathy: decrease in motivation, initiation, interest in life and growth; indifference.

aphasia: loss in ability to speak coherent ideas or understand spoken language.

apraxia: loss of ability to carry out habitual movement or acts that were previously automatic.

astereognosis: inability to recognize objects or shapes by feeling them.

asymmetry: discrepancy in function or appearance between sides of organs.

ataxia: dysfunction in motor coordination and balance.

attention: ability for sustaining focus on task for a period of time to allow for coding and storing of information in memory.

cognition: processes of thinking, understanding, and reasoning.

concentration: ability to remain attentive to a specific task for a sufficient time.

diplopia: seeing two superimposed images of a single object; "double vision."

disinhibition: loss of restraint or decrease in ability to stop oneself from saying or doing something that is typically undesirable.

disorientation: disturbance in recognition of person, place, and/or time and day.

dysarthria: disruption or dysfunction in speech articulation.

emotional lability: intense fluctuations of emotions in response to experiences.

frustration tolerance: amount and degree of frustration; encounter with obstacles one can live with before losing control over affect and thinking.

inflexibility: rigidity in thinking; over reliance on stereotypes; difficulty in recognizing alternative possibilities.

judgment: ability for resolving dilemmas and approaching problems; includes values, morals, and interpretation with respect for interactions.

memory: stored recollections about experiences, events, feelings, dates, etc., from the recent and distant past.

perseveration: over-reliance on or repetition of a specific response or behavior to different tasks.

post-traumatic amnesia: loss in memory for events related to a traumatic event and the period immediately following the trauma.

problem-solving: skills for employing reasoning, judgment, experience, and discernment in resolving problems.

retrograde amnesia: loss of memory for events and periods of time before an injury or accident.

unilateral neglect: unawareness or inattention to one side of the body or the space or events occurring on one side of the body.

visual field deficit: inability to perceive vision in an area of the visual field, such as the right or left field, known as hemianopsia.

Chapter 54

Glossary of Stroke Terms

accreditation: a status awarded to hospitals and other facilities that meet certain standards of excellence in their field.

activities of daily living (ADL): routine activities a person does every day, such as standing, sitting, walking, eating, bathing, and grooming.

acute medical care: medical care that is meant to stabilize one's medical condition and minimize complications; usually received before rehabilitation.

acute rehabilitation: medical services that include both general medical care and medical rehabilitation services.

allowable charges: the maximum amount the Medicare program or other health insurance plans will pay for particular health care services.

aphasia: loss or impairment of the ability to express or understand spoken or written words.

apraxia: loss or impairment of the ability to perform complex muscular movements.

assistive equipment: equipment or devices, such as wheelchairs, braces, walkers, or speech aids, that help a person to perform activities of daily living.

balance billing: charges for doctors' services that exceed Medicare's allowable charges and for which patients are responsible, up to a pre-determined limit.

benefits: services or equipment that a health insurance plan will pay for.

cap: a limit on the amount an insurance plan will pay for a person's health care each year or over a lifetime.

case manager: a professional who works for an insurance company, hospital, or rehabilitation facility to ensure appropriate follow-up to acute care, coordinate care across health care providers and facilities, and make sure that all aspects of treatment comply with the rules of an individual's health plan.

catastrophic limits of coverage: under a health insurance plan, the maximum out-of-pocket expenses a person must pay for medical services or prescription drugs.

certification: a status awarded to facilities that have met minimum health and safety standards and are eligible to accept Medicare payments.

combination plan: a health insurance plan, such as a preferred provider organization (PPO), that combines features of both traditional indemnity policies and managed care plans.

comprehensive outpatient rehabilitation facility (CORF): a rehabilitation facility that provides a full range of rehabilitation services on an outpatient basis.

copayment: a small, fixed-dollar amount (usually $5 or $10) paid by the patient for a doctor's visit, prescription drugs, or other health care services.

covered benefits: health care services that are paid for by an insurance company according to the health insurance policy.

custodial care: care that is provided to help patients take care of their daily needs (eating, bathing, dressing, etc.), which does not require treatment or services from specially trained professionals, such as doctors, therapists, or nurses.

day treatment: rehabilitation care that provides a full range of intensive services, but allows patients to stay at home overnight.

deductible: a dollar amount that the patient must pay before an insurance company begins paying for any services; the amount varies by insurance plan.

disability: a problem with a human function, such as not being able to walk or communicate.

dysarthria: impairment of the ability to produce speech.

dysphagia: impairment of the ability to swallow liquids or solids.

environmental adaptations: conditions or things in a person's environment that enhance independence, such as ramps or elevators.

fee-for-service (FFS): a method of payment for medical services in which a specific fee is charged for each individual service; the method of payment used under traditional indemnity policies.

functional ability: how well a person is able to perform activities of daily living (eating, bathing, dressing, communicating, etc.) without help from someone else.

gatekeeper: a person at a health insurance plan, generally a primary care doctor, who approves treatment (and thus payment) for health care services, such as rehabilitation services.

handicap: a problem caused by one's environment, such as steps that create a barrier for a person in a wheelchair.

health maintenance organization (HMO): (see managed care plan).

hemiparesis: weakness on one side of the body.

hemiplegia: paralysis on one side of the body.

home care: health care services received in one's home from visiting professionals, such as a nurse or a therapist.

impairment: a physical problem with a body or organ function, such as paralysis.

indemnity policy: a traditional health insurance plan through which the patient is treated by his or her choice of physician and pays on a fee-for-service basis.

long-term care facility: (see nursing home).

managed care plan: a health care plan, such as a health maintenance organization, that delivers comprehensive health care services at a reduced price for members who agree to use certain providers and facilities.

Medical Hospital Insurance (Medicare Part A): a part of the Medicare program that covers medical treatment in a hospital, skilled nursing facility, or hospice, as well as medical care a person receives at home from a home health care service.

medical social worker: a medical professional who helps patients solve problems related to their need for medical care by answering questions, providing information, offering counseling, and making referrals to other professionals and resources in the community.

medically stable: a medical term that means a person's condition is not likely to get worse or develop medical complications.

Medicaid: a health insurance program run by individual state governments that provides health coverage primarily for low-income families and people with significant disabilities.

Medicare: a health care insurance program administered by the federal government that provides health insurance for people over age 65, some people with disabilities, and others who qualify.

Medicare Part A: (see Medical Hospital Insurance)

Medicare Part B: (see Supplementary Medical Insurance)

Medigap policy: a health insurance policy purchased through a private insurance company that pays for medical expenses not covered by the Medicare program.

neglect: the act of disregarding stimuli on the side of the body that has been affected by a stroke.

network: a group of health care providers and facilities that participate in a managed care plan or preferred provider organization.

neurologist: a doctor who specializes in the diagnosis and treatment of problems with the nervous system.

nursing home: a facility where patients stay to receive rehabilitation services, long-term care, or skilled nursing care.

occupational therapist (OT): a rehabilitation professional who teaches skills and adaptations that allow people with disabilities to be as independent as possible in their daily activities.

orthoses: devices designed to support or supplement a weakened joint or limb.

out-of-network: providers and facilities that do not participate in a particular managed care plan.

out-of-pocket expenses: the costs of health care services that the patient must pay because they are not paid for through an insurance plan. These include both copayments and deductibles..

outpatient rehabilitation: rehabilitation services provided to a person who lives at home; may be a comprehensive, daily program of multiple services, or only one or two services once or twice a week.

paralysis: the inability to move a part of one's body, such as an arm or a leg.

pastoral care: spiritual support and guidance provided by a chaplain, or other clergyman, to address the emotional and spiritual needs of rehabilitation patients, their families, and members of their rehabilitation team.

physiatrist: a doctor who specializes in physical medicine and rehabilitation.

physical therapist (PT): a rehabilitation professional who works to restore one's movement abilities.

point of service (POS) option: in a managed care plan, the option to pay a higher price for health care services in order to choose providers or facilities outside the plan's network.

preferred provider organization (PPO): a health insurance plan that offers a discounted price for health care services to members who use approved (that is, "network") providers or facilities.

primary care physician: a doctor who provides non-specialist medical care; primary care doctors often are responsible for referring patients to specialists, if needed.

prostheses: artificial limbs or body parts.

quality of life: a person's level satisfaction with all aspects of their world, including self-esteem, personal and family relationships, social activities, financial conditions, employment status, spiritual activities, and anything else that influences satisfaction with life.

rehabilitation services: individual medical or rehabilitation treatments received as part of a program to enhance functional ability. Rehabilitation services include medical and nursing care, rehabilitation therapies such as PT, OT, or SLP, counseling sessions, recreational activities, and anything else prescribed to increase a patient's independence..

skilled nursing facility (SNF): a facility that provides patients with a high level of nursing care and meets certain industry standards.

speech-language pathologist (SLP): a rehabilitation professional who works to restore communication skills.

stroke: a sudden interruption of blood flow to an area of the brain, caused by a blockage (a blood clot) or by bleeding (a cerebral hemorrhage).

stroke club: a local organization that offers programs and support for people with stroke and their families.

subacute rehabilitation: rehabilitation services that include daily nursing services, supervision by a rehabilitation doctor, and medical care as needed; subacute rehabilitation is less intensive and generally lasts longer than acute rehabilitation.

Supplementary Medical Insurance (Medicare Part B): additional health insurance coverage that may be purchased through the Medicare program by people who qualify for Medicare.

transfer between levels of care: the movement of patients between different treatment programs and settings so that they may receive the most appropriate type of care.

Chapter 55

Glossary of Massage Therapy Terms

Massage Therapy (therapeutic massage): a profession in which the practitioner applies manual techniques, and may apply adjunctive therapies, with the intention of positively affecting the health and well-being of a client.

Massage: manual soft tissue manipulation; includes causing movement and/or applying pressure to the body.

Therapy: a series of actions aimed at achieving or increasing health and wellness.

Manual: by use of the hand.

Shiatsu and Acupressure: Oriental-based systems of finger-pressure which treat special points along acupuncture "meridians" (the invisible channels of energy flow in the body).

Reflexology: massage based around a system of points in the hands and feet thought to correspond, or "reflex," to all areas of the body.

Swedish Massage: a system of long strokes, kneading and friction techniques on the more superficial layers of the muscles, combined with active and passive movements of the joints.

Sports Massage: massage therapy focusing on muscle systems relevant to a particular sport.

© 1997 American Massage Therapy Association; reprinted with permission.

AMTA Sports Massage Team: developed by the AMTA to promote sports massage therapy by working with athletes at various national sporting events.

Chapter 56

Glossary of Assistive Technology Terms

assistive devices: Assistive means to help. Therefore, assistive devices help someone perform a given task. For example, a picture board used for communication would be an assistive device.

assistive technology: A generic term including assistive, adaptive and rehabilitative devices and the process used in selecting, locating and using them. Assistive technologies include: mechanical, electronic, and microprocessor based equipment: This includes microcomputers, electronic communication devices and other sophisticated devices. Non-mechanical and non-electronic aids: For example, a ramp to replace steps would fit in this category. Specialized instructional materials, services and strategies include large print for persons with visual impairments.

augmentative communication system: Any system that aids individuals who are not independent verbal communicators. The system can include speech, gestures, sign language, symbols, synthesized speech, dedicated communication aids or microcomputers.

coding system: A process or system of assigning codes, abbreviations or labels to represent a letter, item or message. The system can be arbitrarily or systematically applied. For example, the code, 456 may represent "Turn on the TV," or a picture of a drinking glass may signify, "I want a drink of water." Commonly used coding systems include morse code, abbreviation/expansion and semantic compaction.

dial scan: A device which looks like a clock face without numbers and has only one hand or dial. It is usually battery operated and switch controlled. Pictures or miniature objects are placed around the perimeter of the face. Selection is made when the dial points to the desired object and the switch is pressed or released.

direct selection: Activation of a letter, picture or other item by a single action. Pressing a key on a keyboard, eye gaze selection or use of an optical headpointer, are examples of direct selection.

durable medical equipment: A piece of equipment is considered durable medical equipment if it:

- Can withstand repeated use,

- is primarily and customarily used to service a medical or therapeutic purpose,

- is generally not useful to a person in the absence of illness or injury,

- and is appropriate for use in the home. (This is determined by opinions of medical specialists in the fields of physical medicine and rehabilitation.)

encoding: A selection technique used to specify items from an individual's vocabulary. For example, an individual may select DW on a communication device to say "I want a drink of water."

environmental control unit: A system that enables individuals to control various devices in their environment with single or multiple switches. The control unit may be mounted on a wheelchair for ease of access. Target devices include lights, door openers, televisions and telephones.

expanded keyboard: a keyboard which has keys and/or spaces between the keys larger than the standard microcomputer keyboard.

headwand or headstick: A pointer or extension device that is mounted to a headpiece and extends from the center of the forehead and angles downward. It is usually used in direct selection of an object such as a key on a keyboard or a symbol or word on a board. It is for use by persons with good head control and limited upper and lower body movement. If the pointer extends from the chin, it is referred to as a chinwand or chinstick.

icon: A graphic used to represent a concept or idea. Icons can appear on the computer screen or in print format. For example, a pencil may represent a word processing program.

input device: A method of activating or sending information to a computer or other electronic device. Keyboards, mice and trackballs are common computer input devices.

interdisciplinary team: Individuals involved in assessment and recommendations for persons with disabilities. The team consists of persons from a wide variety of disciplines including, but not limited to, medical experts, educators, speech language pathologists, occupational therapists, rehabilitation engineers, care providers, psychologist, counselors, and social workers.

jack: A jack is used to complete an electrical connection. A plug is inserted into a jack to connect switches to electronic devices.

joystick: A manual device with a moveable control lever that can be tilted in various directions to control computer, wheelchair or other target system.

keyboard emulator: A device that is connected to or resides in a computer and imitates the computer's keyboard in function and performance.

keyguard: A cover, usually made of plastic or plexiglass, which fits directly over the computer's keyboard. Holes in the cover correspond to each key on the keyboard and guide a finger, headstick or mouthstick to facilitate direct key presses. Locking devices which allow keys to operate similarly to a caps lock key are available for keys frequently used in multiple key sequences, such as the shift key, function or command keys.

membrane keyboard: A flat, usually programmable, keyboard with numerous pressure sensitive switches located under a soft surface. After areas of the keyboard have been defined, the user activates them by pressing on the surface.

miniature keyboard: Although smaller than the standard keyboard, a miniature keyboard contains all of the keys and functions. It is useful to persons with limited range of motion and one-handed typists.

moisture guard: A soft plastic cover molded to the shape of the keyboard and placed on the keyboard to protect it from moisture.

mouse: An input device connected to a computer that controls the position of the cursor on the screen. The mouse fits into the user's hand and has a ball encompassed on the underside that is rolled across a flat surface to move the cursor in the same direction as the mouse.

mouse emulator: A device that imitates the function of a mouse. In some instances, software may be used to alter the function of a keyboard to serve as a mouse emulator.

non-transparent access: A method of accessing a computer-based device that requires specialized software to allow it to interface with the computer.

peripheral: Any number of devices connected to a computer to provide input, output, or other functions. Printers, modems, switches, voice synthesizers, and internal memory cards are considered peripherals.

plug: Used in electrical connections, a plug is inserted into a jack to connect switches to electronic devices.

position (seated): The optimal seated position in a wheelchair places the individual's hips, knees and feet at 90 degree angles. The individual should feel secure, comfortable and relaxed.

redefinable keyboard: A keyboard that is defined according to individual users' needs. Keys may be rearranged on the keyboard, or redefined to represent frequently used words, phrases or computer commands.

rehabilitative device: Rehabilitate means to train. Rehabilitative devices are used for testing, exercising and training. For example, a balance beam is a rehabilitative device used to improve coordination.

scanning: A selection technique which presents groups of items to the user. The user then signals with a switch press, gesture or other means when the desired item is being indicated. The scanning may be performed automatically by an electronic system or manually by the communication partner.

selection technique: The means by which the user acquires or gets to and selects items which will be sent to a device.

sip and puff switch: A dual switch that is activated by sipping or puffing on an apparatus resembling a drinking straw.

speech digitizer: A device which allows digitally recorded speech to be analyzed and converted into electronic patterns that can be stored on a computer. Digitized speech may vary in quality from poor to human sounding, depending on the sampling frequency and audio playback system.

speech synthesizer: An electronic device that converts text characters into artificial speech. Speech synthesizers most frequently use pronunciation rules for translating text to speech. The quality of synthetic speech ranges from close to lifelike to robotic sounding speech found in lower end speech synthesizers.

switch: An input device used to control assistive devices and computers. There are a variety of types of switches including pressure switches, pneumatic switches, and voice activated switches. These switches can control adapted toys, environmental control devices, communication devices, and a wide range of computers.

TDD: A Telecommunication Device for the Deaf allows a person to transmit typed messages over the phone lines to another person with a TDD. Most TDD's include a keyboard for typing messages to send and a display and/or printer to receive messages.

touch screen: An input device which allows access to a computer by directly touching the screen.

trackball: An input device which contains a visible sphere mounted in a stationary container. It functions similarly to a mouse, however, the sphere is rotated with the fingers to move the cursor to any position on the screen.

transparent access: A method of using an alternative access system with a computer based device, such that the computer does not detect that the individual is using alternate input.

voice recognition system: An access system designed to replace the standard keyboard as the method of input. The system is "trained" to recognize utterances that are spoken into a microphone. The utterances are translated into computer commands or sequences of alphanumeric characters and used to operate the computer and software.

Chapter 57

Information Sources on Stroke

Organizations

Stroke affects over 500,000 Americans each year. For more information please contact these organizations or visit their Web sites.

Rehabilitation Research and Training Center on Enhancing Quality of Life of Stroke Survivors
Rehabilitation Institute Research Corporation
345 East Superior Street
Chicago, IL 60611
312/908-4637 (V)

Research project created to develop methods to prevent and minimize the medical complications of stroke. Disseminates information to the general public on new advancements in research and stroke care.

National Stroke Association
96 Inverness Drive East, Suite I
Englewood, CO 80112
800/787-6537 (V)
Web Site: http://www.stroke.org

Serves as a national education, information and resource service for stroke survivors, their families and professionals. Provides listings

1998 National Rehabilitation Information Center (NARIC); National Institute on Disability Rehabilitation Research (NIDRR).

of stroke rehabilitation facilities across the country. Web site includes a newsletter, facts and figures and other Internet resources.

The Stroke Connection of The American Heart Association
7272 Greenville Avenue
Dallas, TX 75231
800/553-6321 (V)
Web Site: http://www.amhrt.org/StrokCon

Maintains a listing of over 1000 stroke support groups across the country for referral to stroke survivors, family members and interested professionals. Web site contains heart and stroke guides, up-to-date research news and program information.

National Institute of Neurological Disorders and Stroke
National Institutes of Health
Building 31, Room 8A-06
Bethesda, MD 20892
800/352-9424 (V)
Web Site: http://www.ninds.nih.gov

Conducts research in the causes and treatment of neurological disorders and stroke. Maintains over 100 stroke-related publications. Scientific and technical documents and research reports also available. Web site includes program information, up-to-date research developments, health information and a publications guide.

National Aphasia Association
156 Fifth Street, Suite 707
New York, NY 10010
800/922-4622 (V)
Web Site: http://vvww.aphasia.org

Promotes public awareness by providing information and publications to individuals with aphasia, their family members and professionals. Web site features a pen pal service, an e-mail address exchange, newsletter and support group information.

The Family Caregiver Alliance
425 Bush Street, Suite 500
San Francisco, CA 94108
415/434-3388 (V)
800/524-6686 (California only)

Web Site: http:/twww.caregiver.org

Assists families of adults with chronic or progressive brain disorders, including stroke. Distributes information on caregiving and care of people with cognitive impairments. Web site contains fact sheets, articles, on-line support via e-mail and other resource links.

The National Easter Seal Society
230 West Monroe Street, Suite 1800
Chicago, IL 60606
800/221-6827 (V)
312/726-4258 (TT)
Web Site: http://www.seals.com

Provides multiple services including physical, occupational and speech therapy adult day care and respite care. There are over 400 affiliates across the country; however, all services are not available at all locations. Web site includes program information listed by city and state.

Web Sites

For more online information on stroke, visit the following Web sites:

HealthGuide: Stroke
Basic information
http://www.healthguide.com/stroke/

Brain Injury & Stroke Resources
Comprehensive listing of resources online
http://cmhc.com/guide/brain.htm

Stanford Stroke Center
Stroke information, new treatments
http://www-med.stanford.edu/school/stroke/

Case Management Resource Guide
Search for rehab facilities and numerous other healthcare providers
http://www.cmrg.com

Produced by the National Rehabilitation Information Center (NARIC), a project funded by the National Institute on Disability Rehabilitation Research (NIDRR) under contract #HN93029001. For more Information on NARIC services contact, NARIC, 8456 Colesville Rd.,

Suite 935, Silver Spring, MD 20910. 800-347-2742 (V) 301-495-5626 (TT), Web Site: http://www.naric.com/naric.

Chapter 58

Information Sources on Spinal Cord Injury

Organizations

National Spinal Cord Injury Association

8300 Colesville Road Suite 551
Silver Spring, MD 20910
800/962-9629 (V) 301/588-6959 (V)
Web Site: http://www.spinalcord.org

Serves as a comprehensive information source for anyone effected by spinal cord injury. Referrals and consultations are available through the national office or one of the many state chapters. Web site includes fact sheets, rehabilitation centers by state, chapter and contact information.

National Spinal Cord Injury Hotline

2200 Kernan Drive
Baltimore, MD 21207
800/526-3456 (V)
Web Site: http://user.aol.com/SCI hotline

The 24-hour hotline serves as a network for peer support and offers assistance in locating physicians, services and equipment. Information on accessing resources in one's community is also available. Web site explains the hotline's objectives.

1998 National Rehabilitation Information Center (NARIC); National Institute on Disability and Rehabilitation Research (NIDRR) contract #HN93029001.

Rehabilitation Research and Training Center in Secondary Complications in Spinal Cord Injury
University of Alabama/Birmingham
Department of Physical Medicine and Rehabilitation
Birmingham, AL 35233
205/934-3334 (V) 205/934-4642(TTY)
Web Site: http://www.sci.rehabm.uab.edu/docs/rrtchome.htm

Center's training component disseminates information to the public in the form of videotapes, audiotapes and journal articles. Subjects include urology, pressure sores, spasticity, childbirth and pulmonary complications. Web site contains center and publication information, plus a link to the National Spinal Cord Injury Statistical Center.

Rehabilitation Research and Training Center in Community Integration for Individuals with Spinal Cord Injury
Baylor College of Medicine
Department of Physical Medicine and Rehabilitation
Houston, TX 77030
713/797-5945 (V)

Research project which also serves as a resource guide to videos, pamphlets, booklets and manuals. Topics covered include bowel and bladder management, sexuality, employment, recreation and psychosocial adjustment.

National Institute of Neurological Disorders and Stroke
National Institutes of Health
Bethesda, MD 20892
800/352-9424 (V)
Web Site: http://www.ninds.nih.gov

Provides scientific documents, research reports and publications. Web site includes up-to-date research findings, health information and a publications guide.

National Center for Medical Rehabilitation Research (NCMRR)
National Institutes of Health
Bethesda, MD 20892
301/402-2242 (V)
Web Site: http://silk.nih.gov/silk/NCMRR/

Funds and supports research projects and fosters the development of scientific knowledge needed to enhance the quality of life of persons with disabilities. Web site includes mission statement and information on funding activities.

The Miami Project to Cure Paralysis
University of Miami School of Medicine
P.O. Box 016960
Miami, FL 33101
800/782-6387 (V)
Web Site: http://www.miamiproject.miami.edu

A science and clinical research effort dedicated to finding new treatments and ultimately, a cure for paralysis. Project offers research and rehabilitation information packets. Web site includes project overview, newsletter and latest research findings.

Paralyzed Veterans of America (PVA)
801 18th Street, NW
Washington, DC 20008
800/424-8200 (V) 800/795-4327 (TTY)
Web Site: http://www.pva.org

Advocacy and information association with brochures covering such topics as accessibility, legislation, assistive technology and sports. Web site includes SCI related news, research and treatment guides, chapter information and Internet links.

Websites

For more online information on SCI, visit the following Web sites:

New Mobility Magazine
Interactive site, latest SCI news, jobline, bookstore, chat rooms, other resources
http://www.newmobility.com

Spinal Cord Information Network
Information on a variety of SCI topics from A to Z
http://www.spinalcord.uab.edu

Case Management Resource Guide
Search for rehab facilities and numerous other healthcare providers
http://www.cmrg.com

Chapter 59

Information Sources on Universal and Adaptive Design

Contact these organizations for information on modification of the home or workplace. You may also contact the National Rehabilitation Information Center (NARIC) for home or workplace modification specialists in your area.

National Rehabilitation Information Center (NARIC)
8456 Colesville Rd., Suite 935
Silver Spring, MD 20910
800-347-2742 (V); 301-495-5626 (TT)
Web Site: http://www.naric.com/naric

Organizations

ABLEDATA
8455 Colesville Road, Suite 935
Silver Spring, MD 20910
8001227-0216 (V/TTY)
Web Site http://www.abledata.com

Provides searches for rehabilitation-related products, devices and equipment. The database contains detailed descriptions of thousands of products including price and company information. The database can be searched from the ABLEDATA web site.

1998 National Rehabilitation Information Center (NARIC), National Institute on Disability and Research (NIDRR), #HN970020.

Center for Universal Design
North Carolina State University
P.O. Box 8613
Raleigh, NC 27695
800/647-6777 (V)
919/515-3082 (V/TTY)
Web Site http://www2.ncsu.edu/ncsu/design/cud

Develops publications and instructional materials. Provides information, technical assistance, and referrals on accessible and adaptive design. Web site includes a publications list, glossary and related links.

RESNA Technical Assistance Project
1700 North Moore Street Suite 1540
Arlington, VA 22209
703/524-6686 (V)
Web Site http://www.resna.org/resna.reshome.htm

Administers the assistive technology programs, which provide assistive technology related services to each state. Services include information on financial assistance. Call RESNA or NARIC for details on contacting your states' project.

HUD USER
P.O. Box 6091
Rockville, MD 20850
800/245-2691 (V)
202/877-8339 (TTY)
Web Site: http://www.huduser.org

Source for Federal government reports and research literature on accessible design and housing for people with special needs. Publications can be searched for and ordered from HUD USER or online.

Adaptive Environments Center
374 Congress Street, Suite 301
Boston, MA 02110
617/695-1225 (V/TTY)
Web Site http://www.adaptenv.org

Offers resource materials on design, accessibility standards, guidelines, and legislation. Web site includes a publications list, ADA resource information and related links.

Barrier Free Environments
410 Oberlin Road, Suite 400
Raleigh, NC 27605
919/839-6381 (V)

Provides design and consulting services on accessibility of the home or work environment. Publications on accessible housing design and product information are available.

National Kitchen and Bath Association
687 Willow Grove Street
Hackettstown, NJ 07840
908/852-0033 (V)
Web Site http://www.nkba.org

Offers books on universal kitchen and bath planning and provides assistance in locating services. Web site has design guidelines and a professional locating section.

Paralyzed Veterans of America
801 18th Street, NW
Washington, DC 20008
800/424-8200 (V)
800/795-4327 (TTY)
Web Site http://www.pva.org

Provides publications covering such topics as accessibility, assistive technology and adaptive design. Web site includes design guidelines for the kitchen and bath.

Websites

Please visit these Web sites for more information:

IDEA Center at the School of Architecture & Planning at SUNY Buffalo
http://www.arch.buffalo.edu/~ idea

Remodeling Online
http://www.remodeling.hw.net

National Association of the Remodeling Industry
http://www.nari.org

Making Your Home More Accessible
http://www.gnt.net/~mombee

Chapter 60

Information Sources for Children with Special Needs

The federal government provides a variety of community-based services for children with special needs. Programs vary by state. Contact your state's health agency for information on the Maternal and Child Health Bureau. Contact your state's education department for information on early intervention and special education programs. If you cannot locate these numbers, please call the National Rehabilitation Information Center (NARIC) for assistance:

National Rehabilitation Information Center (NARIC)
8456 Colesville Rd., Suite 935
Silver Spring, MD 20910
800-347-2742 (V); 301-495-5626 (TT)
Web Site: http://www.naric.com/naric

Organizations

RESNA Technical Assistance Project
1700 North Moore Street, Suite 1540
Arlington, VA 22209
703/524-6686 (V)
Web Site http://www.resna.org

Administers the assistive technology programs, which provide assistive technology related services to each state. Services include

1998 National Institute on Disability and Rehabilitation Research; National Rehabilitation Information Center (NARIC), #HN970020.

information on financial assistance. Call RESNA or NARIC for details on contacting your state's project. Web site has information on each project plus other documents.

Beach Center on Families and Disability
University of Kansas
3111 Haworth Hall
Lawrence, KS 66045
785/864-7600 (V/TTY)
Web Site http://www.Isi.ukans.edu/beach/beachhp.htm

Disseminates the results of research studies involving families and disabilities. Provides referrals to local and national resources. Web site contains research briefs, newsletters and links to other organizations.

Alliance for Technology Access/National Office
2175 E. Francisco Boulevard, Suite L
San Rafael, CA 94901
415/455-4575 (V)
415/455-0491 (TTY)
Web Site http://www.ataccess.org

A nationwide network of community-based centers. Provides information and support services to children with disabilities, relative to the use of computer and assistive technology. Call the national office for information on a center in your area. Web site contains information on centers, newsletters and links.

Technical Assistance Alliance for Parent Centers
4826 Chicago Avenue
Minneapolis, MN 55417
888/248-0822 (V)
612/827-7770 (M)
Web Site http://taalliance.org

Administers the Parent Training and Information (PTI) programs which assist parents of children with disabilities. Parents can obtain information about services, resources, educational planning, and more. Call for the location of the PTI program in your state. Web site includes program information and articles concerning legislative issues.

HEATH Resource Center
One Dupont Circle, NW Suite 800
Washington, DC 20036
800/544-3284 (V/TTY)
Web Site http://www.acenet.edu

Operates the National Clearinghouse on Postsecondary Education for
Individuals with Disabilities which provides information relative to educational programs, financial aid, accommodation, and counseling. Web
site contains a publications list, fact sheets and general information.

National Parent to Parent Support and Information System
P.O. Box 907
Blue Ridge, GA 30513
800/651-1151 (V/TTY)
Web Site http://www.nppsis.org

Links families of children with special needs through one-to-one parent contacts. Also provides information, resources, and referrals. Web
site contains a database of nationwide parent-to-parent programs.

Disability Rights Education and Defense Fund
2212 Sixth Street
Berkeley, CA 94710
800/466-4232 (V/TTY)
Web Site http://www.dredf.org

Dedicated to furthering the civil rights of persons with disabilities.
Helps parents secure educational and related services as laws dictate.
Provides advocacy training to individuals or groups. Answers legal
questions. Web Site includes mission statement and ADA related information.

National Information Clearinghouse for Infants with Dis-abilities and Life-Threatening Conditions
Center for Developmental Disabilities
University of South Carolina
Columbia, SC 29208
800/922-9234 (V/TTY)

Offers information and referrals to appropriate providers of services
for infants and young children with disabilities. Disseminates related
fact sheets and articles.

National Information Center for Children and Youth with Disabilities (NICHCY)
P.O. Box 1492
Washington, DC 20013
800/695-0285 (V/TTY)
Web Site http://www.nichcy.org

Maintains an extensive database of information on services, options, and issues pertinent to children with disabilities. Offers consultation and answers relevant questions. Provides fact sheets and other written information. Web site includes a publications list and Internet links.

National Easter Seal Society
230 West Monroe Street, Suite 1800
Chicago, IL 60606
800/221-6827 (V)
312/726-4258 (TTY)
Web Site http://www.seals.com

Provides multiple services for children, including physical therapy and speech therapy. Also offers assistive technology related services. There are over 400 affiliates nationwide. Contact the national office for details on services available in your area. Web site lists services by city and state.

Websites

For more online information, please visit the following web sites:

Internet Resources for Special Children
http://www.irsc.org

Website for Sick and Disabled Kids
http://www.mania.apple.com

Advocacy and Support for Families
http://www.familyvoices.org

Chapter 61

Web Links for Adaptive Toys and Games

Adaptive: Capable of being readily altered to accommodate the needs of people with varying abilities.

Toys are often adapted for widespread use.

Links you may want to explore:

- **AssisTech**—offers a low-tech mobility kit, which enables anyone to easily convert an off-the-shelf, ride-in kid's vehicle to operate with a switch. In addition, the company features a full line of fun puppetry "stuff" for kids with and without disabilities, including switch-run puppetstands.

    URL: http://www.assisttech.com/text.html

- **Dragon Fly Toy Company**—a catalog that contains adapted battery operated toys, adapted art equipment, textured material toys for children who are blind, adapted playground equipment, and books for children and parents.

    URL: http://www.dftoys.com/

- **JESANA Ltd.: For Children with Special Needs**—a catalog that carries products and toys for children with disabilities.

    URL: http://www.jesana.com/

- **The Official TACK-TILES Website**—A braille teaching tool invented by a parent to teach literacy to his visually impaired multi-handicapped son. Now in effective use throughout the U.S., and Canada.

    URL: http://www.tack-tiles.com/

- **Unicorn Quest**—The Kid's Typing Tutor Game for One or Two Hands. Unicorn Quest is a DOS typing tutor game for children.

    URL: http://www.splam.com/down/pc/unicornquest.html

Acknowledgement: Definitions and descriptions were provided by Anthony Langton at the South Carolina Vocational Rehabilitation Department

Chapter 62

National Institute on Disability and Rehabilitation Research

The National Institute on Disability and Rehabilitation Research (NIDRR) is part of the Office of Special Education and Rehabilitative Services (OSERS) in the U.S. Department of Education.

NIDRR contributes to the independence of persons of all ages who have disabilities by seeking improved systems, products, and practices in the rehabilitation process. It does this through grants, contracts, and cooperative agreements with universities, Indian tribes, research groups, nonprofit organizations, some profit-making companies, and individuals. Recipients of funds range from graduate student fellows to university consortia.

Rehabilitation Research and Training Centers (RRTCs)

This is NIDRR's largest program. Each center focuses on a particular aspect of the behavioral, medical or vocational rehabilitation of people with disabilities. Some centers concentrate on a specific disabling condition, such as: deafness, low vision, spinal cord injury, or long-term mental illness. Others study activity areas important in the lives of people with disabilities, including independent living, housing, service delivery, and information systems. Knowledge contributed by the RRTCs has greatly influenced the fields of rehabilitation medicine,

1992 The National Institute on Disability and Rehabilitation Research, U.S. Department of Education, 400 Maryland Avenue, S.W., Washington, D.C. 20202-2572, Telephone: (202) 205-9151 (Voice); (202) 205-9136 (TDD); Grant Information Line: (202) 205-8207.

psychosocial rehabilitation, integration, vocational strategies, and architecture.

Rehabilitation Engineering Centers (RECS)

These centers seek solutions to disability-related problems through technology. Areas of study include sensory loss, mobility impairment, chronic pain, communication difficulties, the adaptation of assistive devices, and technology transfer.

Field Initiated Research

These projects allow NIDRR to fund activities that blend well with its overall mandate but which fall outside the usual range of priorities. Institutions of higher education, nonprofit organizations, and profit-making businesses are eligible to apply for these grants.

Research and Demonstration Projects

To supplement the work of the RRTCs and RECS, the Institute supports research and demonstration projects that seek solutions to specific problems encountered by individuals with disabilities and the professionals who work with them. Some of these have included model care systems for traumatic brain injury, the creation of a specialized dataset for the collection of clinical and scientific information, and job development and placement for agricultural workers with disabilities.

Research Fellowships

Fellowships named for the late Mary E. Switzer are building future research capacity. NIDRR makes these grants on two levels. Distinguished Fellowships are awarded to individuals of doctorate or comparable academic status who have had seven or more years' experience relevant to rehabilitation research. Merit Fellowships are given to persons in earlier stages of their research careers.

Research Training and Career Development Grants

These grants train physicians, therapists of various types, rehabilitation engineers, and other professionals in research methods and statistical analysis.

Dissemination and Utilization Grants

Through this type of grant, the Institute places information derived from research as well as the products of its grants and contracts in the hands of policy makers, rehabilitation practitioners, educators, technology developers, and persons with disabilities.

Innovation Grants

One-year grants, for a maximum of $50,000, support inventive approaches to old and newly identified problems. These projects test new concepts, evaluate prototype aids and devices, develop and test rehabilitation training curricula and disseminate specific research findings.

Technology Assistance

NIDRR supports consumer-driven state plans for the delivery of assistive technology. Some grants also explore innovative ways of financing these devices.

Small Business Innovative Research Grants

New products useful to persons with disabilities and the rehabilitation field are encouraged through grants to small businesses. This three-phase program takes an idea from development to market readiness.

International Program

NIDRR's legislation encourages active outreach to other countries with similar rehabilitation concerns. NIDRR cooperates in jointly funded programs with India and Yugoslavia. It has also taken part in several projects with the USSR in cooperation with the Department of State and other international agencies. NIDRR also conducts a worldwide program for the exchange of experts and information on rehabilitation.

Interagency Activity

The Director of NIDRR chairs a statutory committee that provides a forum and a resource for all federal entities conducting or supporting rehabilitation research. The Interagency Committee on Disability Research promotes networking, information sharing, and cooperative efforts among its members and the programs they fund.

Regional Disability and Business Technical Assistance Centers

The Americans with Disabilities Act opens new opportunities for persons with disabilities. It also places new responsibilities on employers, transit and telecommunication systems, state and local governments and public accommodations. To assist in all these areas, NIDRR funds Regional Disability and Business Technical Assistance Centers. These centers will provide technical assistance, training and resource referral on all aspects of the ADA. Their work will be complemented by two other NIDRR ADA programs: four Materials Development Projects and two National Peer Training Projects.

For additional information, contact:

The National Institute on Disability and Rehabilitation Research, U.S. Department of Education, 400 Maryland Avenue, S.W., Washington, D.C. 20202-2572 Telephone: (202) 205-9151 (Voice) (202) 205-9136 (TDD) Grant Information Line: (202) 205-8207.

Index

Index

Page numbers followed by 'n' indicate a footnote. Page numbers in *italics* indicate a table or illustration.

canes 155, 200
  stroke rehabilitation 361
cap, defined 454
CAPTE *see* Physical Therapy Education, Commission on Accreditation in (CAPTE)
cardiac rehabilitation 371–400
Cardiac Rehabilitation: Exercise Training, Education, Counseling, and Behavioral Interventions 382
"Cardiac rehabilitation after myocardial infarction: Combined experience..." 394
Cardiac Rehabilitation Guideline 382
"Cardiac rehabilitation participation predicts lower rehospitalization costs" 393
cardiomyopathy 386
cardiopulmonary exercise tests 423–24
Cardiovascular and Pulmonary Rehabilitation, American Association of
  national program directory 376
  rehabilitation centers 381–82
caregivers
  adaptive equipment 171–88
  emotional stress 251–54
  stroke rehabilitation 362–63
CARF *see* Rehabilitation Facilities, Commission on Accreditation of (CARF)
Carlson, D. 5
Carter, Jerry 286
Case Management Resource Guide, web site 469, 473
"A case-management system for coronary risk factor modification after acute myocardial infarction" 398
"Case-management system for coronary risk factor modification after acute myocardial infarction" *(Annual Internal Medicine)* 398
case manager, defined 454
Case Western Reserve University, neural prostheses research 291
catastrophic limits of coverage, defined 454
catheters
  defined 447
  Foley catheter, defined 447
  Swan-Ganz catheter, defined 448

Census Bureau, culturally sensitive rehabilitation 59
Center for Rehabilitation Technology Services 163, 164
central venous pressure (CVP) line, defined 447
Cerebral Palsy Research Foundation of Kansas, Inc. 227–28
certification
  see also accreditation
  art therapists 147
  audiologists 241
  dance/movement therapy 138–39
  defined 454
  physiatrists 12–13
  physical medicine 21–22
  physical therapists 85
  recreation therapists 151
  rehabilitation facilities 29–30
  sports massage 125
certified occupational therapy assistants (COTAS) 105–6
Chen, Van T. 204
chest physical therapy, described 418
chest tubes, defined 447
CHF *see* congestive heart failure (CHF)
child care 180–81, 183–84, 185–86, 187–88
child development programs 36
Child Health and Human Development, National Institute of
  contact information 406
  Total Hip Joint Replacement Conference 304
children
  broken bones 341
  family rehabilitation issues 248
  idiopathic scoliosis 92
  massage therapy 131–35
  physical therapy 82
  robotic aids 223–24
  special needs information sources 479–82
  toys and games information sources 483–84
  wheelchairs 192
Children & Youth with Disabilities, National Information Center for, contact information 482

driver training, spinal cord injury 293
drug abuse, brain injury 256
durable medical equipment, defined 462
dysarthria
  defined 452, 455
  stroke 349
  traumatic brain injury 403
dysphagia
  defined 455
  stroke 350
  traumatic brain injury 403
dyspnea 417–21
  measurement tests 425–26
dysreflexia, spinal cord injury 283

E

Easter Seal Rehabilitation Center of Will-Grundy Counties 109
Easter Seal Society, National
  contact information 367, 469, 482
  neural prostheses research 291
eating disorders, massage therapy 133
ECG *see* electrocardiogram (ECG: EKG)
Ecological Assessment 162
Edelstein, Joan E. 211
Edlich, Richard F. 199n, 204
education programs
  adaptive equipment 175–78
  art therapists 146–47
  cardiac rehabilitation 374, 380
  dance/movement therapists 138–39
  occupational therapy 111, 112–13
  physical therapists 86, 88, 92–93, 100
EEG *see* electroencephalogram (EEG)
EKG *see* electrocardiogram (ECG: EKG)
eldercare, art therapy 146
Eldercare Locator, contact information 238, 254
electrical stimulation
  bone fractures 343–44
  physical therapy 81
electrocardiogram (ECG: EKG), described 450
electroencephalogram (EEG), described 450

electromyography (EMG) 14
embolus 387
emergency services, rehabilitation facilities 34–35
EMG *see* electromyography (EMG)
emotional concerns
  burns 438
  cardiac rehabilitation 387–89
  dance/movement therapy 137
  depression
    cardiac rehabilitation 395–96
    caregivers 253
    massage therapy 133–34
    prostheses 214, 217
    stroke 350–51
    therapeutic massage 130
  spinal cord injury 282, 293
  stress 251–54
    caregivers 251–54
    drama therapy 142
    massage therapy 120
    spouses 246–47
  stroke 350–51
emotional lability, defined 452
employment issues
  industrial rehabilitation 111–18
  physical therapists 99–100
encoding, defined 462
endorphin blockers, spinal cord injury 288
endotrachial tube, defined 447
Energy, US Department of, home modification and repair 236
Engh, Charles A. 302
environmental adaptations, defined 455
Environmental Controls 162
environmental control unit, defined 462
environmental modifications, adaptive equipment 175
ergonomics
  occupational therapists 115
  physical therapists 87
Ergonomics, Board of Certification of Professional (BCPE) 115
Establishing an Adaptive Computer Lab in a Post-Secondary Setting: Ideas and Resources 161

I

Lioresal 284
Littman, A. B. 393
"Living With Heart Disease: Is It Heart Failure?" 377
Locust, Carol 59
Loman, Susan 138
long-term oxygen therapy 413
Lovophed 283
Low, K. G. 397
low back pain, physical therapy 82
lower extremity exercise training, described 418–19
Low-Income Home Energy Assistance Program (LIHEAP) 236
lumbar puncture, defined 450
lung transplantation, pulmonary rehabilitation 414, 431

M

Maalox, described 449
Mackey, Francis G. 23
Macrodantin 284
Macro International Inc. 198
magnetic resonance imaging (MRI)
  described 450
  knee problems 324–25
magnifiers 155
Making Your Home More Accessible 478
malnutrition, burns 433
managed care plans
  see also health maintenance organizations (HMO)
  defined 455–56
  massage therapy 123–24
"Managing Unstable Angina" 377
Mannitol, described 449
manual, defined 459
Manual Mobility: Finding the Right Wheels (videotape) 197
manual therapy techniques, physical therapists 87
Marcotte, Paula 125
Massachusetts Institute of Technology 231
massage, defined 459
massage therapist locator service 125

massage therapy 119–35
  see also therapeutic massage
  benefits 121–22
  defined 459
  described 124
  insurance coverage 123–24
  research 122–23
Massage Therapy Association, American (AMTA)
  alternative treatments study 130
  benefits of massage 123
  contact information 125, 128, 130
  grants for researchers 129
  massage therapist locator 125
  massage therapy 120, 126
  massage therapy profession 121
  massage therapy study 119
Massage Training Accreditation, Commission on (COMTA) 125
Matheis-Kraft, Carol 151, 157
mats, spinal cord injury 292
maximum sustainable ventilatory capacity (MSVC) 422–23
Mayfield, Jennifer 207
McCormack, Douglas 209
McDermott, Kenneth 342
McDowell, Fletcher H. 232
McFarland, Samuel R. 196
MCL *see* medial collateral ligament (MCL)
McLanahan, Sandra 122
McMenamin, Peter 277
Mead, Marjorie 77
Meals on Wheels 365
medial collateral ligament (MCL) 323
  injuries 330–31
Medicaid
  described 456
  health care coverage for low-income people 354
  home health services 272
  home modification and repair 236
  rehabilitation services 271–72
  vocational rehabilitation coverage 268
medical history
  knee problems 324
  physical therapists 93

517

Health Reference Series
COMPLETE CATALOG

AIDS Sourcebook, 1st Edition

Basic Information about AIDS and HIV Infection, Featuring Historical and Statistical Data, Current Research, Prevention, and Other Special Topics of Interest for Persons Living with AIDS, Along with Source Listings for Further Assistance

Edited by Karen Bellenir and Peter D. Dresser. 831 pages. 1995. 0-7808-0031-1. $78.

"One strength of this book is its practical emphasis. The intended audience is the lay reader . . . useful as an educational tool for health care providers who work with AIDS patients. Recommended for public libraries as well as hospital or academic libraries that collect consumer materials." — *Bulletin of the MLA, Jan '96*

"This is the most comprehensive volume of its kind on an important medical topic. Highly recommended for all libraries." — *Reference Book Review, '96*

"Very useful reference for all libraries."
— *Choice, Oct '95*

"There is a wealth of information here that can provide much educational assistance. It is a must book for all libraries and should be on the desk of each and every congressional leader. Highly recommended."
— *AIDS Book Review Journal, Aug '95*

"Recommended for most collections."
— *Library Journal, Jul '95*

AIDS Sourcebook, 2nd Edition

Basic Consumer Health Information about Acquired Immune Deficiency Syndrome (AIDS) and Human Immunodeficiency Virus (HIV) Infection, Featuring Updated Statistical Data, Reports on Recent Research and Prevention Initiatives, and Other Special Topics of Interest for Persons Living with AIDS, Including New Antiretroviral Treatment Options, Strategies for Combating Opportunistic Infections, Information about Clinical Trials, and More; Along with a Glossary of Important Terms and Resource Listings for Further Help and Information

Edited by Karen Bellenir. 751 pages. 1999. 0-7808-0225-X. $78.

Allergies Sourcebook

Basic Information about Major Forms and Mechanisms of Common Allergic Reactions, Sensitivities, and Intolerances, Including Anaphylaxis, Asthma, Hives and Other Dermatologic Symptoms, Rhinitis, and Sinusitis, Along with Their Usual Triggers Like Animal Fur, Chemicals, Drugs, Dust, Foods, Insects, Latex, Pollen, and Poison Ivy, Oak, and Sumac; Plus Information on Prevention, Identification, and Treatment

Edited by Allan R. Cook. 611 pages. 1997. 0-7808-0036-2. $78.

Alternative Medicine Sourcebook

Basic Consumer Health Information about Alternatives to Conventional Medicine, Including Acupressure, Acupuncture, Aromatherapy, Ayurveda, Bioelectromagnetics, Environmental Medicine, Essence Therapy, Food and Nutrition Therapy, Herbal Therapy, Homeopathy, Imaging, Massage, Naturopathy, Reflexology, Relaxation and Meditation, Sound Therapy, Vitamin and Mineral Therapy, and Yoga, and More

Edited by Allan R. Cook. 737 pages. 1999. 0-7808-0200-4. $78.

Alzheimer's, Stroke & 29 Other Neurological Disorders Sourcebook, 1st Edition

Basic Information for the Layperson on 31 Diseases or Disorders Affecting the Brain and Nervous System, First Describing the Illness, Then Listing Symptoms, Diagnostic Methods, and Treatment Options, and Including Statistics on Incidences and Causes

Edited by Frank E. Bair. 579 pages. 1993. 1-55888-748-2. $78.

"Nontechnical reference book that provides reader-friendly information."
— *Family Caregiver Alliance Update, Winter '96*

"Should be included in any library's patient education section." — *American Reference Books Annual, '94*

"Written in an approachable and accessible style. Recommended for patient education and consumer health collections in health science center and public libraries." — *Academic Library Book Review, Dec '93*

"It is very handy to have information on more than thirty neurological disorders under one cover, and there is no recent source like it." — *RQ, Fall '93*

Alzheimer's Disease Sourcebook, 2nd Edition

Basic Consumer Health Information about Alzheimer's Disease, Related Disorders, and Other Dementias, Including Multi-Infarct Dementia, AIDS-Related Dementia, Alcoholic Dementia, Huntington's Disease, Delirium, and Confusional States; Along with Reports Detailing Current Research Efforts in Prevention and Treatment, Long-Term Care Issues, and Listings of Sources for Additional Help and Information

Edited by Karen Bellenir. 524 pages. 1999. 0-7808-0223-3. $78.

Arthritis Sourcebook

Basic Consumer Health Information about Specific Forms of Arthritis and Related Disorders, Including Rheumatoid Arthritis, Osteoarthritis, Gout, Polymyalgia Rheumatica, Psoriatic Arthritis, Spondyloarthropathies, Juvenile Rheumatoid Arthritis, and Juvenile Ankylosing Spondylitis; Along with Information about Medical, Surgical, and Alternative Treatment Options, and Including Strategies for Coping with Pain, Fatigue, and Stress

Edited by Allan R. Cook. 550 pages. 1998. 0-7808-0201-2. $78.

"... accessible to the layperson."
— *Reference and Research Book News, Feb '99*

Back & Neck Disorders Sourcebook

Basic Information about Disorders and Injuries of the Spinal Cord and Vertebrae, Including Facts on Chiropractic Treatment, Surgical Interventions, Paralysis, and Rehabilitation, Along with Advice for Preventing Back Trouble

Edited by Karen Bellenir. 548 pages. 1997. 0-7808-0202-0. $78.

"The strength of this work is its basic, easy-to-read format. Recommended."
— *Reference and User Services Quarterly, Winter '97*

Blood & Circulatory Disorders Sourcebook

Basic Information about Blood and Its Components, Anemias, Leukemias, Bleeding Disorders, and Circulatory Disorders, Including Aplastic Anemia, Thalassemia, Sickle-Cell Disease, Hemochromatosis, Hemophilia, Von Willebrand Disease, and Vascular Diseases; Along with a Special Section on Blood Transfusions and Blood Supply Safety, a Glossary, and Source Listings for Further Help and Information

Edited by Karen Bellenir and Linda M. Shin. 554 pages. 1998. 0-7808-0203-9. $78.

"Recent and recommended reference source."
— *Booklist, Feb '99*

"An important reference sourcebook written in simple language for everyday, non-technical users. "
— *Reviewer's Bookwatch, Jan '99*

Brain Disorders Sourcebook

Basic Consumer Health Information about Strokes, Epilepsy, Amyotrophic Lateral Sclerosis (ALS/Lou Gehrig's Disease), Parkinson's Disease, Brain Tumors, Cerebral Palsy, Headache, Tourette Syndrome, and More; Along with Statistical Data, Treatment and

Rehabilitation Options, Coping Strategies, Reports on Current Research Initiatives, a Glossary, and Resource Listings for Additional Help and Information

Edited by Karen Bellenir. 481 pages. 1999. 0-7808-0229-2. $78.

Burns Sourcebook

Basic Consumer Health Information about Various Types of Burns and Scalds, Including Flame, Heat, Cold, Electrical, Chemical, and Sun Burns; Along with Information on Short-Term and Long-Term Treatments, Tissue Reconstruction, Plastic Surgery, Prevention Suggestions, and First Aid

Edited by Allan R. Cook. 604 pages. 1999. 0-7808-0204-7. $78.

Cancer Sourcebook, 1st Edition

Basic Information on Cancer Types, Symptoms, Diagnostic Methods, and Treatments, Including Statistics on Cancer Occurrences Worldwide and the Risks Associated with Known Carcinogens and Activities

Edited by Frank E. Bair. 932 pages. 1990. 1-55888-888-8. $78.

"Written in nontechnical language. Useful for patients, their families, medical professionals, and librarians."
— *Guide to Reference Books, '96*

"Designed with the non-medical professional in mind. Libraries and medical facilities interested in patient education should certainly consider adding the Cancer Sourcebook to their holdings. This compact collection of reliable information ... is an invaluable tool for helping patients and patients' families and friends to take the first steps in coping with the many difficulties of cancer."
— *Medical Reference Services Quarterly, Winter '91*

"Specifically created for the nontechnical reader ... an important resource for the general reader trying to understand the complexities of cancer."
— *American Reference Books Annual, '91*

"This publication's nontechnical nature and very comprehensive format make it useful for both the general public and undergraduate students."
— *Choice, Oct '90*

New Cancer Sourcebook, 2nd Edition

Basic Information about Major Forms and Stages of Cancer, Featuring Facts about Primary and Secondary Tumors of the Respiratory, Nervous, Lymphatic, Circulatory, Skeletal, and Gastrointestinal Systems, and Specific Organs; Statistical and Demographic Data; Treatment Options; and Strategies for Coping

Edited by Allan R. Cook. 1,313 pages. 1996. 0-7808-0041-9. $78.

"This book is an excellent resource for patients with newly diagnosed cancer and their families. The dialogue is simple, direct, and comprehensive. Highly recommended for patients and families to aid in their understanding of cancer and its treatment."
— *Booklist Health Sciences Supplement, Oct '97*

"The amount of factual and useful information is extensive. The writing is very clear, geared to general readers. Recommended for all levels."
— *Choice, Jan '97*

Cancer Sourcebook, 3rd Edition

Basic Consumer Health Information about Major Forms and Stages of Cancer, Featuring Facts about Primary and Secondary Tumors of the Respiratory, Nervous, Lymphatic, Circulatory, Skeletal, and Gastrointestinal Systems, and Specific Organs; Along with Statistical and Demographic Data, Treatment Options, Strategies for Coping, a Glossary, and a Directory of Sources for Additional Help and Information

Edited by Edward J. Prucha. 1,100 pages. 1999. 0-7808-0227-6. $78.

Cancer Sourcebook for Women, 1st Edition

Basic Information about Specific Forms of Cancer That Affect Women, Featuring Facts about Breast Cancer, Cervical Cancer, Ovarian Cancer, Cancer of the Uterus and Uterine Sarcoma, Cancer of the Vagina, and Cancer of the Vulva; Statistical and Demographic Data; Treatments, Self-Help Management Suggestions, and Current Research Initiatives

Edited by Allan R. Cook and Peter D. Dresser. 524 pages. 1996. 0-7808-0076-1. $78.

". . . written in easily understandable, non-technical language. Recommended for public libraries or hospital and academic libraries that collect patient education or consumer health materials."
— *Medical Reference Services Quarterly, Spring '97*

"Would be of value in a consumer health library. . . . written with the health care consumer in mind. Medical jargon is at a minimum, and medical terms are explained in clear, understandable sentences."
— *Bulletin of the MLA, Oct '96*

"The availability under one cover of all these pertinent publications, grouped under cohesive headings, makes this certainly a most useful sourcebook."
— *Choice, Jun '96*

"Presents a comprehensive knowledge base for general readers. Men and women both benefit from the gold mine of information nestled between the two covers of this book. Recommended."
— *Academic Library Book Review, Summer '96*

"This timely book is highly recommended for consumer health and patient education collections in all libraries." — *Library Journal, Apr '96*

Cancer Sourcebook for Women, 2nd Edition

Basic Consumer Health Information about Specific Forms of Cancer That Affect Women, Including Cervical Cancer, Ovarian Cancer, Endometrial Cancer, Uterine Sarcoma, Vaginal Cancer, Vulvar Cancer, and Gestational Trophoblastic Tumor; and Featuring Statistical Information, Facts about Tests and Treatments, a Glossary of Cancer Terms, and an Extensive List of Additional Resources

Edited by Edward J. Prucha. 600 pages. 1999. 0-7808-0226-8. $78.

Cardiovascular Diseases & Disorders Sourcebook, 1st Edition

Basic Information about Cardiovascular Diseases and Disorders, Featuring Facts about the Cardiovascular System, Demographic and Statistical Data, Descriptions of Pharmacological and Surgical Interventions, Lifestyle Modifications, and a Special Section Focusing on Heart Disorders in Children

Edited by Karen Bellenir and Peter D. Dresser. 683 pages. 1995. 0-7808-0032-X. $78.

". . . comprehensive format provides an extensive overview on this subject." — *Choice, Jun '96*

". . . an easily understood, complete, up-to-date resource. This well executed public health tool will make valuable information available to those that need it most, patients and their families. The typeface, sturdy non-reflective paper, and library binding add a feel of quality found wanting in other publications. Highly recommended for academic and general libraries. "
— *Academic Library Book Review, Summer '96*

Communication Disorders Sourcebook

Basic Information about Deafness and Hearing Loss, Speech and Language Disorders, Voice Disorders, Balance and Vestibular Disorders, and Disorders of Smell, Taste, and Touch

Edited by Linda M. Ross. 533 pages. 1996. 0-7808-0077-X. $78.

"This is skillfully edited and is a welcome resource for the layperson. It should be found in every public and medical library."
— *Booklist Health Sciences Supplement, Oct '97*

Congenital Disorders Sourcebook

Basic Information about Disorders Acquired during Gestation, Including Spina Bifida, Hydrocephalus, Cerebral Palsy, Heart Defects, Craniofacial Abnormalities, Fetal Alcohol Syndrome, and More, Along with Current Treatment Options and Statistical Data

Edited by Karen Bellenir. 607 pages. 1997. 0-7808-0205-5. $78.

"Recent and recommended reference source."
— Booklist, Oct '97

Consumer Issues in Health Care Sourcebook

Basic Information about Health Care Fundamentals and Related Consumer Issues, Including Exams and Screening Tests, Physician Specialties, Choosing a Doctor, Using Prescription and Over-the-Counter Medications Safely, Avoiding Health Scams, Managing Common Health Risks in the Home, Care Options for Chronically or Terminally Ill Patients, and a List of Resources for Obtaining Help and Further Information

Edited by Karen Bellenir. 618 pages. 1998. 0-7808-0221-7. $78.

"The editor has researched the literature from government agencies and others, saving readers the time and effort of having to do the research themselves. Recommended for public libraries."
— Reference and Users Services Quarterly, Spring '99

"Recent and recommended reference source."
— Booklist, Dec '98

Contagious & Non-Contagious Infectious Diseases Sourcebook

Basic Information about Contagious Diseases like Measles, Polio, Hepatitis B, and Infectious Mononucleosis, and Non-Contagious Infectious Diseases like Tetanus and Toxic Shock Syndrome, and Diseases Occurring as Secondary Infections Such as Shingles and Reye Syndrome, Along with Vaccination, Prevention, and Treatment Information, and a Section Describing Emerging Infectious Disease Threats

Edited by Karen Bellenir and Peter D. Dresser. 566 pages. 1996. 0-7808-0075-3. $78.

Death & Dying Sourcebook

Basic Consumer Health Information for the Layperson about End-of-Life Care and Related Ethical and Legal Issues, Including Chief Causes of Death, Autopsies, Pain Management for the Terminally Ill, Life Support Systems, Insurance, Euthanasia, Assisted Suicide, Hospice Programs, Living Wills, Funeral Planning, Counseling, Mourning, Organ Donation, and Physician Training; Along with Statistical Data, a Glossary, and Listings of Sources for Further Help and Information

Edited by Annemarie S. Muth. 641 pages. 1999. 0-7808-0230-6. $78.

Diabetes Sourcebook, 1st Edition

Basic Information about Insulin-Dependent and Noninsulin-Dependent Diabetes Mellitus, Gestational Diabetes, and Diabetic Complications, Symptoms, Treatment, and Research Results, Including Statistics on Prevalence, Morbidity, and Mortality, Along with Source Listings for Further Help and Information

Edited by Karen Bellenir and Peter D. Dresser. 827 pages. 1994. 1-55888-751-2. $78.

"...very informative and understandable for the layperson without being simplistic. It provides a comprehensive overview for laypersons who want a general understanding of the disease or who want to focus on various aspects of the disease." *— Bulletin of the MLA, Jan '96*

Diabetes Sourcebook, 2nd Edition

Basic Consumer Health Information about Type 1 Diabetes (Insulin-Dependent or Juvenile-Onset Diabetes), Type 2 (Noninsulin-Dependent or Adult-Onset Diabetes), Gestational Diabetes, and Related Disorders, Including Diabetes Prevalence Data, Management Issues, the Role of Diet and Exercise in Controlling Diabetes, Insulin and Other Diabetes Medicines, and Complications of Diabetes Such as Eye Diseases, Periodontal Disease, Amputation, and End-Stage Renal Disease; Along with Reports on Current Research Initiatives, a Glossary, and Resource Listings for Further Help and Information

Edited by Karen Bellenir. 688 pages. 1998. 0-7808-0224-1. $78.

"Recent and recommended reference source."
— Booklist, Feb '99

Diet & Nutrition Sourcebook, 1st Edition

Basic Information about Nutrition, Including the Dietary Guidelines for Americans, the Food Guide Pyramid, and Their Applications in Daily Diet, Nutritional Advice for Specific Age Groups, Current Nutritional Issues and Controversies, the New Food Label and How to Use It to Promote Healthy Eating, and Recent Developments in Nutritional Research

Edited by Dan R. Harris. 662 pages. 1996. 0-7808-0084-2. $78.

"Useful reference as a food and nutrition sourcebook for the general consumer."
— Booklist Health Sciences Supplement, Oct '97

"Recommended for public libraries and medical libraries that receive general information requests on nutrition. It is readable and will appeal to those interested in learning more about healthy dietary practices."
— Medical Reference Services Quarterly, Fall '97

Diet & Nutrition Sourcebook, 2nd Edition

Basic Consumer Health Information about Dietary Guidelines, Recommended Daily Intake Values, Vitamins, Minerals, Fiber, Fat, Weight Control, Dietary Supplements, and Food Additives; Along with Special Sections on Nutrition Needs throughout Life and Nutrition for People with Such Specific Medical Concerns as Allergies, High Blood Cholesterol, Hypertension, Diabetes, Celiac Disease, Seizure Disorders, Phenylketonuria (PKU), Cancer, and Eating Disorders, and Including Reports on Current Nutrition Research and Source Listings for Additional Help and Information

Edited by Karen Bellenir. 650 pages. 1999. 0-7808-0228-4. $78.

Digestive Diseases & Disorders Sourcebook

Basic Consumer Health Information about Diseases and Disorders that Impact the Upper and Lower Digestive System, Including Celiac Disease, Constipation, Crohn's Disease, Cyclic Vomiting Syndrome, Diarrhea, Diverticulosis and Diverticulitis, Gallstones, Heartburn, Hemorrhoids, Hernias, Indigestion (Dyspepsia), Irritable Bowel Syndrome, Lactose Intolerance, Ulcers, and More; Along with Information about Medications and Other Treatments, Tips for Maintaining a Healthy Digestive Tract, a Glossary, and Directory of Digestive Diseases Organizations

Edited by Karen Bellenir. 335 pages. 1999. 0-7808-0327-2. $48.

Disabilities Sourcebook

Basic Consumer Health Information about Physical and Psychiatric Disabilities, Including Descriptions of Major Causes of Disability, Assistive and Adaptive Aids, Workplace Issues, and Accessibility Concerns; Along with Information about the Americans with Disabilities Act, a Glossary, and Resources for Additional Help and Information

Edited by Dawn D. Matthews. 600 pages. 1999. 0-7808-0389-2. $78.

Domestic Violence & Child Abuse Sourcebook

Basic Information about Spousal/Partner, Child, and Elder Physical, Emotional, and Sexual Abuse, Teen Dating Violence, and Stalking, Including Information about Hotlines, Safe Houses, Safety Plans, and Other Resources for Support and Assistance, Community Initiatives, and Reports on Current Directions in Research and Treatment; Along with a Glossary, Sources for Further Reading, and Governmental and Non-Governmental Organizations Contact Information

Edited by Helene Henderson. 600 pages. 1999. 0-7808-0235-7. $78.

Ear, Nose & Throat Disorders Sourcebook

Basic Information about Disorders of the Ears, Nose, Sinus Cavities, Pharynx, and Larynx, Including Ear Infections, Tinnitus, Vestibular Disorders, Allergic and Non-Allergic Rhinitis, Sore Throats, Tonsillitis, and Cancers That Affect the Ears, Nose, Sinuses, and Throat, Along with Reports on Current Research Initiatives, a Glossary of Related Medical Terms, and a Directory of Sources for Further Help and Information

Edited by Karen Bellenir and Linda M. Shin. 576 pages. 1998. 0-7808-0206-3. $78.

"Overall, this sourcebook is helpful for the consumer seeking information on ENT issues. It is recommended for public libraries."
— *American Reference Books Annual, '99*

"Recent and recommended reference source."
— *Booklist, Dec '98*

Endocrine & Metabolic Disorders Sourcebook

Basic Information for the Layperson about Pancreatic and Insulin-Related Disorders Such as Pancreatitis, Diabetes, and Hypoglycemia; Adrenal Gland Disorders Such as Cushing's Syndrome, Addison's Disease, and Congenital Adrenal Hyperplasia; Pituitary Gland Disorders Such as Growth Hormone Deficiency, Acromegaly, and Pituitary Tumors; Thyroid Disorders Such as Hypothyroidism, Graves' Disease, Hashimoto's Disease, and Goiter; Hyperparathyroidism; and Other Diseases and Syndromes of Hormone Imbalance or Metabolic Dysfunction, Along with Reports on Current Research Initiatives

Edited by Linda M. Shin. 574 pages. 1998. 0-7808-0207-1. $78.

"Recent and recommended reference source."
— *Booklist, Dec '98*

Environmentally Induced Disorders Sourcebook

Basic Information about Diseases and Syndromes Linked to Exposure to Pollutants and Other Substances in Outdoor and Indoor Environments Such as Lead, Asbestos, Formaldehyde, Mercury, Emissions, Noise, and More

Edited by Allan R. Cook. 620 pages. 1997. 0-7808-0083-4. $78.

"Recent and recommended reference source."
— Booklist, Sept '98

"This book will be a useful addition to anyone's library."
— Choice Health Sciences Supplement, May '98

". . . a good survey of numerous environmentally induced physical disorders . . . a useful addition to anyone's library."
— Doody's Health Science Book Reviews, Jan '98

". . . provide[s] introductory information from the best authorities around. Since this volume covers topics that potentially affect everyone, it will surely be one of the most frequently consulted volumes in the Health Reference Series." — Rettig on Reference, Nov '97

Ethical Issues in Medicine Sourcebook

Basic Information about Controversial Treatment Issues, Genetic Research, Reproductive Technologies, and End-of-Life Decisions, Including Topics Such as Cloning, Abortion, Fertility Management, Organ Transplantation, Health Care Rationing, Advance Directives, Living Wills, Physician-Assisted Suicide, Euthanasia, and More; Along with a Glossary and Resources for Additional Information

Edited by Helene Henderson. 600 pages. 1999. 0-7808-0237-3. $78.

Fitness & Exercise Sourcebook

Basic Information on Fitness and Exercise, Including Fitness Activities for Specific Age Groups, Exercise for People with Specific Medical Conditions, How to Begin a Fitness Program in Running, Walking, Swimming, Cycling, and Other Athletic Activities, and Recent Research in Fitness and Exercise

Edited by Dan R. Harris. 663 pages. 1996. 0-7808-0186-5. $78.

"A good resource for general readers."
— Choice, Nov '97

"The perennial popularity of the topic . . . make this an appealing selection for public libraries."
— Rettig on Reference, Jun/Jul '97

Food & Animal Borne Diseases Sourcebook

Basic Information about Diseases That Can Be Spread to Humans through the Ingestion of Contaminated Food or Water or by Contact with Infected Animals and Insects, Such as Botulism, E. Coli, Hepatitis A, Trichinosis, Lyme Disease, and Rabies, Along with Information Regarding Prevention and Treatment Methods, and a Special Section for International Travelers Describing Diseases Such as Cholera, Malaria, Travelers' Diarrhea, and Yellow Fever, and Offering Recommendations for Avoiding Illness

Edited by Karen Bellenir and Peter D. Dresser. 535 pages. 1995. 0-7808-0033-8. $78.

"Targeting general readers and providing them with a single, comprehensive source of information on selected topics, this book continues, with the excellent caliber of its predecessors, to catalog topical information on health matters of general interest. Readable and thorough, this valuable resource is highly recommended for all libraries."
— Academic Library Book Review, Summer '96

"A comprehensive collection of authoritative information." — Emergency Medical Services, Oct '95

Food Safety Sourcebook

Basic Consumer Health Information about the Safe Handling of Meat, Poultry, Seafood, Eggs, Fruit Juices, and Other Food Items, and Facts about Pesticides, Drinking Water, Food Safety Overseas, and the Onset, Duration, and Symptoms of Foodborne Illnesses, Including Types of Pathogenic Bacteria, Parasitic Protozoa, Worms, Viruses, and Natural Toxins; Along with the Role of the Consumer, the Food Handler, and the Government in Food Safety; a Glossary, and Resources for Additional Help and Information

Edited by Dawn D. Matthews. 339 pages. 1999. 0-7808-0326-4. $48.

Forensic Medicine Sourcebook

Basic Consumer Information for the Layperson about Forensic Medicine, Including Crime Scene Investigation, Evidence Collection and Analysis, Expert Testimony, Computer-Aided Criminal Identification, Digital Imaging in the Courtroom, DNA Profiling, Accident Reconstruction, Autopsies, Ballistics, Drugs and Explosives Detection, Latent Fingerprints, Product Tampering, and Questioned Document Examination; Along with Statistical Data, a Glossary of Forensics Terminology, and Listings of Sources for Further Help and Information

Edited by Annemarie S. Muth. 574 pages. 1999. 0-7808-0232-2. $78.

Gastrointestinal Diseases & Disorders Sourcebook

Basic Information about Gastroesophageal Reflux Disease (Heartburn), Ulcers, Diverticulosis, Irritable Bowel Syndrome, Crohn's Disease, Ulcerative Colitis, Diarrhea, Constipation, Lactose Intolerance, Hemorrhoids, Hepatitis, Cirrhosis, and Other Digestive Problems, Featuring Statistics, Descriptions of Symptoms, and Current Treatment Methods of Interest for Persons Living with Upper and Lower Gastrointestinal Maladies

Edited by Linda M. Ross. 413 pages. 1996. 0-7808-0078-8. $78.

"... very readable form. The successful editorial work that brought this material together into a useful and understandable reference makes accessible to all readers information that can help them more effectively understand and obtain help for digestive tract problems." — *Choice, Feb '97*

Genetic Disorders Sourcebook

Basic Information about Heritable Diseases and Disorders Such as Down Syndrome, PKU, Hemophilia, Von Willebrand Disease, Gaucher Disease, Tay-Sachs Disease, and Sickle-Cell Disease, Along with Information about Genetic Screening, Gene Therapy, Home Care, and Including Source Listings for Further Help and Information on More Than 300 Disorders

Edited by Karen Bellenir. 642 pages. 1996. 0-7808-0034-6. $78.

"Provides essential medical information to both the general public and those diagnosed with a serious or fatal genetic disease or disorder." — *Choice, Jan '97*

"Geared toward the lay public. It would be well placed in all public libraries and in those hospital and medical libraries in which access to genetic references is limited." — *Doody's Health Sciences Book Review, Oct '96*

Head Trauma Sourcebook

Basic Information for the Layperson about Open-Head and Closed-Head Injuries, Treatment Advances, Recovery, and Rehabilitation, Along with Reports on Current Research Initiatives

Edited by Karen Bellenir. 414 pages. 1997. 0-7808-0208-X. $78.

Health Insurance Sourcebook

Basic Information about Managed Care Organizations, Traditional Fee-for-Service Insurance, Insurance Portability and Pre-Existing Conditions Clauses, Medicare, Medicaid, Social Security, and Military Health Care, Along with Information about Insurance Fraud

Edited by Wendy Wilcox. 530 pages. 1997. 0-7808-0222-5. $78.

"Particularly useful because it brings much of this information together in one volume." — *Medical Reference Services Quarterly, Fall '98*

"The layout of the book is particularly helpful as it provides easy access to reference material. A most useful addition to the vast amount of information about health insurance. The use of data from U.S. government agencies is most commendable. Useful in a library or learning center for healthcare professional students." — *Doody's Health Sciences Book Reviews, Nov '97*

Healthy Aging Sourcebook

Basic Consumer Health Information about Maintaining Health through the Aging Process, Including Advice on Nutrition, Exercise, and Sleep, Help in Making Decisions about Midlife Issues and Retirement, and Guidance Concerning Practical and Informed Choices in Health Consumerism; Along with Data Concerning the Theories of Aging, Different Experiences in Aging by Minority Groups, and Facts about Aging Now and Aging in the Future; and Featuring a Glossary, a Guide to Consumer Help, Additional Suggested Reading, and Practical Resource Directory

Edited by Jenifer Swanson. 536 pages. 1999. 0-7808-0390-6. $78.

Heart Diseases & Disorders Sourcebook, 2nd edition

Basic Consumer Health Information about Heart Attacks, Angina, Rhythm Disorders, Heart Failure, Valve Disease, Congenital Heart Disorders, and More, Including Descriptions of Surgical Procedures and Other Interventions, Medications, Cardiac Rehabilitation, Risk Identification, and Prevention Tips; Along with Statistical Data, Reports on Current Research Initiatives, a Glossary of Cardiovascular Terms, and Resource Directory

Edited by Karen Bellenir. 600 pages. 1999. 0-7808-0238-1. $78.

Immune System Disorders Sourcebook

Basic Information about Lupus, Multiple Sclerosis, Guillain-Barré Syndrome, Chronic Granulomatous Disease, and More, Along with Statistical and Demographic Data and Reports on Current Research Initiatives

Edited by Allan R. Cook. 608 pages. 1997. 0-7808-0209-8. $78.

Infant & Toddler Health Sourcebook

Basic Consumer Health Information about the Physical and Mental Development of Newborns, Infants, and Toddlers, Including Neonatal Concerns, Nutritional Recommendations, Immunization Schedules, Common Pediatric Disorders, Assessments and Milestones, Safety Tips, and Advice for Parents and Other Caregivers; Along with a Glossary of Terms and Resource Listings for Additional Help

Edited by Jenifer Swanson. 600 pages. 1999. 0-7808-0246-2. $78.

■

Kidney & Urinary Tract Diseases & Disorders Sourcebook

Basic Information about Kidney Stones, Urinary Incontinence, Bladder Disease, End Stage Renal Disease, Dialysis, and More, Along with Statistical and Demographic Data and Reports on Current Research Initiatives

Edited by Linda M. Ross. 602 pages. 1997. 0-7808-0079-6. $78.

■

Learning Disabilities Sourcebook

Basic Information about Disorders Such as Dyslexia, Visual and Auditory Processing Deficits, Attention Deficit/Hyperactivity Disorder, and Autism, Along with Statistical and Demographic Data, Reports on Current Research Initiatives, an Explanation of the Assessment Process, and a Special Section for Adults with Learning Disabilities

Edited by Linda M. Shin. 579 pages. 1998. 0-7808-0210-1. $78.

"Readable . . . provides a solid base of information regarding successful techniques used with individuals who have learning disabilities, as well as practical suggestions for educators and family members. Clear language, concise descriptions, and pertinent information for contacting multiple resources add to the strength of this book as a useful tool." — Choice, Feb '99

"Recent and recommended reference source."
— Booklist, Sept '98

■

Liver Disorders Sourcebook

Basic Consumer Health Information about the Liver and How It Works; Liver Diseases, Including Cancer, Cirrhosis, Hepatitis, and Toxic and Drug Related Diseases; Tips for Maintaining a Healthy Liver; Laboratory Tests, Radiology Tests, and Facts about Liver Transplantation; Along with a Section on Support Groups, a Glossary, and Resource Listings

Edited by Joyce Brennfleck Shannon. 600 pages. 1999. 0-7808-0383-3. $78.

■

Medical Tests Sourcebook

Basic Consumer Health Information about Medical Tests, Including Periodic Health Exams, General Screening Tests, Tests You Can Do at Home, Findings of the U.S. Preventive Services Task Force, X-ray and Radiology Tests, Electrical Tests, Tests of Blood and Other Body Fluids and Tissues, Scope Tests, Lung Tests, Genetic Tests, Pregnancy Tests, Newborn Screening Tests, Sexually Transmitted Disease Tests, and Computer Aided Diagnoses; Along with a Section on Paying for Medical Tests, a Glossary, and Resource Listings

Edited by Joyce Brennfleck Shannon. 691 pages. 1999. 0-7808-0243-8. $78.

■

Men's Health Concerns Sourcebook

Basic Information about Health Issues That Affect Men, Featuring Facts about the Top Causes of Death in Men, Including Heart Disease, Stroke, Cancers, Prostate Disorders, Chronic Obstructive Pulmonary Disease, Pneumonia and Influenza, Human Immunodeficiency Virus and Acquired Immune Deficiency Syndrome, Diabetes Mellitus, Stress, Suicide, Accidents and Homicides; and Facts about Common Concerns for Men, Including Impotence, Contraception, Circumcision, Sleep Disorders, Snoring, Hair Loss, Diet, Nutrition, Exercise, Kidney and Urological Disorders, and Backaches

Edited by Allan R. Cook. 738 pages. 1998. 0-7808-0212-8. $78.

"Recent and recommended reference source."
— Booklist, Dec '98

■

Mental Health Disorders Sourcebook, 1st Edition

Basic Information about Schizophrenia, Depression, Bipolar Disorder, Panic Disorder, Obsessive-Compulsive Disorder, Phobias and Other Anxiety Disorders, Paranoia and Other Personality Disorders, Eating Disorders, and Sleep Disorders, Along with Information about Treatment and Therapies

Edited by Karen Bellenir. 548 pages. 1995. 0-7808-0040-0. $78.

"This is an excellent new book . . . written in easy-to-understand language."
— Booklist Health Science Supplement, Oct '97

". . . useful for public and academic libraries and consumer health collections."
— Medical Reference Services Quarterly, Spring '97

"The great strengths of the book are its readability and its inclusion of places to find more information. Especially recommended." — RQ, Winter '96

". . . a good resource for a consumer health library."
— Bulletin of the MLA, Oct '96

"The information is data-based and couched in brief, concise language that avoids jargon. . . . a useful reference source." — *Readings, Sept '96*

"The text is well organized and adequately written for its target audience." — *Choice, Jun '96*

". . . provides information on a wide range of mental disorders, presented in nontechnical language." — *Exceptional Child Education Resources, Spring '96*

"Recommended for public and academic libraries." — *Reference Book Review, '96*

Mental Health Disorders Sourcebook, 2nd Edition

Basic Consumer Health Information about Anxiety Disorders, Depression and Other Mood Disorders, Eating Disorders, Personality Disorders, Schizophrenia, and More, Including Disease Descriptions, Treatment Options, and Reports on Current Research Initiatives; Along with Statistical Data, Tips for Maintaining Mental Health, a Glossary, and Directory of Sources for Additional Help and Information

Edited by Karen Bellenir. 600 pages. 1999. 0-7808-0240-3. $78.

Ophthalmic Disorders Sourcebook

Basic Information about Glaucoma, Cataracts, Macular Degeneration, Strabismus, Refractive Disorders, and More, Along with Statistical and Demographic Data and Reports on Current Research Initiatives

Edited by Linda M. Ross. 631 pages. 1996. 0-7808-0081-8. $78.

Oral Health Sourcebook

Basic Information about Diseases and Conditions Affecting Oral Health, Including Cavities, Gum Disease, Dry Mouth, Oral Cancers, Fever Blisters, Canker Sores, Oral Thrush, Bad Breath, Temporomandibular Disorders, and other Craniofacial Syndromes, Along with Statistical Data on the Oral Health of Americans, Oral Hygiene, Emergency First Aid, Information on Treatment Procedures and Methods of Replacing Lost Teeth

Edited by Allan R. Cook. 558 pages. 1997. 0-7808-0082-6. $78.

"Unique source which will fill a gap in dental sources for patients and the lay public. A valuable reference tool even in a library with thousands of books on dentistry. Comprehensive, clear, inexpensive, and easy to read and use. It fills an enormous gap in the health care literature." — *Reference and User Services Quarterly, Summer '98*

"Recent and recommended reference source." — *Booklist, Dec '97*

Osteoporosis Sourcebook

Basic Consumer Health Information about Primary and Secondary Osteoporosis, Juvenile Osteoporosis, Related Conditions, and Other Such Bone Disorders as Fibrous Dysplasia, Myeloma, Osteogenesis Imperfecta, Osteopetrosis, and Paget's Disease; Along with Information about Risk Factors, Treatments, Traditional and Non-Traditional Pain Management, and Including a Glossary and Resource Directory

Edited by Allan R. Cook. 600 pages. 1999. 0-7808-0239-X. $78.

Pain Sourcebook

Basic Information about Specific Forms of Acute and Chronic Pain, Including Headaches, Back Pain, Muscular Pain, Neuralgia, Surgical Pain, and Cancer Pain, Along with Pain Relief Options Such as Analgesics, Narcotics, Nerve Blocks, Transcutaneous Nerve Stimulation, and Alternative Forms of Pain Control, Including Biofeedback, Imaging, Behavior Modification, and Relaxation Techniques

Edited by Allan R. Cook. 667 pages. 1997. 0-7808-0213-6. $78.

"The text is readable, easily understood, and well indexed. This excellent volume belongs in all patient education libraries, consumer health sections of public libraries, and many personal collections." — *American Reference Books Annual, '99*

"A beneficial reference." — *Booklist Health Sciences Supplement, Oct '98*

"The information is basic in terms of scholarship and is appropriate for general readers. Written in journalistic style . . . intended for non-professionals. Quite thorough in its coverage of different pain conditions and summarizes the latest clinical information regarding pain treatment." — *Choice, Jun '98*

"Recent and recommended reference source." — *Booklist, Mar '98*

Pediatric Cancer Sourcebook

Basic Consumer Health Information about Leukemias, Brain Tumors, Sarcomas, Lymphomas, and Other Cancers in Infants, Children, and Adolescents, Including Descriptions of Cancers, Treatments, and Coping Strategies; Along with Suggestions for Parents, Caregivers, and Concerned Relatives, a Glossary of Cancer Terms, and Resource Listings

Edited by Edward J. Prucha. 587 pages. 1999. 0-7808-0245-4. $78.

Physical & Mental Issues in Aging Sourcebook

Basic Consumer Health Information on Physical and Mental Disorders Associated with the Aging Process, Including Concerns about Cardiovascular Disease, Pulmonary Disease, Oral Health, Digestive Disorders, Musculoskeletal and Skin Disorders, Metabolic Changes, Sexual and Reproductive Issues, and Changes in Vision, Hearing, and Other Senses; Along with Data about Longevity and Causes of Death, Information on Acute and Chronic Pain, Descriptions of Mental Concerns, a Glossary of Terms, and Resource Listings for Additional Help

Edited by Jenifer Swanson. 660 pages. 1999. 0-7808-0233-0. $78.

Pregnancy & Birth Sourcebook

Basic Information about Planning for Pregnancy, Maternal Health, Fetal Growth and Development, Labor and Delivery, Postpartum and Perinatal Care, Pregnancy in Mothers with Special Concerns, and Disorders of Pregnancy, Including Genetic Counseling, Nutrition and Exercise, Obstetrical Tests, Pregnancy Discomfort, Multiple Births, Cesarean Sections, Medical Testing of Newborns, Breastfeeding, Gestational Diabetes, and Ectopic Pregnancy

Edited by Heather E. Aldred. 737 pages. 1997. 0-7808-0216-0. $78.

"A well-organized handbook. Recommended."
— Choice, Apr '98

"Recent and recommended reference source."
— Booklist, Mar '98

"Recommended for public libraries."
— American Reference Books Annual, '98

Public Health Sourcebook

Basic Information about Government Health Agencies, Including National Health Statistics and Trends, Healthy People 2000 Program Goals and Objectives, the Centers for Disease Control and Prevention, the Food and Drug Administration, and the National Institutes of Health, Along with Full Contact Information for Each Agency

Edited by Wendy Wilcox. 698 pages. 1998. 0-7808-0220-9. $78.

"Recent and recommended reference source."
— Booklist, Sept '98

"This consumer guide provides welcome assistance in navigating the maze of federal health agencies and their data on public health concerns."
— SciTech Book News, Sept '98

Rehabilitation Sourcebook

Basic Consumer Health Information about Rehabilitation for People Recovering from Heart Surgery, Spinal Cord Injury, Stroke, Orthopedic Impairments, Amputation, Pulmonary Impairments, Traumatic Injury, and More, Including Physical Therapy, Occupational Therapy, Speech/Language Therapy, Massage Therapy, Dance Therapy, Art Therapy, and Recreational Therapy; Along with Information on Assistive and Adaptive Devices, a Glossary, and Resources for Additional Help and Information

Edited by Dawn D. Matthews. 531 pages. 1999. 0-7808-0236-5. $78.

Respiratory Diseases & Disorders Sourcebook

Basic Information about Respiratory Diseases and Disorders, Including Asthma, Cystic Fibrosis, Pneumonia, the Common Cold, Influenza, and Others, Featuring Facts about the Respiratory System, Statistical and Demographic Data, Treatments, Self-Help Management Suggestions, and Current Research Initiatives

Edited by Allan R. Cook and Peter D. Dresser. 771 pages. 1995. 0-7808-0037-0. $78.

"Designed for the layperson and for patients and their families coping with respiratory illness. . . . an extensive array of information on diagnosis, treatment, management, and prevention of respiratory illnesses for the general reader."
— Choice, Jun '96

"A highly recommended text for all collections. It is a comforting reminder of the power of knowledge that good books carry between their covers."
— Academic Library Book Review, Spring '96

"This sourcebook offers a comprehensive collection of authoritative information presented in a nontechnical, humanitarian style for patients, families, and caregivers."
— Association of Operating Room Nurses, Sept/Oct '95

Sexually Transmitted Diseases Sourcebook

Basic Information about Herpes, Chlamydia, Gonorrhea, Hepatitis, Nongonoccocal Urethritis, Pelvic Inflammatory Disease, Syphilis, AIDS, and More, Along with Current Data on Treatments and Preventions

Edited by Linda M. Ross. 550 pages. 1997. 0-7808-0217-9. $78.

Skin Disorders Sourcebook

Basic Information about Common Skin and Scalp Conditions Caused by Aging, Allergies, Immune Reactions, Sun Exposure, Infectious Organisms, Parasites, Cosmetics, and Skin Traumas, Including Abrasions, Cuts, and Pressure Sores, Along with Information on Prevention and Treatment

Edited by Allan R. Cook. 647 pages. 1997. 0-7808-0080-X. $78.

". . . comprehensive easily read reference book."
— *Doody's Health Sciences Book Reviews, Oct '97*

Sleep Disorders Sourcebook

Basic Consumer Health Information about Sleep and Its Disorders, Including Insomnia, Sleepwalking, Sleep Apnea, Restless Leg Syndrome, and Narcolepsy; Along with Data about Shiftwork and Its Effects, Information on the Societal Costs of Sleep Deprivation, Descriptions of Treatment Options, a Glossary of Terms, and Resource Listings for Additional Help

Edited by Jenifer Swanson. 439 pages. 1998. 0-7808-0234-9. $78.

"Recent and recommended reference source."
— *Booklist, Feb '99*

Sports Injuries Sourcebook

Basic Consumer Health Information about Common Sports Injuries, Prevention of Injury in Specific Sports, Tips for Training, and Rehabilitation from Injury; Along with Information about Special Concerns for Children, Young Girls in Athletic Training Programs, Senior Athletes, and Women Athletes, and a Directory of Resources for Further Help and Information

Edited by Heather E. Aldred. 624 pages.1999. 0-7808-0218-7. $78.

Substance Abuse Sourcebook

Basic Health-Related Information about the Abuse of Legal and Illegal Substances Such as Alcohol, Tobacco, Prescription Drugs, Marijuana, Cocaine, and Heroin; and Including Facts about Substance Abuse Prevention Strategies, Intervention Methods, Treatment and Recovery Programs, and a Section Addressing the Special Problems Related to Substance Abuse during Pregnancy

Edited by Karen Bellenir. 573 pages. 1996. 0-7808-0038-9. $78.

"A valuable addition to any health reference section. Highly recommended."
— *The Book Report, Mar/Apr '97*

". . . a comprehensive collection of substance abuse information that's both highly readable and compact. Families and caregivers of substance abusers will find the information enlightening and helpful, while teachers, social workers and journalists should benefit from the concise format. Recommended."
— *Drug Abuse Update, Winter '96-'97*

Women's Health Concerns Sourcebook

Basic Information about Health Issues That Affect Women, Featuring Facts about Menstruation and Other Gynecological Concerns, Including Endometriosis, Fibroids, Menopause, and Vaginitis; Reproductive Concerns, Including Birth Control, Infertility, and Abortion; and Facts about Additional Physical, Emotional, and Mental Health Concerns Prevalent among Women Such as Osteoporosis, Urinary Tract Disorders, Eating Disorders, and Depression, Along with Tips for Maintaining a Healthy Lifestyle

Edited by Heather Aldred. 567 pages. 1997. 0-7808-0219-5. $78.

"Handy compilation. There is an impressive range of diseases, devices, disorders, procedures, and other physical and emotional issues covered . . . well organized, illustrated, and indexed." — *Choice, Jan '98*

Workplace Health & Safety Sourcebook

Basic Information about Musculoskeletal Injuries, Cumulative Trauma Disorders, Occupational Carcinogens and Other Toxic Materials, Child Labor, Workplace Violence, Histoplasmosis, Transmission of HIV and Hepatitis-B Viruses, and Occupational Hazards Associated with Various Industries, Including Mining, Confined Spaces, Agriculture, Construction, Electrical Work, and the Medical Professions, with Information on Mortality and Other Statistical Data, Preventative Measures, Reproductive Risks, Reducing Stress for Shiftworkers, Noise Hazards, Industrial Back Belts, Reducing Contamination at Home, Preventing Allergic Reactions to Rubber Latex, and More; Along with Public and Private Programs and Initiatives, a Glossary, and Sources for Additional Help and Information

Edited by Helene Henderson. 600 pages. 1999. 0-7808-0231-4. $78.

Health Reference Series Cumulative Index

A Comprehensive Index to 42 Volumes of the Health Reference Series, 1990-1998

1,500 pages. 1999. 0-7808-0382-5. $78.